# Illustrated Guide to
# Medical
# Terminology

## SECOND EDITION

# Illustrated Guide to
# Medical Terminology

SECOND EDITION

## Juanita J. Davies

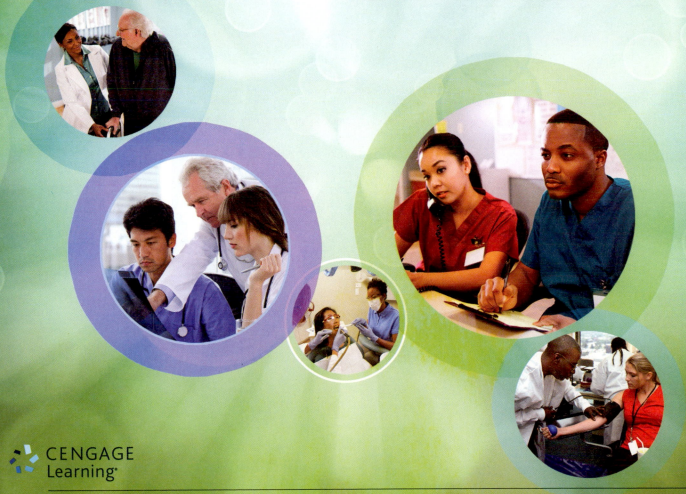

CENGAGE
Learning®

Australia • Brazil • Mexico • Singapore • United Kingdom • United States

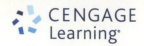

*Illustrated Guide to Medical Terminology,*
**Second Edition**
**Juanita J. Davies**

SVP, GM Skills & Global Product Management:
Dawn Gerrain

Product Director: Matthew Seeley

Senior Director, Development:
Marah Bellegarde

Product Development Manager:
Juliet Steiner

Senior Content Developer: Darcy M. Scelsi

Product Assistant: Deborah Handy

Vice President, Marketing Services:
Jennifer Ann Baker

Marketing Director: Michelle McTighe

Senior Production Director: Wendy Troeger

Production Director: Andrew Crouth

Content Project Manager: Tom Heffernan

Managing Art Director: Jack Pendleton

Cover Image Credits: ©bikeriderlondon;
©Monkey Business Images/Shutterstock.com,
©dlewsis33; ©stevecoleimages; ©STILLFX;
©Wavebreak/iStock.com

Additional Chapter Opener Image Credits:
©Sebastian Kaulitzki; ©VictorOley; ©Alex
Luengo; ©CLIPAREA l Custom media;
©martan; ©RomanenkoAlexey; ©Creations;
©Lightspring; ©Horoscope; ©eAlisa; ©3Dalia;
©Nerthuz/Shutterstock.com

For product information and technology assistance, contact us at
**Cengage Learning Customer & Sales Support, 1-800-354-9706.**

For permission to use material from this text or product,
submit all requests online at **www.cengage.com/permissions.**
Further permissions questions can be e-mailed to
**permissionrequest@cengage.com.**

Library of Congress Control Number: 2014959547

Book Only ISBN: 978-1-285-17442-6

**Cengage Learning**
20 Channel Center Street
Boston, MA 02210
USA

Cengage Learning is a leading provider of customized learning solutions with employees residing in nearly 40 different countries and sales in more than 125 countries around the world. Find your local representative at **www.cengage.com.**

Cengage Learning products are represented in Canada by Nelson Education, Ltd.

To learn more about Cengage Learning, visit **www.cengage.com**

Purchase any of our products at your local college store or at our preferred online store **www.cengagebrain.com**

**Notice to the Reader**

Publisher does not warrant or guarantee any of the products described herein or perform any independent analysis in connection with any of the product information contained herein. Publisher does not assume, and expressly disclaims, any obligation to obtain and include information other than that provided to it by the manufacturer. The reader is expressly warned to consider and adopt all safety precautions that might be indicated by the activities described herein and to avoid all potential hazards. By following the instructions contained herein, the reader willingly assumes all risks in connection with such instructions. The publisher makes no representations or warranties of any kind, including but not limited to, the warranties of fitness for particular purpose or merchantability, nor are any such representations implied with respect to the material set forth herein, and the publisher takes no responsibility with respect to such material. The publisher shall not be liable for any special, consequential, or exemplary damages resulting, in whole or part, from the readers' use of, or reliance upon, this material.

Printed in the United States of America
Print Number: 01    Print Year: 2015

Dedication
To Jim

# CONTENTS

# PREFACE

## Development of the Text

Most learners find the structure of the body and its diseases very interesting to learn. However, over the years, I observed many of my students struggle with the written material to be learned. My colleagues said the same thing—they sensed frustration in many learners. More and more frequently, I found myself thinking that a comprehensive book with extensive illustrations and very simple writing would be very useful. That's what led me to write *Illustrated Guide to Medical Terminology*. I wanted to make it easy and enjoyable for every student to learn anatomy, physiology, medical terminology, and pathology.

The theme of this book is "Read, Look, and Listen so you can Speak and Write." This means that you first read the text and then look at diagrams corresponding to what you have read. Often you are asked to write the names of parts on the diagrams. Then, you complete the review exercises and listen to terms from the chapter pronounced (the audio pronunciations can be found on the Student Companion Website). You are asked to say the terms and then write them down. This process of reading the text, looking at the diagrams, writing in the structure names, completing the review exercises, listening to and repeating the correct pronunciation of terms, and finally writing the terms down on paper is the best way to learn. *Illustrated Guide to Medical Terminology, 2e* is ideal for visual and auditory learners, as well as learners whose first language is not English. I hope it serves you well.

## Text Organization

*Illustrated Guide to Medical Terminology, 2e* is organized based on the body-system approach. After more than 30 years of teaching, I feel confident that this is the most effective and learner-friendly way to teach terminology.

Chapter 1 outlines the proper way to analyze terms. Chapter 2 presents basic body organization and introduces the common anatomical roots. Chapter 3 introduces suffixes, and Chapter 4 presents prefixes. Chapter 5 explains how the body is organized. The remaining 14 chapters are each devoted to a single body system.

## Chapter Organization

Each chapter begins with a very brief chapter outline in point form. This is followed by the learning objectives for the chapter, also in point form, and a brief introduction. In the body system chapters, an illustration of the body system to be studied immediately follows the introduction. The purpose is to provide a broad overview of the body system before details are presented. Each chapter has diagrams illustrating body structure, function, and disease. The text associated with the diagrams is as simple as possible. Regular review is accomplished by the use of sidebars that contain brief summaries. Memory devices designed to enhance learning are also included.

Vocabulary building is presented throughout each chapter. Near the end of each chapter is a list of common system-specific terms and their pronunciation. This list, used together with the accompanying audio files, accomplishes the objective of having the learner listen to the correct pronunciation in order to speak and write the medical terms correctly. Quizzes with answers included throughout each chapter allow learners to test themselves on the content presented before moving on to new content in the chapter.

## Features Designed to Enhance Learning

This is the most comprehensive of the short-course medical terminology books on the market. The writing is simple and straightforward, even though the content is quite challenging. Despite the brevity of the textual material, each chapter tells a story so that the learner can chunk the information, which allows for ease of learning.

Be sure to read the **How to Use This Book** section on page XXV for detailed descriptions and images of the many features specifically developed to enhance your learning of medical terminology.

## New to This Edition

Chapter 1
- Significantly rewritten

Chapter 2
- Minor changes

Chapter 3
- New terms added to Learning the Terms

Chapter 4
- New terms added to Learning the Terms

Chapter 5
- Content on body planes rewritten

Chapter 6
- Additional topics added: subcutaneous tissue, accessory structures
- New terms added to Learning the Terms
- Pathology added: bruises, lesions, skin infections
- New images: cutaneous lesions

Chapter 7
- New terms added to Learning the Terms
- Pathology added: abnormal curvatures, fractures
- Added table of bones, common names, and adjectives
- New images skull, abnormal spinal curvatures, and fractures

Chapter 8
- New terms added to Learning the Terms
- Pathology added: carpal tunnel syndrome

Chapter 9
- Additional topics added: synapse, protective coverings
- New terms added to Learning the Terms
- Pathology added: amyotrophic lateral sclerosis, levels of consciousness, poliomyelitis, sciatica, types of seizures
- New images: protective coverings

Chapter 10
- Additional topics added: accessory structures
- New terms added to Learning the Terms
- Pathology added: otiitis media, otosclerosis
- New images: flow of aqueous humor, accessory structures, extraocular muscles, normal versus abnormal vision

Chapter 11
- Additional topics added: teeth, salivary glands
- New terms added to Learning the Terms
- Pathology added: cleft palate, cleft lip, cirrhosis of liver, diverticulosis hemorrhoids, hiatal hernia intestinal obstruction
- New images: structures of the tooth, salivary glands, stomach, hiatal hernia, intestinal obstruction, diverticulosis

Chapter 12
- Additional topics added: Major arteries and veins
- New terms added to Learning the Terms

- Pathology added: arrhythmia, types of strokes, congestive heart failure, murmur, valvular disorders
- New images: electrocardiography, common arteries, common veins, cardiac catheterization, angioplasty, coronary artery bypass surgery

Chapter 13
- New terms added to Learning the Terms

Chapter 14
- No changes

Chapter 15
- New terms added to Learning the Terms
- Pathology added: allergic rhinitis, cystic fibrosis, deviated nasal septum, epistaxis, pneumoconiosis, tuberculosis

Chapter 16
- New terms added to Learning the Terms
- Pathology added: nephrotic syndrome
- New images: vesicovaginal fistula, extracorporeal shockwave lithotripsy

Chapter 17
- New terms added to Learning the Terms

Chapter 18
- Additional topics added: obstetrics
- New terms added to Learning the Terms
- Pathology added: breast cancer revised, cervical cancer, abortion, abruptio placenta, infertility, placenta previa, pre-eclampsia, premature infant, stillbirth uterine inertia

Chapter 19
- Additional topics added: thymus
- New terms added to Learning the Terms
- Pathology revised

# Resources to Accompany This Book

## Student Companion Website

The Student Companion Website contains the following resources to aid you with study and learning the medical terminology in your course:

- Audio files for pronunciation of terms
- PowerPoint presentations
- Animations and videos to help further comprehension of content areas

To set up your Student Companion account:

- Log into https://login.cengage.com
- Click on **New Student User** and follow the instructions for completing your account setup.
- If you already have a student account, simply login and add the book to your bookshelf.

## Instructor Companion Website

The Instructor Companion Website contains the following resources to aid you in planning your course and implementing class activities:

- Syllabus
- Instructor Manual
- Handouts
- PowerPoint presentations
- Animations and videos
- Answer key to review questions in the text
- Testbank powered by Cognero

To set up your Instructor Companion account:

- Go to https://login.cengage.com/cb/
- Choose **Create a New Faculty Account**.
- Next you will need to select your **Institution**.
- Complete your personal **Account Information**.
- Accept the **License Agreement**.
- Choose **Register**.
- Your account will be pending validation—you will receive an e-mail notification when the validation process is complete.
- If you are unable to find your Institution, complete an **Account Request Form**.

Once your account is set up or if you already have an account:

- Go to https://login.cengage.com/cb/
- Enter your e-mail address and password and select **Sign In**.
- Search for your book by author, title, or ISBN.
- Select the book and click **Continue**.
- You will receive a list of available resources for the title you selected.
- Choose the resources you would like and click **Add to My Bookshelf**.

# ABOUT THE AUTHOR

Juanita Davies has taught anatomy and medical terminology for over 30 years. She has also written extensively on the subject of medical terminology. Her early work includes *A Programmed Learning Approach to Medical Terminology* and a computerized testbank containing 15,000 questions. Her first book with Delmar, *Modern Medical Language*, is a combination of anatomy, medical terminology, pathology, signs and symptoms, diagnostic procedures, and treatment. Her second book, *Essentials of Medical Terminology*, combines anatomy with medical terminology. Her third book, *A Quick Reference to Medical Terminology*, is a basic handbook on medical terminology.

# ACKNOWLEDGMENTS

This book would not have been possible without the help of many people. This second edition was initiated by Matt Seeley, Acquisitions Editor at Cengage Learning. Darcy Selci, Senior Content editor, gave me wonderful practical advice throughout this project, and always remembered a discussion point, no matter how many months went by from discussion to implementation. Thanks to Jack Pendleton, Senior Art Director, who brought about the colorful art and design. To all of my professional colleagues who reviewed this book, I sincerely thank you. A special thank you to my friend Nancy Johnson, who gave me wise counsel and insight on this project.

Thank you to my husband, Jim, who spent many hours reading the manuscript. Your critiques were thorough, your suggestions imaginative.

## Reviewers

Cengage Learning and the author would like to thank the following individuals for their valuable input:

**Jennie Diaz-Ontiveros**, CCMA
Medical Assistant Instructor
Tri-Cities Regional Occupational Program
Whittier, California

**Cassie Gentry**, MEd, RHI, CHP
Chair, Department of Health Related
    Professions
Program Director/Professor, Health
    Information Technology
Community College of Southern Nevada
Las Vegas, Nevada

**Krista L. Hoekstra**, RN, BSN
Practical Nursing Instructor
Hennepin Technical College
Brooklyn Park, Minnesota

**Francine R. Page,** LPN
Instructor, Medical Office Technology
    Program
Health, Environmental, Natural &
    Physical Science Division
Pikes Peak Community College
Colorado Springs, Colorado

**June M. Petillo**, MBA, RMC
Associate Professor and Director of
    Medical Billing and Coding
Goodwin College
East Hartford, Connecticut

# HOW TO USE THIS BOOK

## Learner-Friendly Approach

The approach is simple—"Read, Look, and Listen in order to Speak and Write." This means that you first read the text and then look at diagrams corresponding to the text. You are often asked to write the names of parts on the diagrams. At the end of each chapter, complete the review exercises. Go to the Student Companion Website and listen to terms from the chapter pronounced. Say the terms aloud and then write them down. This process of reading the text, looking at the diagrams, writing in the structure names, completing the review exercises, listening to and repeating the correct pronunciation of terms, and finally writing the terms down on paper maximizes your learning experience.

## Full-Color Illustrations

An illustration of the body system to be studied immediately follows the chapter introduction to provide a broad overview of the system before learning the details. Writing labels on the diagrams helps reinforce learning. Numerous diagrams illustrate body structure, function, and disease with the associated content presented as simply as possible.

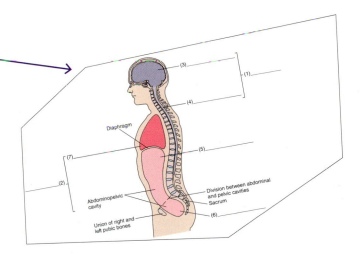

## Pronunciations

Pronunciations are presented phonetically beside every new term and are repeated throughout the chapter.

## Learning the Terms

Learning medical language is based on repetition. In each chapter, roots, suffixes, and prefixes are often repeated to reinforce learning. After each word element is introduced, it is followed by several examples of terms using that word element. This helps you remember the terms because you learn them in clusters using the same word element.

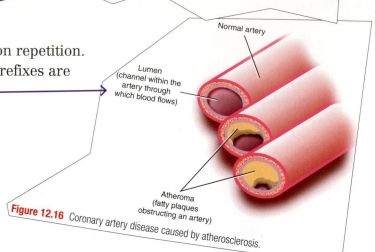

| ROOT ather/o | | MEANING fatty debris |
|---|---|---|
| *Term* | *Term Analysis* | *Definition* |
| **atheroma** (ath-er-OH-mah) | -oma = mass; tumor | name given to the fatty mass (plaque) that accumulates on the wall of an artery. The fatty mass contains cholesterol. |
| **atherosclerosis** (ath-er-oh-skleh-ROH-sis) | -sclerosis = hardening | hardening and narrowing of an artery due to an atheroma (Figure 12-16) |

Normal artery

Lumen (channel within the artery through which blood flows)

Atheroma (fatty plaques obstructing an artery)

**Figure 12.16** Coronary artery disease caused by atherosclerosis.

## Dorsal Cavity

The dorsal cavity is subdivided into two parts: the cranial cavity and vertebral cavity. The cranial cavity is inside the skull. The brain is contained in the cranial cavity. The vertebral cavity is inside the vertebral column, or spine. The spinal cord (a group of nerves) is contained in the vertebral cavity.

## Ventral Cavity

The ventral cavity contains many internal organs including the heart, lungs, kidneys, digestive organs, and others. These internal organs are also called **viscera** (**VIS**-er-ah). A large muscle called the **diaphragm** (**DYE**-ah-fram) divides the ventral cavity into upper and lower cavities. The upper cavity is called the thoracic cavity. The lower cavity is the **abdominopelvic** (ab-**dom**-ih-noh-**PEL**-vick) cavity.

The thoracic cavity contains the heart and lungs. The abdominopelvic cavity is divided into two smaller cavities: the abdominal cavity and the pelvic cavity. The abdominal cavity is above the pelvic cavity. It contains organs such as the liver, intestines, stomach, and kidneys. The pelvic cavity contains some reproductive organs, the urinary bladder, and parts of the intestine.

**In Brief**   The **dorsal cavity** is subdivided into the cranial and vertebral cavities. The **ventral cavity** is subdivided into the thoracic and abdominopelvic cavities.

## In Brief

Regular review of what you have learned is accomplished through the use of sidebars that contain brief definitions of terms found on the same page.

**PRACTICE FOR LEARNING: Directional Terms**

1. Write the opposite meaning of the following directional terms. The first one is done for you.

   **a.** anterior posterior _____

   **b.** lateral _____

   **c.** proximal _____

   **d.** deep _____

   **e.** prone _____

   **f.** dorsum _____

2. Choose the correct answer from the choices in parentheses.

   **g.** The neck is (inferior/superior) to the chin.

   **h.** Your mouth is (medial/lateral) to your ear.

   **i.** You have stepped on a sharp object. The bottom of your foot starts to bleed. You have cut the (plantar/dorsum) area of your foot.

## Practice for Learning

Brief reviews ensure that you have mastered the content presented and are ready to move on to the next section of material.

## Helping You Remember

Suggestions are provided to help you remember a difficult term or concept presented in the chapter.

**Directional Terms**

As stated above, we need directional terms to describe the position of body parts, particularly in relation to each other. Directional terms are also useful in communicating the location of diseases when they appear in the body.

All of the directional terms are listed in Table 5-1. To help you remember them, they are grouped in opposite pairs. For example, the terms "superior" and "inferior" are grouped because they are opposites: superior means "above," and inferior means "below." Figures 5-2 A–F illustrate the use of the terms.

**Helping You Remember**   To remember the meaning of supine, notice that supine has "up" as part of the word.

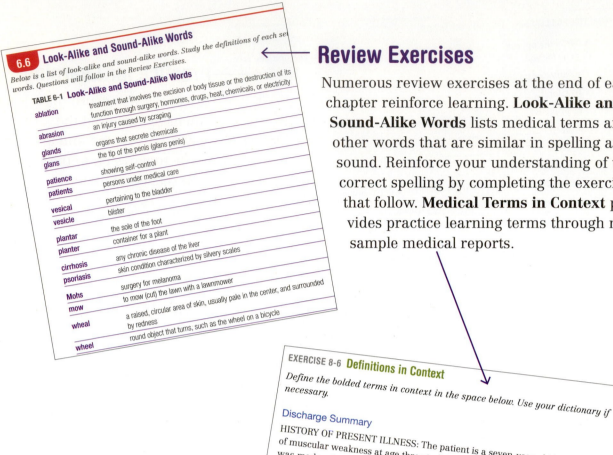

**6.6   Look-Alike and Sound-Alike Words**

*Below is a list of look-alike and sound-alike words. Study the definitions of each set of words. Questions will follow in the Review Exercises.*

**TABLE 6-1  Look-Alike and Sound-Alike Words**

| | |
|---|---|
| ablation | treatment that involves the excision of body tissue or the destruction of its function through surgery, hormones, drugs, heat, chemicals, or electricity |
| abrasion | an injury caused by scraping |
| glands | organs that secrete chemicals |
| glans | the tip of the penis (glans penis) |
| patience | showing self-control |
| patients | persons under medical care |
| vesical | pertaining to the bladder |
| vesicle | blister |
| plantar | the sole of the foot |
| planter | container for a plant |
| cirrhosis | any chronic disease of the liver |
| psoriasis | skin condition characterized by silvery scales |
| Mohs | surgery for melanoma |
| mow | to mow (cut) the lawn with a lawnmower |
| wheal | a raised, circular area of skin, usually pale in the center, and surrounded by redness |
| wheel | round object that turns, such as the wheel on a bicycle |

# Review Exercises

Numerous review exercises at the end of each chapter reinforce learning. **Look-Alike and Sound-Alike Words** lists medical terms and other words that are similar in spelling and sound. Reinforce your understanding of the correct spelling by completing the exercises that follow. **Medical Terms in Context** provides practice learning terms through mock sample medical reports.

**EXERCISE 8-6  Definitions in Context**

*Define the bolded terms in context in the space below. Use your dictionary if necessary.*

**Discharge Summary**

HISTORY OF PRESENT ILLNESS: The patient is a seven-year-old boy who showed signs of muscular weakness at age three to four years. The diagnosis of **muscular dystrophy** was made when a muscle **biopsy** confirmed **degeneration** of muscle fibers. He is still walking and was started on drug **therapy** four months ago.

PHYSICAL EXAMINATION: On examination, the patient is a pleasant young fellow. He has **proximal** muscle weakness. He has **hypertrophy** and some shortening of the **Achilles tendon**. General physical examination is within normal limits.

COURSE IN HOSPITAL: While in the hospital, an **intravenous** line was started, and blood samples were taken for tests during a 24-hour period. The course in hospital was uneventful.

ssible Diagn                  r Dystrophy

**Pronunciation and Spelling Exercises** in each chapter helps you learn the common system-specific terms and their pronunciation.

**5.9   Pronunciation and Spelling**

1. Listen to each word on the audio file provided on the Student Companion Website.
2. Pronounce each word carefully.
3. Spell each word in the space provided.

| Word | Pronunciation | Spelling |
|---|---|---|
| epigastric | **ep**-ih-**GAS**-trick | |
| hypogastric | **high**-poh-**GAS**-trick | |
| iliac | **ILL**-ee-ack | |
| abdominal | ab-**DOM**-ih-nal | |
| cranial | **KRAY**-nee-al | |
| dorsal | **DOR**-sal | |
| inguinal | **ING**-gwih-nal | |
| | nee-al | |

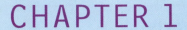

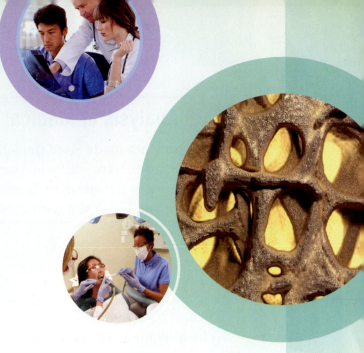

## CHAPTER 1

# Basic Word Structure

## Chapter Outline

*This chapter will help you learn the basics of medical word structure. It is divided into the following sections:*

## Learning Objectives

*After studying this chapter and completing the review exercises, you should be able to:*

1. Define a root, suffix, and prefix.
2. Distinguish between roots, suffixes, and prefixes in a medical word.
3. Learn the basic rules of medical word structure.
4. Write the meaning of the roots, suffixes, and prefixes found in this chapter.
5. Build medical words.
6. Define medical words.

## Introduction

Medical words are made of parts. You need to learn what the parts are and what they mean in order to easily learn medical words. This chapter will teach you how to do that.

## 1.1    Analysis of Medical Word Parts

Medical words are made up of the following word parts: roots, suffixes, and prefixes. Not all medical words have all three parts, but we will start by looking at an example that does. The word is peri**neur**itis (**per**-ih-nyoo-**RYE**-tis). It means inflammation around a nerve. When you break the word into its word parts you will have the following:

- peri-
- neur
- -itis

The first part, **peri**-, is the prefix. Whenever a prefix stands alone in this text, it is followed by a hyphen, as can be seen in the above example. Common prefixes are studied in Chapter 4.

The root in this example is **neur**. A root is usually (but not always) a body part. An introduction to roots is in Chapter 2.

The last part of the example is the suffix, **-itis**. Whenever a suffix stands alone in this text it is preceded by a hyphen. You will learn the suffixes in Chapter 3.

Once you learn roots, suffixes, and prefixes you will be able to define words you have not seen before by simply analyzing the word using the method described in the next section.

### How to Define Medical Words

This is the way to define medical words:

1. *Identify* the suffix first, then the prefix (if there is one), and then the root. Remember that most words have only two parts, so do not think you will find all three all the time. A few words only have one part.

2. *Define* the medical word by starting at the suffix. Find out what it means. Then go to the beginning of the word. It will be either a prefix or a root. Find out what it means. If there is another part, it will be a root. Once you have all the meanings, put them together.

---

**In Brief**

**Word Parts**

- root
- suffix
- prefix

**Defining Words**

Define the suffix first.

Then define the first part of the word, then the second part (if there is one).

**PRACTICE FOR LEARNING: Analysis of Medical Word Parts**

Identify and write the part of **perineuritis** indicated below. The answers are provided, but try to do the exercise first without looking at them.

**1.** Suffix _____ (means **inflammation**)

**2.** Prefix _____ (means **around**)

**3.** Root _____ (means **nerve**)

**4.** Now write the meaning of **perineuritis** _____

> Answers: 1. -itis. 2. peri-. 3. neur. 4. inflammation around the nerve.

## 1.2  Basic Word Structure

### Roots

A root is the main part of a medical word. It often refers to a body part. Examples used in this chapter are:

- **aden** means **gland**
- **arthr** means **joint**
- **col** means **colon**
- **hemat** means **blood**
- **neur** means **nerve**
- **oste** means **bone**

### Combining Vowel

Previously, you learned the word **peri**neuritis. In that example, the suffix **-itis** joined the root **neur** quite easily. Sometimes roots and suffixes do not go together as well. For example, if the root **hemat** was combined with the suffix **-logy**, the word would be spelled **hematlogy**. Try pronouncing this word. You will find it difficult. To make this word easier to pronounce, the letter "o" is added to the end of the root to make the word **hematology** (**hee**-mah-**TOL**-eh-jee). The "o" is called a **combining vowel**. As you can see, with the combining vowel added, the word is much easier to pronounce.

The combining vowel is usually "o." It can be used to connect a root to a suffix (as in the above example) or to join two roots. When connecting a root to a suffix, the combining vowel is used only when the suffix starts with a consonant, such as in the word "hematology" above. If the suffix starts with a vowel (a, e, i, o, u) the combining vowel is **not** needed. For example, in the word **arthritis** (ar-**THRIGH**-tis), we do not add the combining vowel to *arthr* because the suffix -*itis* starts with a vowel.

As stated above, the combining vowel can also be used to joint two roots. For example, in the word "osteoarthritis," the combining vowel joins the roots *oste* and *arthr.*

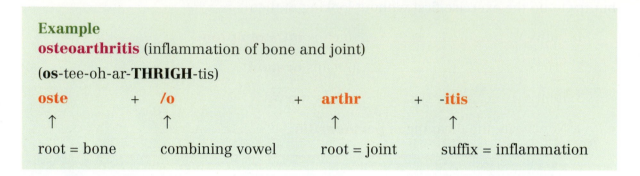

**Example**
**osteoarthritis** (inflammation of bone and joint)
(**os**-tee-oh-ar-**THRIGH**-tis)

| oste | + | /o | + | arthr | + | -itis |
|------|---|----|---|-------|---|-------|
| ↑ | | ↑ | | ↑ | | ↑ |
| root = bone | | combining vowel | | root = joint | | suffix = inflammation |

**In Brief**

**Vowels**
a, e, i, o, u

**Consonants**
letters that are not vowels

**Combining vowel**
usually "o"

**Used when**
- Combining two roots
- Combining a root with a suffix beginning with a consonant

PRACTICE FOR LEARNING: **Roots and Combining Vowels**

**1.** Define a root

**2.** Define a combining vowel.

**3.** In the word **hematology**,

    **a.** _____ is the root.

    **b.** _____ is the combining vowel.

    **c.** _____ is the suffix.

**4.** A combining vowel is used when the suffix starts with a _____

**5.** A combining vowel is **not** used when the suffix starts with a _____

Answers: 1. The root is the main part of a medical word. It is often a body part.
2. A combining vowel is a single letter, usually "o," added onto the end of the root.
3. (a) hemat = root, (b) "o" = combining vowel, (c) -logy = suffix. 4. consonant. 5. vowel.

## Combining Forms

You have already learned what a combining vowel is. The **combining form** is the name given to a root that is followed by a combining vowel. For example, the root *arthr,* written in its combining form, is:

arthr/o

The root is separated from the combining vowel by a slash (/). This is the standard way to write a combining form. It means that the combining vowel might be used in building medical words. Where the combining vowel is not needed for pronunciation, it is not used. In medical language, the root standing alone is almost always written in the combining form. So you should expect to see a root like **aden** written as **aden/o** almost all of the time.

**In Brief**

**Combining form**
root + combining vowel

**Example**
hemat/o

PRACTICE FOR LEARNING: **Combining Forms**

**1.** Define a combining form. Give an example.

_____

_____

**2.** What is the difference between the combining vowel and the combining form?

_____

_____

_____

_____

Answers: 1. A combining form is the name given to a root that is followed by a combining vowel. Example: arthr/o is one example of many. 2. A combining vowel is a single letter, usually "o," added onto the end of a root. A combining form is the name given to a root plus combining vowel.

## Suffixes

A suffix is the last part of a word. It can be attached to a root or a prefix. Whenever a suffix stands alone in this book, a hyphen comes before it.

### When the Suffix Starts with a Vowel, the Combining Vowel Is Dropped

**Example**
**arthralgia** (joint pain)
(ar-**THRAL**-jee-ah)

**arthr** + **-algia**
↑ ↑
root = joint suffix = pain

### When the Suffix Starts with a Consonant, the Combining Vowel Is **Not** Dropped

**Example**
**colostomy** (new opening in the colon)
(koh-**LOSS**-toh-mee)

**col** + **/o** + **-stomy**
↑ ↑ ↑
root = colon + combining vowel + suffix = new opening

## Prefixes

A prefix is the first part of a medical word. It can be attached to the beginning of the root or sometimes a suffix. Whenever a prefix stands alone in this book, it is followed by a hyphen.

### Prefix Joining with a Root

**Example**
**polyadenoma** (tumor of many glands)
(**pahl**-ee-ah-deh-**NOH**-mah)

**poly-** + **aden** + **-oma**
↑ ↑ ↑
prefix = many root = gland suffix = tumor; mass

### Prefix Joining with a Suffix

**Example**
**dysphasia** (difficulty speaking)
(dis-**FAY**-zhee-ah)

**dys-** + **-phasia**
↑ ↑
prefix = difficulty suffix = speech

**PRACTICE FOR LEARNING:** Suffixes and Prefixes

1. Underline the suffix in the following words:

   a. adenoma

   b. hematology

   c. osteoarthritis

   d. dysphasia

2. Underline the prefix in the following words:

   a. dysphasia

   b. polyadenoma

> Answers: 1. (a) -oma, (b) -logy, (c) -itis, (d) -phasia. 2. (a) dys-, (b) poly-.

## 1.3   New Roots, Suffixes, and Prefixes

Use the following suggestions for learning word parts (roots, suffixes, and prefixes):

1. Pronounce the term repeatedly until it is easy for you.

2. Write it down. Ensure the spelling is correct.

3. Also write the definition. If possible, relate the word to a word, thought, or picture that will help you remember it.

**Helping You Remember**

Many students find that using memory tricks helps them remember. That works with medical terminology too. It can really help if you learn to mentally connect a word or word part with a feeling or a mental picture, especially if it is something that has personal meaning to you. For example, the first suffix below, *-algia*, means "pain." The best way to remember that suffix is to think of a particular pain you have experienced every time you see the suffix. So if someone who has broken a leg thinks of that every time she sees *-algia*, she will never forget it. Use memory tricks whenever you can.

| ROOTS | MEANING |
|-------|---------|
| aden/o | gland |
| arthr/o | joint |
| hemat/o | blood |
| col/o | colon |
| neur/o | nerve |
| oste/o | bone |

| SUFFIX | MEANING |
|--------|---------|
| -algia; -dynia | pain |
| -itis | inflammation |
| -logy | study of |
| -oma | tumor; mass |
| -phasia | speech |

| PREFIX | MEANING |
|--------|---------|
| dys- | difficult; pain; bad |
| peri- | around |
| poly- | many |

## 1.4 Review Exercises

### EXERCISE 1-1 Vocabulary

*Build the medical word by filling in the blank with the correct word part or parts.*

Example: adenitis                  inflammation of a gland

1. _____ itis        inflammation of a joint

2. _____ logy      study of blood

3. aden _____      tumor of a gland

4. _____ oma       tumor of bone

5. _____ oma       tumor of many glands

6. _____ itis                    inflammation of bones and joints

7. col _____                     new opening in the colon

8. _____ neur _____  inflammation around a nerve

9. _____ phasia                  difficult speech

10. arthr _____                  joint pain

## EXERCISE 1-2   Definitions

*Define the following words:*

**1. arthritis**

_____

**2. adenoma**

_____

**3. polyadenoma**

_____

**4. osteoarthritis**

_____

**5. hematology**

_____

## EXERCISE 1-3   Word Parts

*Fill in the blanks with the correct word.*

1. The three main parts of a medical word are the _____,
   _____, and _____.

2. The word part usually found at the end of a medical word is the
   _____.

3. When you define a medical word, you usually start at the _____,
   and then define the _____.

4. The combining form in "hematology" is _____.

5. The difference between the combining form and combining vowel is
   _____.

**EXERCISE 1-4  Word Parts**

*Circle True if the statement is true. Circle False if the statement is false.*

1. The word "adenoma" has no suffix.                                    True    False

2. In the word "hematology," the combining form is used because
   the suffix starts with a consonant.                                 True    False

3. Usually, a combining vowel is not used between two roots.           True    False

4. The prefix *poly-* means "many."                                    True    False

**EXERCISE 1-5  Definitions (Medical to English)**

*Give the meaning of the following word parts:*

1. **hemat/o**

   _____

2. **arthr/o**

   _____

3. **aden/o**

   _____

4. **oste/o**

   _____

5. **-logy**

   _____

6. **-itis**

   _____

7. **-oma**

   _____

8. **-phasia**

   _____

9. **dys-**

   _____

10. **poly-**

    _____

## EXERCISE 1-6 Definitions (English to Medical)

*I. Write the root for the following:*

**1. bone**

_____

**2. joint**

_____

**3. blood**

_____

**4. gland**

_____

*II. Write the suffix for the following:*

**1. inflammation**

_____

**2. speech**

_____

**3. study of**

_____

**4. tumor**

_____

*III. Write the prefix for the following:*

**1. difficult**

_____

**2. many**

_____

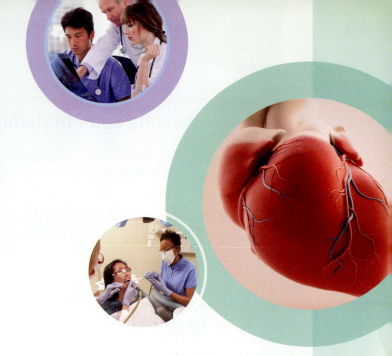

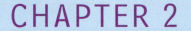

# CHAPTER 2

# Basic Body Structure

## Chapter Outline

*This chapter will help you understand how the body is organized. Basic anatomical roots are also learned. It is divided into the following sections:*

- **2.1** Anatomy and Physiology
- **2.2** Levels of Organization
- **2.3** Body Systems
- **2.4** Common Anatomical Roots
- **2.5** Review Exercises

## Learning Objectives

*After studying this chapter and completing the review exercises, you should be able to:*

1. Define anatomy and physiology.
2. Describe how the body is organized.
3. Define cells, tissues, organs, and systems.
4. Name 12 body systems and the common organs found in each system.
5. Define roots pertaining to the body systems.

## Introduction

This chapter starts by introducing you to some basic concepts related to the study of the human body. It will prepare you to learn the roots you need to know for this and the following chapters on suffixes and prefixes.

The roots in this chapter are grouped according to body systems. You will find it much easier to remember each root if you associate it with a mental picture of the organ it refers to. The roots you encounter in this chapter will give you a foundation for building medical terms. Note that the roots in the tables of this chapter are expressed in their combining forms, as described in Chapter 1.

## 2.1  Anatomy and Physiology

Two terms often used in this text are **anatomy** (ah-**NAT**-oh-mee) and **physiology** (**fiz**-ee-**OL**-oh-jee). Anatomy is the study of the structure or parts of the body. Physiology is the study of how a body part functions. For example, the biceps brachii (**BYE**-seps **BRAY**-kee-eye) muscle is located on top of the upper arm (Figure 2-1). It is made up of cells that are long and slender. These cells are called muscle fibers. The function of the biceps brachii is to flex the lower arm by pulling on the bones of the forearm.

## 2.2  Levels of Organization

All life consists of microscopic living structures called cells. They perform various functions throughout the body. All cells are similar in structure, but not identical. Each cell has a **cell membrane**, which acts as a barrier separating the inside of the cell from its surroundings. The inside of the cell is called the **cytoplasm** (**SIGH**-toh-plaz-um). The cytoplasm contains small organs called organelles. These organelles carry on life's functions as mentioned below.

The central portion of the cell is the **nucleus** (**NOO**-klee-us). The nucleus contains DNA. Human DNA contains thousands of genes, which are responsible for transmitting hereditary characteristics such as the shape of the body and color of the hair. **Chromosomes** (**KROH**-moh-zohms) are structures in the nucleus that carry the DNA

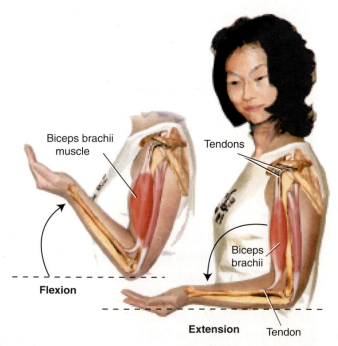

Biceps brachii muscle

Tendons

Biceps brachii

**Flexion**

**Extension**     Tendon

**Figure 2-1**  The biceps brachii muscle flexes the lower arm by pulling on the bones of the forearm. Tendons attach muscle to bone.

and likewise the genetic information of each cell. DNA analysis is used to identify individuals and to prove genetic relationships.

The body's cells carry on all of the functions of life such as:

- Taking in food and oxygen
- Producing heat and energy
- Eliminating wastes
- Responding to changes in the environment
- Reproducing

Trillions of cells make up the cellular level, which is the first level of organization of the body.

The next level is called **tissues**. Similar cells working together to perform a specific function combine to make up tissues. For example, muscle cells form muscle tissue. Nerve cells form nervous tissue. A **histologist** (hiss-**TOL**-oh-jist) is someone who specializes in the study of tissues. The major tissue types are:

- **Epithelial** (**ep**-ih-**THEE**-lee-al) **tissue:** Epithelial tissue covers external surfaces of the body, lines body structures, and forms glands. The skin is an example of an organ that is made up of epithelial tissue. Mucous membrane is also made up of epithelial tissue. It is found lining the digestive, respiratory, reproductive, and urinary tracts.

- **Connective tissue:** Connective tissue functions to support and shape the body structures and keeps them in place. Tendons and ligaments, blood, bone, cartilage, and fat are examples of connective tissue.

- **Muscle tissue:** Muscle tissue takes its name from its location in the body; for example, in the heart it is called **cardiac** muscle tissue. Within organs, such as the stomach and intestines, it is called **visceral** (**VIS**-er-al) muscle tissue. Muscle associated with bones is called **skeletal** muscle tissue. All muscles, no matter where their location, create movement of some kind. Muscle cells are not round, but long and slender. For this reason, muscle cells are often referred to as fibers. See Figure 2-1.

- **Nervous tissue:** This tissue makes up nerves that conduct electrical impulses throughout the body. The brain, spinal cord, and nerves are made up of nervous tissue.

The next level of organization is the **organs**. Tissues of all types combine to make up organs such as the **muscles**, **nerves**, **liver**, and **heart**.

Related organs make up body systems, such as the muscular and nervous systems. All of the body systems combine to form the human being. These levels of organization are in Figure 2-2.

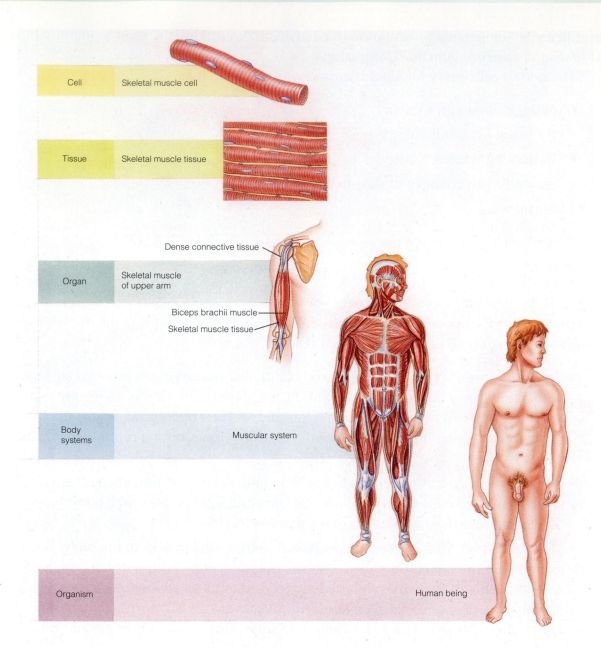

**Figure 2-2** Levels of organization.

**In Brief**   **Cells → Tissues → Organs → Body Systems → Human Being**

**PRACTICE FOR LEARNING: Anatomy and Physiology**

Choose the correct answer from the choices in parentheses.

1. The study of body structure is (anatomy/physiology).

2. The third structural level of body organization is (tissues/organs/cells/body systems).

3. Tissue that holds body structures together is (epithelial/connective).

4. Tissue covering the external surfaces of the body is (epithelial/connective).

5. A specialist in the study of tissue is a (histologist/physiologist/geneticist).

6. Muscles in the esophagus are made up of (cardiac/skeletal/visceral) muscle tissue.

7. Mucous membrane is made up of (connective/epithelial/muscle) tissue.

8. The cell nucleus contains genetic structures known as (chromosomes/cytoplasm).

9. DNA and the body's genes are found on structures called (chromosomes/cytoplasm).

10. Muscular tissue in the stomach and intestine are known as (cardiac/skeletal/visceral) tissue.

> **Answers: 1. anatomy. 2. organs. 3. connective. 4. epithelial. 5. histologist. 6. visceral. 7. epithelial. 8. chromosomes. 9. chromosomes. 10. visceral.**

## 2.3 Body Systems

The following body systems make up the human body: integumentary, skeletal, muscular, nervous, eyes and ears, endocrine, cardiovascular and blood, lymphatic and immune, respiratory, digestive, urinary, male reproductive, and female reproductive. These systems work together to perform all of the necessary functions of life. Figures 2-3 to 2-14 illustrate the most common features of all of these systems. A list of the common anatomical roots of each system is given for each figure.

## 2.4  Common Anatomical Roots

### Body as a Whole

| ROOT | MEANING |
|------|---------|
| axill/o | armpit |
| bi/o | life |
| cephal/o | head |
| cervic/o | neck |
| cyt/o | cell |
| hist/o; histi/o | tissue |
| lip/o; adip/o | fat |
| path/o | disease |
| viscer/o | internal organs |

### Integumentary System

| ROOT | MEANING |
|------|---------|
| cili/o; pil/o | hair |
| derm/o; dermat/o; cutane/o | skin |
| onych/o; ungu/o | nail |

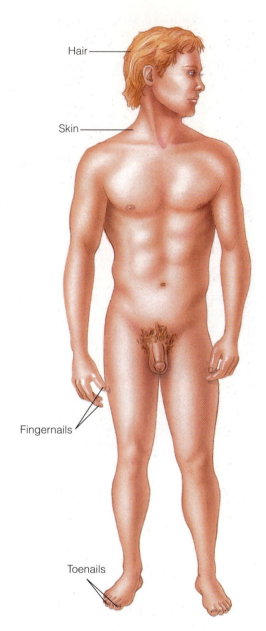

**Integumentary system
(The Skin)**

**Figure 2-3**  The skin and related structures.
Common structures: skin, hair, and nails.

## Skeletal System

| ROOT | MEANING |
|---|---|
| arthr/o | joint |
| chondr/o | cartilage |
| oste/o | bone |

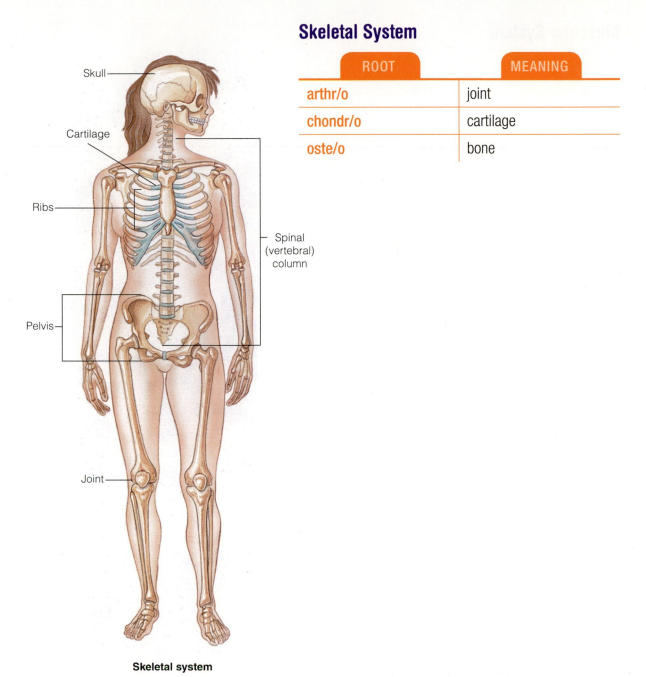

Skeletal system

**Figure 2-4** Skeletal system. Common structures: joints, cartilage, and bones.

## Muscular System

| ROOT | MEANING |
|------|---------|
| my/o; muscul/o | muscle |
| tend/o; tendin/o | tendon |

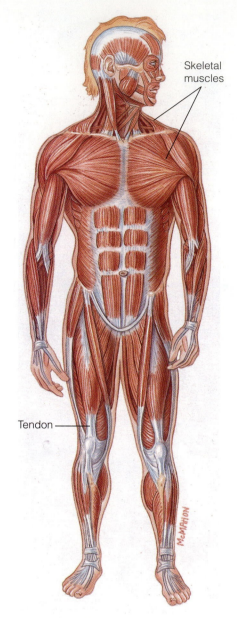

**Muscular system**

**Figure 2-5** Muscular system. Common structures: muscles and tendons.

## Nervous System, Eyes, Ears

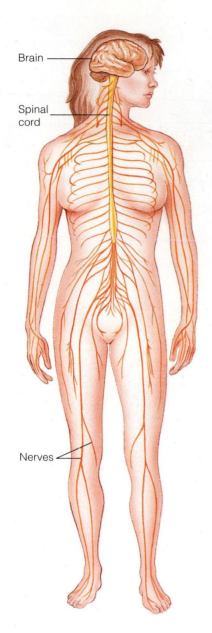

Brain

Spinal cord

Nerves

**Nervous system**

**Figure 2-6**  Nervous system, eyes, and ears. Common structures: brain, spinal cord, nerves, eyes, and ears.

| ROOT | MEANING |
|------|---------|
| blephar/o | eyelid |
| cerebr/o; encephal/o | brain |
| myel/o | spinal cord (also bone marrow) |
| neur/o | nerve |
| ophthalm/o; ocul/o | eye |
| ot/o | ear |

## Endocrine System

| ROOT | MEANING |
|------|---------|
| aden/o | gland |
| adren/o | adrenal gland |
| pituitar/o | pituitary gland |
| thyroid/o | thyroid gland |

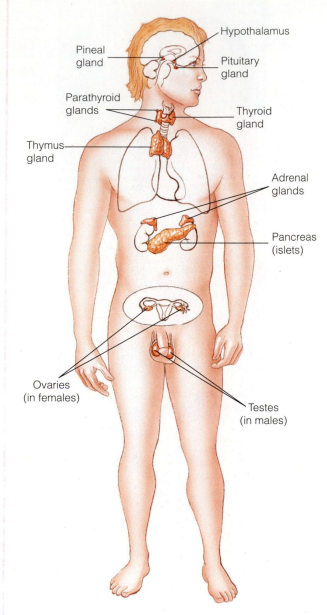

**Endocrine system**

**Figure 2-7** Endocrine system. Common structures: pineal gland, hypothalamus, pituitary gland, thyroid gland, thymus gland, pancreas, ovaries, testes, adrenal glands, and parathyroid glands.

## Cardiovascular System and Blood

| ROOT | MEANING |
|------|---------|
| adenoid/o | adenoids |
| angi/o; vascul/o; vas/o | vessel |
| arteri/o | artery |
| cardi/o | heart |
| hem/o; hemat/o | blood |
| ven/o; phleb/o | vein |

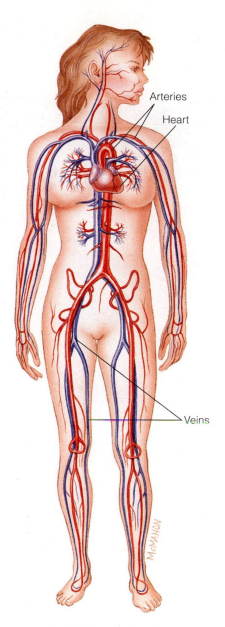

Arteries

Heart

Veins

McMAHON

**Cardiovascular system**

**Figure 2-8**  Cardiovascular system and blood. Common structures: heart, arteries, veins, and blood.

## Lymphatic and Immune Systems

| ROOT | MEANING |
|------|---------|
| adenoid/o | adenoids |
| lymph/o | clear fluid in lymphatic vessels |
| lymphaden/o | lymph gland; lymph node |
| lymphangi/o | lymph vessel |
| splen/o | spleen |
| tonsill/o | tonsil |

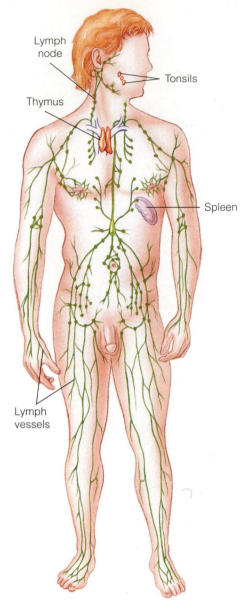

**Lymphatic and immune systems**

**Figure 2-9** Lymphatic and immune systems. Common structures: tonsils, lymph nodes, spleen, lymph vessels, and thymus.

## Respiratory System

| ROOT | MEANING |
| --- | --- |
| **bronch/o** | bronchus |
| **laryng/o** | larynx; voice box |
| **naso; rhin/o** | nose |
| **pharyng/o** | pharynx; throat |
| **phren/o** | diaphragm |
| **pneum/o; pneumon/o; pulmon/o** | lung |
| **thorac/o** | chest |
| **trache/o** | trachea; windpipe |

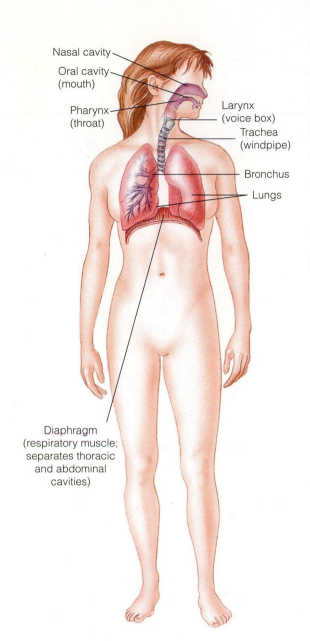

Nasal cavity
Oral cavity (mouth)
Pharynx (throat)
Larynx (voice box)
Trachea (windpipe)
Bronchus
Lungs
Diaphragm (respiratory muscle; separates thoracic and abdominal cavities)

**Respiratory system**

**Figure 2-10**  Respiratory system. Common structures: oral cavity, nasal cavity, pharynx, larynx, trachea, bronchus, lungs, and diaphragm.

## Digestive System

| ROOT | MEANING |
|------|---------|
| abdomin/o | abdomen |
| an/o | anus |
| cheil/o | lips |
| col/o | colon; large intestine |
| enter/o | small intestine |
| esophag/o | esophagus |
| gastr/o | stomach |
| gloss/o; lingu/o | tongue |
| hepat/o | liver |
| or/o; stomat/o | mouth |
| pharyng/o | pharynx; throat (also part of the respiratory tract) |
| rect/o | rectum |

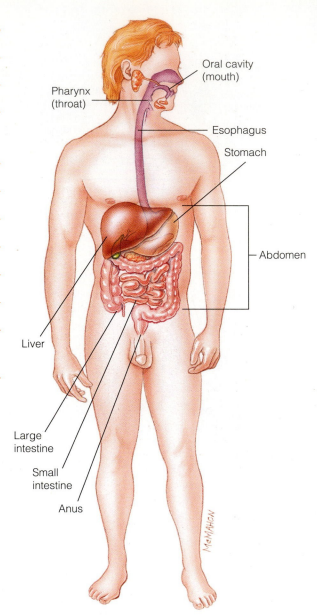

Oral cavity (mouth)
Pharynx (throat)
Esophagus
Stomach
Abdomen
Liver
Large intestine
Small intestine
Anus

**Digestive system**

**Figure 2-11** Digestive system. Common structures: oral cavity, pharynx, esophagus, stomach, small intestine, large intestine, anus, abdomen, and liver.

## Urinary System

| ROOT | MEANING |
|------|---------|
| cyst/o | bladder |
| ren/o; nephr/o | kidney |
| ureter/o | ureters |
| urethr/o | urethra |

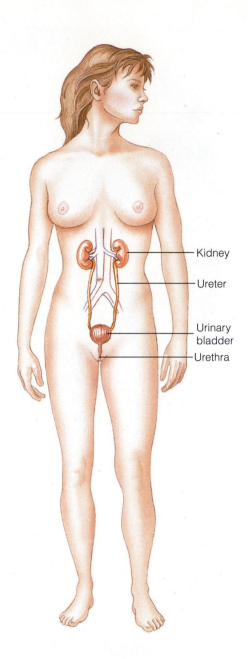

Kidney

Ureter

Urinary
bladder

Urethra

**Urinary system**

**Figure 2-12** Urinary system. Common structures:
kidneys, ureters, urinary bladder, and urethra.

## Male Reproductive System

| ROOT | MEANING |
|---|---|
| orchid/o; test/o | testicle; testis |
| prostat/o | prostate |
| vas/o | ductus deferens; vas deferens |

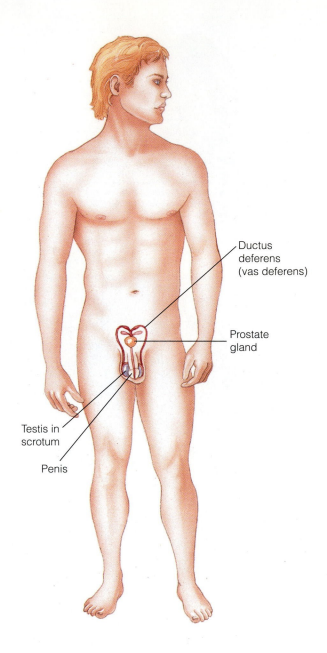

Ductus deferens (vas deferens)

Prostate gland

Testis in scrotum

Penis

**Male Reproductive system**

**Figure 2-13** Male reproductive system. Common structures: prostate gland, testes, penis, and ductus deferens.

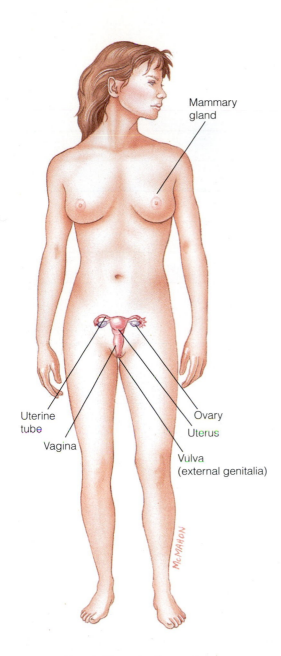

Female Reproductive system

**Figure 2-14** Female reproductive system. Common structures: mammary gland, uterine tubes, ovaries, uterus, vagina, and vulva (external genitalia).

## Female Reproductive System

| ROOT | MEANING |
|------|---------|
| colp/o; vagin/o | vagina |
| gynec/o | female |
| mast/o; mamm/o | breast |
| oophor/o; ovari/o | ovary |
| salping/o | fallopian tube; uterine tube |
| uter/o; hyster/o; metr/o | uterus |
| vulv/o | vulva; external genitalia |

## 2.5   Review Exercises

### EXERCISE 2-1   Definitions

*Give the meaning of the following roots.*

1. **abdomin/o** _____

2. **aden/o** _____

3. **adren/o** _____

4. **angi/o** _____

5. **arteri/o** _____

6. **arthr/o** _____

7. **bi/o** _____

8. **bronch/o** _____

9. **cardi/o** _____

10. **cephal/o** _____

11. **cerebr/o** _____

12. **cervic/o** _____

13. **chondr/o** _____

14. **cili/o** _____

15. **col/o** _____

16. **colp/o** _____

17. **cutane/o** _____

18. **cyst/o** _____

19. **cyt/o** _____

20. **dermat/o** _____

21. **encephal/o** _____

22. **enter/o** _____

23. **esophag/o** _____

24. **gastr/o** _____

25. **gloss/o** _____

26. **gynec/o** _____

27. **hem/o** _____

28. **hepat/o** _____

29. **hist/o** _____

30. **hyster/o** _____

31. **laryng/o** _____

32. **lingu/o** _____

33. **lip/o** _____

34. **lymphaden/o** _____

35. **lymphangi/o** _____

36. **mamm/o** _____

37. **mast/o** _____

38. **my/o** _____

39. **myel/o** _____

40. **nas/o** _____

41. **nephr/o** _____

42. **neur/o** _____

43. **ocul/o** _____

44. **onych/o** _____

45. **oophor/o** _____

46. **ophthalm/o** _____

47. **or/o** _____

48. **orchid/o** _____

49. **oste/o** _____

50. **ot/o** _____

51. **ovari/o** _____

52. **path/o** _____

53. **pharyng/o** _____

**54. phleb/o** _____

**55. pil/o** _____

**56. pneum/o** _____

**57. prostat/o** _____

**58. ren/o** _____

**59. rhin/o** _____

**60. salping/o** _____

**61. splen/o** _____

**62. stomat/o** _____

**63. tend/o** _____

**64. test/o** _____

**65. thorac/o** _____

**66. tonsill/o** _____

**67. trache/o** _____

**68. ungu/o** _____

**69. ureter/o** _____

**70. urethr/o** _____

**71. vagin/o** _____

**72. vas/o** _____

**73. vascul/o** _____

**74. ven/o** _____

**75. viscer/o** _____

**76. vulv/o** _____

**EXERCISE 2-2  Roots**

*Give the root for each of the following.*

**1. fat** _____

**2. life** _____

**3. head** _____

   **4. neck** _____

   **5. cell** _____

   **6. tissue** _____

   **7. disease** _____

   **8. internal organs** _____

   **9. hair** _____

 **10. skin** _____

 **11. nail** _____

 **12. joint** _____

 **13. cartilage** _____

 **14. bone** _____

 **15. muscle** _____

 **16. tendon** _____

 **17. brain** _____

 **18. spinal cord** _____

 **19. nerve** _____

 **20. eye** _____

 **21. ear** _____

 **22. gland** _____

 **23. adrenal gland** _____

 **24. pituitary gland** _____

 **25. thyroid gland** _____

 **26. vessel** _____

 **27. artery** _____

 **28. heart** _____

 **29. blood** _____

 **30. vein** _____

 **31. lymph node** _____

 **32. lymph vessel** _____

**33. spleen** _____

**34. tonsil** _____

## EXERCISE 2-3  Short Answers

*Answer the following in the space provided.*

**1.** Define anatomy and physiology.

_____

_____

**2.** Name at least 12 body systems and at least two organs in each.

_____

_____

_____

_____

_____

_____

_____

_____

_____

_____

_____

_____

_____

# Common Suffixes

## Chapter Outline

## Learning Objectives

*After studying this chapter and completing the exercises, you should be able to do the following:*

1. Spell and define common suffixes.
2. Identify suffixes used to convert medical nouns to adjectives.
3. Pronounce, spell, define, and write medical terms found in this chapter.

## Introduction

In Chapter 1 you learned two important points to remember about suffixes:

- The suffix is always at the end of a medical word.
- The suffix is the first word part to look at when you try to understand a medical word.

This chapter starts by listing new roots and prefixes. The next section introduces you to the most common suffixes. Each suffix and its meaning are listed first, followed by words using the suffix. These examples will help you remember the meaning of the suffixes. When you have learned them, you will be able to understand a great number of medical words.

## 3.1 New Roots, Suffixes, and Prefixes

Use these additional roots, prefixes, and suffixes when studying the terms in this chapter.

| ROOT | MEANING |
|------|---------|
| acr/o | top; extremities |
| all/o | referring to another |
| electr/o | electric |
| home/o | same; constant |
| iatr/o | physician |
| idi/o | individual; distinct |
| radi/o | x-rays |
| tom/o | to cut |

| PREFIX | MEANING |
|--------|---------|
| dia- | through; complete |
| pro- | before |

## 3.2 Learning the Terms

Use the following suggestions for learning medical terms:

1. Pronounce the term repeatedly until it is easy for you.

2. Write it down. Ensure the spelling is correct.

3. Also write the definition. If possible relate the word to a word, thought, or picture that will help you remember it.

4. Analyze the term with the method taught in this text.

| SUFFIX -algia (see also -dynia) | | MEANING pain |
|---------------------------------|---------------|--------------|
| Term | Term Analysis | Definition |
| cephalgia (sef-**AL**-jee-ah) | cephal/o = head | headache; pain in the head |
| otalgia (oh-**TAL**-jee-ah) | ot/o = ear | earache; pain in the ear |

| SUFFIX -cyte | | MEANING cell |
| --- | --- | --- |
| Term | Term Analysis | Definition |
| adipocyte (**AD**-ih-poh-sight) | adip/o = fat | fat cell |

| SUFFIX -dynia | | MEANING pain |
| --- | --- | --- |
| Term | Term Analysis | Definition |
| gastrodynia (**gas**-troh-**DIN**-ee-ah) | gastr/o = stomach | Pain in the stomach. Also known as gastralgia (gas-**TRAL**-jee-ah). |
| mastodynia (**mas**-toh-**DIN**-ee-ah) | mast/o = breast | breast pain |

| SUFFIX -ectomy | | MEANING surgical removal; excision |
| --- | --- | --- |
| Term | Term Analysis | Definition |
| hysterectomy (**hiss**-ter-**ECK**-toh-mee) | hyster/o = uterus | surgical removal or excision of the uterus |
| mastectomy (mas-**TECK**-toh-mee) | mast/o = breast | surgical removal or excision of the breast |

| SUFFIX -emesis | | MEANING vomiting |
| --- | --- | --- |
| Term | Term Analysis | Definition |
| hematemesis (**hee**-mah-**TEM**-eh-sis) | hemat/o = blood | vomiting of blood |
| emetic (eh-**MET**-ick) | -ic = pertaining | an agent such as a drug that causes vomiting |

| SUFFIX -genic | | MEANING producing; produced by |
| --- | --- | --- |
| Term | Term Analysis | Definition |
| allogenic (**al**-oh-**JEN**-ick) | all/o = referring to another | originating within another. In an allogenic heart transplant, the heart would be harvested from an individual of the same species but different genetic background. |
| iatrogenic (eye-**at**-roh-**JEN**-ick) | iatr/o = physician | adverse (harmful) side effects from treatment by physicians |

| SUFFIX -gnosis | | MEANING knowledge |
| --- | --- | --- |
| Term | Term Analysis | Definition |
| **diagnosis** (**dye**-ag-**NOH**-sis) | dia- = through; complete | determining what disease or condition is present through a study of the signs and symptoms, and laboratory, x-ray, and other diagnostic procedures<br><br>*Example: After complete investigation, a diagnosis of osteoarthritis was made.* |
| **prognosis** (prahg-**NOH**-sis) | pro- = before | forecast of the outcome of the disease<br><br>*Example: The patient is admitted for a hip replacement because of osteoarthritis. His **prognosis** is good.* |

**Note:** The prognosis is either good or bad. If the patient is likely to recover from the disease, the prognosis is good. If the patient is not likely to recover from the disease, the prognosis is bad.

| SUFFIX -gram | | MEANING record (written record or image) |
| --- | --- | --- |
| Term | Term Analysis | Definition |
| **angiogram** (**AN**-jee-oh-**gram**) | angi/o = vessel | record (image) of a blood vessel is produced using x-rays and contrast medium (Figure 3-1). |

**Note 1:** An image is produced of the body structure, thereby creating a record of that structure.

**Note 2:** Contrast medium is a dye that is placed into the patient's body to improve the visibility of the x-ray.

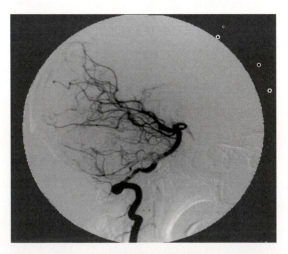

**Figure 3-1** Angiogram. The blood vessels, in black, are highlighted because a contrast medium was used to improve visibility.

| Term | Term Analysis | Definition |
|---|---|---|
| **mammogram**<br>(**MAM**-oh-gram) | mamm/o = breast | record (image) of the breast is produced using x-rays (Figure 3-2). |

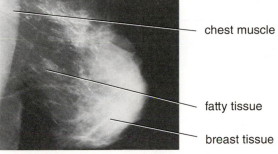

chest muscle

fatty tissue

breast tissue

**Figure 3-2**  Mammogram: record of the breast.

| Term | Term Analysis | Definition |
|---|---|---|
| **myelogram**<br>(**MY**-eh-loh-gram) | myel/o = spinal cord | record (image) of the spinal cord taken by x-rays |
| **venogram**<br>(**VEE**-noh-gram) | ven/o = vein | record (image) of a vein is produced using x-rays and contrast medium |

| SUFFIX<br>**-graph** | | MEANING<br>**instrument used to record** | |
|---|---|---|---|
| **Term** | **Term Analysis** | **Definition** | |
| **cardiograph**<br>(**KAR**-dee-oh-**graf**) | cardi/o = heart | instrument used to record the heart's activity | |
| **electrocardiograph**<br>(ee-**leck**-troh-**KAR**-dee-oh-**graf**) | electr/o = electric<br>cardi/o = heart | instrument used to record the electrical activity of the heart (Figure 3-3A and 3-3B) | |

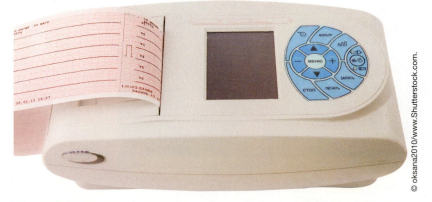

© oksana2010/www.Shutterstock.com.

**Figure 3-3A**  Electrocardiograph: instrument that records the electrical activity of the heart.

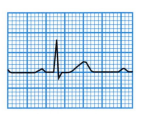

**Figure 3-3B**
Electrocardiogram: record of the electrical activity of the heart.

| SUFFIX -graphy | | MEANING process of recording; process of producing images |
|---|---|---|
| *Term* | *Term Analysis* | *Definition* |
| **cardiography** (**Kar**-dee-**OG**-rah-fee) | cardi/o = heart | process of recording the heart's activity |
| **computed tomography** (kom-**PYOO**-ted) (toh-**MOG**-rah-fee) | tom/o = to cut | an x-ray beam rotates around the patient taking multiple images of an organ at different depths (Figure 3-4A, and C). The information is computer analyzed and converted to a picture of the body part. |

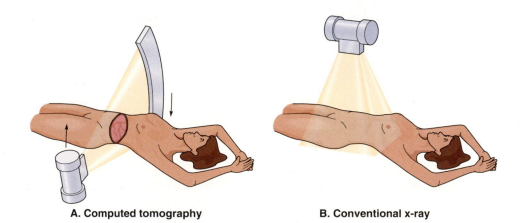

**A. Computed tomography**          **B. Conventional x-ray**

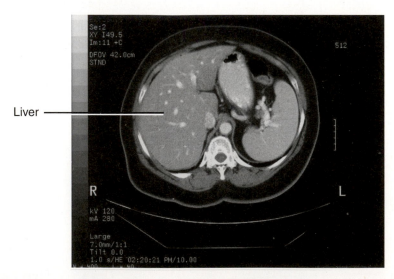

Liver —

**Figure 3-4** A. CT scan has an x-ray beam rotating around the patient. Images are taken of the organ at various depths. B. Conventional x-ray. The x-ray beam travels through the body from anterior to posterior (AP view). C. Abdominal CT scan showing the liver.

| Term | Term Analysis | Definition |
|---|---|---|
| **mammography** (mam-**OG**-rah-fee) | mamm/o = breast | process of producing images of the breast (See Figure 3-5) |

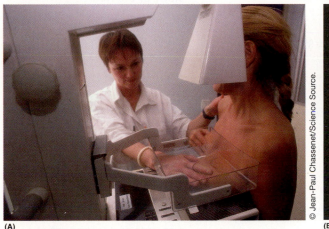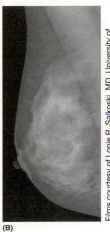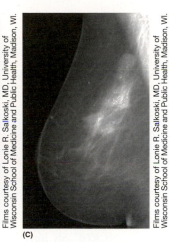

**Figure 3-5** A. Mammography. B. Normal mammogram. C. Mammogram showing visible breast cancer.

| Term | Term Analysis | Definition |
|---|---|---|
| **myelography** (**my**-eh-**LOG**-rah-fee) | myel/o = spinal cord | producing images of the spinal cord (using x-rays) |
| **radiography** (**ray**-dee-**OG**-rah-fee) | radi/o = x-rays | process of producing images using x-rays |

**Note:** Radiography is a general term. It refers to images that are taken of any internal body structure using x-rays.

**In Brief**

-**gram** = record
-**graph** = instrument used to record
-**graphy** = process of recording

| SUFFIX -itis | | MEANING inflammation |
|---|---|---|
| Term | Term Analysis | Definition |
| **enteritis** (**en**-ter-**EYE**-tis) | enter/o = small intestine | inflammation of the small intestine |
| **stomatitis** (**sto**-mah-**TYE**-tis) | stomat/o = mouth | inflammation of the mouth |
| **tonsillitis** (**ton**-sih-**LYE**-tis) | tonsill/o = tonsil | inflammation of the tonsils |

| SUFFIX -logy | | MEANING study of |
|---|---|---|
| Term | Term Analysis | Definition |
| cardiology (**kar**-dee-**OL**-oh-jee) | cardi/o = heart | study of the heart |
| dermatology (**der**-mah-**TOL**-oh-jee) | dermat/o = skin | study of the skin |

| SUFFIX -logist | | MEANING specialist; one who studies |
|---|---|---|
| Term | Term Analysis | Definition |
| gynecologist (**guy**-neh-**KOL**-oh-**jist**) | gynec/o = woman | specialist in the study of the diseases and treatment of female disorders |
| ophthalmologist (**ahf**-thal-**MOL**-eh-jist) | ophthalm/o = eye | specialist in the study of the diseases and treatment of eye disorders |

| SUFFIX -malacia | | MEANING softening |
|---|---|---|
| Term | Term Analysis | Definition |
| adenomalacia (**ad**-eh-noh-mah-**LAY**-shee-ah) | aden/o = gland | abnormal softening of a gland |
| osteomalacia (**os**-tee-oh-mah-**LAY**-shee-ah) | oste/o = bone | softening of bone |

| SUFFIX -megaly | | MEANING enlargement |
|---|---|---|
| Term | Term Analysis | Definition |
| visceromegaly (**VIS**-er-oh-**meg**-ah-lee) | viscer/o = internal organs | enlarged internal organs |

| SUFFIX -oma | | MEANING tumor; mass |
| --- | --- | --- |
| *Term* | *Term Analysis* | *Definition* |
| **adenocarcinoma** (**ad**-eh-o-**kar**-sih-**NOH**-mah) | aden/o = gland carin/o = cancer | cancer of glandular tissue |
| adenoma (**ad**-eh-**NOH**-mah) | aden/o = gland | tumor of a gland |
| **osteoma** (**os**-tee-**OH**-mah) | oste/o = bone | tumor of bone |
| **hematoma** (**hem**-ah-**TOH**-mah) | hemat/o = blood | mass or collection of blood outside a blood vessel; a bruise |

| SUFFIX -osis | | MEANING abnormal condition |
| --- | --- | --- |
| *Term* | *Term Analysis* | *Definition* |
| nephrosis (neh-**FROH**-sis) | nephr/o = kidney | abnormal condition of the kidney |

| SUFFIX -pathy | | MEANING disease |
| --- | --- | --- |
| *Term* | *Term Analysis* | *Definition* |
| **nephropathy** (neh-**FROP**-pah-thee) | nephr/o = kidney | disease of the kidney |
| **neuropathy** (new-**ROP**-pah-thee) | neur/o = nerve | disease of the nerve |

| SUFFIX -phobia | | MEANING fear |
| --- | --- | --- |
| *Term* | *Term Analysis* | *Definition* |
| **acrophobia** (**ack**-roh-**FOH**-bee-ah) | acr/o = top; extremities | fear of heights |

| SUFFIX -plasty | | MEANING surgical reconstruction |
| --- | --- | --- |
| *Term* | *Term Analysis* | *Definition* |
| **rhinoplasty** (**RYE**-noh-**plas**-tee) | rhin/o = nose | surgical reconstruction of the nose; nose job |
| **arthroplasty** (**AR**-throh-**plas**-tee) | arthr/o = joint | surgical reconstruction of a joint |

| SUFFIX -ptosis | | MEANING drooping; sagging |
| --- | --- | --- |
| Term | Term Analysis | Definition |
| nephroptosis (**nef**-rop-**TOH**-sis) | nephr/o = kidney | drooping kidney |

| SUFFIX -ptysis | | MEANING spitting |
| --- | --- | --- |
| Term | Term Analysis | Definition |
| hemoptysis (hee-**MOP**-tih-sis) | hem/o = blood | spitting up of blood |

| SUFFIX -rrhage; -rrhagia | | MEANING bursting forth |
| --- | --- | --- |
| Term | Term Analysis | Definition |
| hemorrhage (**HEM-**or-idj) | hem/o = blood | bursting forth of blood; bleeding |
| gastrorrhagia (**gas**-troh-**RAY**-jee-ah) | gastr/o = stomach | bleeding from the stomach |

| SUFFIX -rrhaphy | | MEANING to suture (to sew) |
| --- | --- | --- |
| Term | Term Analysis | Definition |
| colporrhaphy (kol-**POR**-ah-fee) | colp/o = vagina | suturing the wall of the vagina (Figure 3-6) |

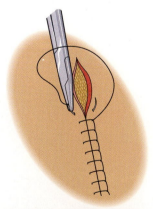

**Continuous sutures**

**Figure 3-6** To suture (sew). The edges of the wound are brought together by suturing.

| SUFFIX -rrhea | | MEANING flow; discharge |
|---|---|---|
| Term | Term Analysis | Definition |
| otorrhea (oh-toh-REE-ah) | ot/o = ear | discharge from the ear |

| SUFFIX -rrhexis | | MEANING rupture |
|---|---|---|
| Term | Term Analysis | Definition |
| splenorrhexis (splee-nor-ECKS-sis) | splen/o = spleen | ruptured spleen |

**In Brief**

-rrhage = burst forth
-rrhaphy = suture
-rrhea = flow; discharge
-rrhexis = rupture

| SUFFIX -sclerosis | | MEANING hardening |
|---|---|---|
| Term | Term Analysis | Definition |
| arteriosclerosis (ar-teer-ee-oh-skleh-ROH-sis) | arteri/o = artery | hardening of the arteries |

| SUFFIX -scope | | MEANING instrument used to view inside a body cavity or organ |
|---|---|---|
| Term | Term Analysis | Definition |
| arthroscope (AR-throh-skope) | arthr/o = joint | instrument used to view the inside of a joint cavity |
| gastroscope (GAS-troh-skope) | gastr/o = stomach | instrument used to view the inside of the stomach |

**In Brief**

-scope = instrument used to view inside a body cavity or organ
-scopy = process of viewing inside a body cavity or organ

| SUFFIX -scopy | | MEANING the process of viewing inside a body cavity or organ |
|---|---|---|
| *Term* | *Term Analysis* | *Definition* |
| **endoscopy** (en-**DOS**-koh-pee) | endo- = within | process of visually examining the inside of a body cavity or organ using an endoscope (Figure 3-7) |

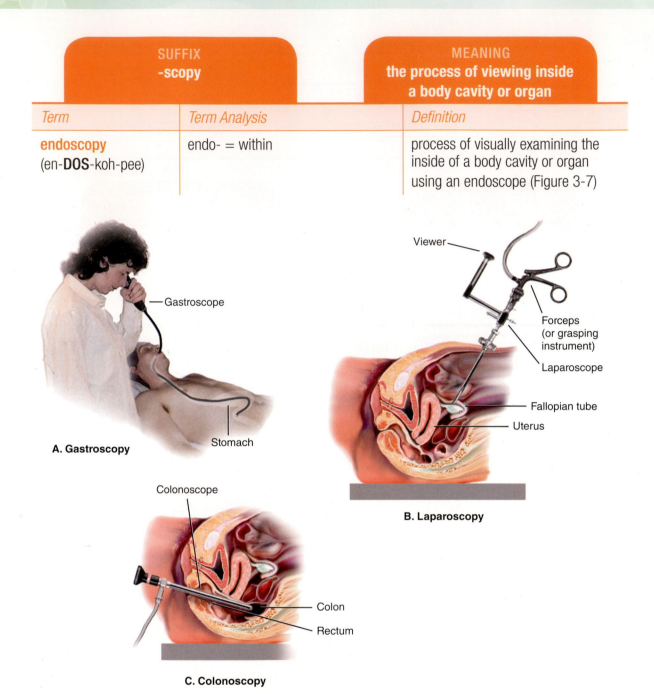

**Figure 3-7** Endoscopies. A. Gastroscopy. B. Laparoscopy. C. Colonoscopy.

**Note:** Endoscopy is a general term. Specific endoscopies are named after the organ being studied. See the following terms as examples.

| | | |
|---|---|---|
| **bronchoscopy** (brong-**KOS**-koh-pee) | bronch/o = bronchus | process of viewing inside the bronchus |
| **laparoscopy** (lap-ah-**ROS**-koh-pee) | lapar/o = abdomen | process of viewing the abdomen (refer to Figure 3-7B) |

| SUFFIX -spasm | | MEANING sudden involuntary muscle contraction |
| --- | --- | --- |
| *Term* | *Term Analysis* | *Definition* |
| laryngospasm (lah-**RING**-go-**spaz**-um) | laryng/o = larynx | sudden muscular spasm of the larynx |

| SUFFIX -stasis | | MEANING stable; stopping; controlling |
| --- | --- | --- |
| *Term* | *Term Analysis* | *Definition* |
| hemostasis (**hee**-moh-**STAY**-sis) | hem/o = blood | stopping of bleeding |
| homeostasis (**hoh**-mee-oh-**STAY**-sis) | home/o = same | balanced yet varied state |

| SUFFIX -stenosis | | MEANING narrowing |
| --- | --- | --- |
| *Term* | *Term Analysis* | *Definition* |
| arteriostenosis (ar-**teer**-ee-oh-steh-**NOH**-sis) | arteri/o = artery | narrowing of an artery |

| SUFFIX -stomy | | MEANING surgical creation of a new opening |
| --- | --- | --- |
| *Term* | *Term Analysis* | *Definition* |
| colostomy (koh-**LOSS**-toh-mee) | col/o = colon | surgical creation of a new opening in the colon |
| tracheostomy (**tray**-kee-**OS**-toh-mee) | trache/o = trachea; windpipe | surgical creation of a new opening into the trachea |

| SUFFIX -tomy | | MEANING to cut; incision |
| --- | --- | --- |
| *Term* | *Term Analysis* | *Definition* |
| tenotomy (teh-**NOT**-oh-mee) | ten/o = tendon | to cut the tendon; incision of the tendon |
| tracheotomy (**tray**-kee-**OT**-toh-mee) | trache/o = trachea; windpipe | to cut the trachea; incision of the trachea |

**Note:** Incision means to cut into.

| In Brief | **-stomy** = surgical creation of a new opening |
|----------|------------------------------------------------|
|          | **-tomy** = to cut |
|          | **incision** means to cut into |
|          | **excision** means to cut out |

| SUFFIX | | MEANING |
|--------|-|---------|
| **-trophy** | | **growth; nourishment** |
| *Term* | *Term Analysis* | *Definition* |
| **atrophy** (**AH**-troh-fee) | a- = no; not | wasting away of the muscle (Figure 3-8A) |
| **hypertrophy** (high-**PER**-troh-fee) | hyper- = excessive | excessive growth or enlargement of an organ or part (Figure 3-8B) |

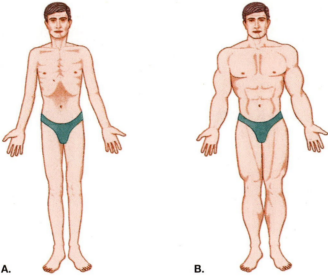

A.                              B.

**Figure 3-8** Differences in muscle size. A. Atrophy. B. Hypertrophy.

## Suffixes Used as Adjectives

| SUFFIX | | MEANING |
|--------|-|---------|
| **-ac; -ous; -ic; -al** **-ary; -ar; -eal** | | **pertaining to** |
| *Term* | *Term Analysis* | *Definition* |
| **cardiac** (**KAR**-dee-ack) | cardi/o = heart | pertaining to the heart |
| **chondral** (**KON-**dral) | chondr/o = cartilage | pertaining to cartilage |

| Term | Term Analysis | Definition |
|------|---------------|------------|
| **cutaneous** (kyoo-**TAY**-nee-us) | cutane/o = skin | pertaining to the skin |
| **gastric** (**GAS**-trik) | gastr/o = stomach | pertaining to the stomach |
| **idiopathic** (**id**-ee-oh-**PATH**-ick) | idi/o = one's own; distinct path/o = disease | unknown cause. *Example: idiopathic disease.* |
| **mammary** (**MAM**-ah-ree) | mamm/o = breast | pertaining to the breast |
| **muscular** (**MUS**-kyou-lar) | muscul/o = muscle | pertaining to muscle |
| **natal** (**NAY**-tal) | nat/o = birth | pertaining to birth |
| **pharyngeal** (far-**IN**-jee-al) | pharyng/o = throat; pharynx | pertaining to the throat |
| **septic** (**SEHP**-tick) | sept/o = infection | pertaining to infection |
| **venous** (**VEE**-nus) | ven/o = vein | pertaining to a vein |

**Note:** Although there are some exceptions, the suffixes meaning "pertaining to" are not interchangeable with a given root. For example, you can say muscul**ar**, but not muscul**al**, muscul**ic**, or muscul**ous**. You can say cardi**ac** but not cardi**ous** or cardi**ary**.

## 3.3  Review Exercises

### EXERCISE 3-1  Matching Word Elements with Meaning

*Match the word part in Column A with its meaning in Column B*

| | Column A | Column B |
|---|----------|----------|
| _____ | **1.** -algia | A. specialist |
| _____ | **2.** -ectomy | B. tumor; mass |
| _____ | **3.** -logy | C. nourishment |
| _____ | **4.** -logist | D. excision; surgical removal |
| _____ | **5.** -ous | E. surgical reconstruction |
| _____ | **6.** -scopy | F. pertaining to |

| | | | |
|---|---|---|---|
| _____ | **7.** -scope | G. | pain |
| _____ | **8.** -plasty | H. | instrument used to view inside an organ |
| _____ | **9.** -oma | I. | study of |
| _____ | **10.** -trophy | J. | process of viewing inside an organ |

## EXERCISE 3-2   Definitions

*Give the meaning of the following suffixes.*

**a**. **-trophy** _____

**b.** **-algia** _____

**c. -tomy** _____

**d. -ectomy** _____

**e. -gram** _____

**f. -logist** _____

**g. -scope** _____

**h. -itis** _____

**i. -plasty** _____

**j. -logy** _____

**k. -ous** _____

**l. -oma** _____

**m. -ic** _____

**n. -al** _____

**o. -scopy** _____

**p. -osis** _____

## EXERCISE 3-3   Identifying and Defining Word Parts

*In the words listed below, separate the medical term into its word parts with a slash (/). Then, define the term in the space provided. The first question is answered for you.*

**a. aden/oma** tumor of a gland

**b. otalgia** _____

**c. dermatologist** _____

d. **hysterectomy** _____

e. **cardiology** _____

f. **myelogram** _____

g. **tonsillitis** _____

h. **cutaneous** _____

i. **hypertrophy** _____

j. **rhinoplasty** _____

k. **arthroscopy** _____

l. **arthroscope** _____

m. **tracheotomy** _____

n. **natal** _____

o. **septic** _____

## EXERCISE 3-4 Adjectival Suffix

*Match the root with the correct adjectival ending, then complete the sentences below.*

| ROOT | ADJECTIVAL SUFFIX |
|------|-------------------|
| muscul- | -al |
| nat- | -ic |
| sept- | -ous |
| cutane- | -ar |

1. I pulled a muscle. I now have _____ pain.

2. I have red marks on my skin. The doctor said it was a _____ rash.

3. I am going to have a baby. I am going to pre- _____ classes.

4. Throw the infectious material away. Put it in the garbage for _____ material.

## EXERCISE 3-5 Spelling

*Circle the word that is correctly spelled in each group below.*

1. cephalalga        cefalalgia        cephalgia
2. hysterectomy        histerectomy
3. tonsillitis        tonsilitis
4. cardology        cardiology
5. ophthalmologist        opthalmologist        ophtalmologist
6. nephrosis        nephrosus
7. tracheotomy        traechotomy
8. hypertrophe        hypertrophy
9. enteritis        enteritus
10. mylogram        myelogram

## EXERCISE 3-6 Definitions

*Define the following terms.*

1. **adenoma** _____

2. **arthroplasty** _____

3. **arthroscope** _____

4. **bronchoscopy** _____

5. **cardiology** _____

6. **cephalgia** _____

7. **dermatology** _____

8. **enteritis** _____

9. **gastroscope** _____

10. **laparoscopy** _____

11. **gynecologist** _____

12. **hematoma** _____

13. **hypertrophy** _____

14. **hysterectomy** _____

15. **mastectomy** _____

**16. myelogram** _____

**17. nephropathy** _____

**18. nephrosis** _____

**19. neuropathy** _____

**20. ophthalmologist** _____

**21. osteoma** _____

**22. otalgia** _____

**23. rhinoplasty** _____

**24. stomatitis** _____

**25. tenotomy** _____

**26. tonsillitis** _____

**27. tracheotomy** _____

**28. tracheostomy** _____

**29. excision** _____

**30. incision** _____

## 3.4 Pronunciation and Spelling

*To practice your pronunciation:*

1. Listen to each word on the audio file provided on the Student Companion Website.

2. Pronounce each word carefully.

3. Spell each word in the space provided.

| Word | Pronunciation | Spelling |
| --- | --- | --- |
| acrophobia | **ack**-roh-**FOH**-bee-ah | |
| adenocarcinoma | **ad**-eh-no-**kar**-sih-**NOH**-mah | |
| adenomalacia | **ad**-eh-noh-mah-**LAY**-shee-ah | |
| adenoma | **ad**-eh-**NOH**-mah | |
| allogenic | **al**-oh-**JEN**-ick | |
| arteriosclerosis | ar-**teer**-ee-oh-skleh-**ROH**-sis | |

| Word | Pronunciation | Spelling |
|------|---------------|----------|
| arthroscope | **AR**-throh-skohp | |
| arthroscopy | ar-**THROS**-koh-pee | |
| cardiac | **KAR**-dee-ack | |
| cardiology | **kar**-dee-**OL**-oh-jee | |
| chondral | **KON**-dral | |
| colostomy | koh-**LOSS**-toh-mee | |
| cutaneous | kyoo-**TAY**-nee-us | |
| dermatology | **der**-mah-**TOL**-oh-jee | |
| electrocardiograph | ee-**leck**-troh-**KAR**-dee-oh-**graf** | |
| emetic | eh-**MET**-ick | |
| enteritis | **en**-ter-**EYE**-tis | |
| gastric | **GAS**-trik | |
| gastrodynia | **gas**-troh-**DIN**-ee-ah | |
| gastroscopy | gas-**TROS**-koh-pee | |
| gynecologist | **guy**-neh-**KOL**-oh-jist | |
| hematemesis | **hee**-mah-**TEM**-eh-sis | |
| hematoma | **hem**-ah-**TOH**-mah | |
| hemoptysis | hee-**MOP**-tih-sis | |
| hemostasis | **hee**-moh-**STAY**-sis | |
| homeostasis | **hoh**-mee-oh-**STAY**-sis | |
| hypertrophy | high-**PER**-troh-fee | |
| hysterectomy | **hiss**-ter-**ECK**-toh-mee | |
| iatrogenic | eye-**at**-roh-**JEN**-ick | |
| idiopathic | **id**-ee-oh-**PATH**-ick | |
| laryngospasm | lah-**RING**-go-**spaz**-um | |
| mastectomy | mas-**TECK**-toh-mee | |
| mastodynia | **mas**-toh-**DIN**-ee-ah | |
| muscular | **MUS**-kyoo-lar | |
| myelogram | **MY**-eh-loh-gram | |

| Word | Pronunciation | Spelling |
|------|---------------|----------|
| myelography | **my**-eh-**LOG**-rah-fee | |
| natal | **NAY**-tal | |
| nephropathy | nef-**ROP**-pah-thee | |
| nephroptosis | **nef**-rop-**TOH**-sis | |
| nephrosis | neh-**FROH**-sis | |
| neuropathy | new-**ROP**-pah-thee | |
| ophthalmologist | **ahf**-thal-**MOL**-eh-jist | |
| osteomalacia | **os**-tee-oh-mah-**LAY**-shee-ah | |
| osteoma | **os**-tee-**OH**-mah | |
| otalgia | **oh**-**TAL**-gee-ah | |
| pharyngeal | far-**IN**-jee-al | |
| prognosis | prahg-**NOH**-sis | |
| radiography | **ray**-dee-**OG**-rah-fee | |
| stomatitis | **sto**-mah-**TYE**-tis | |
| tenotomy | teh-**NOT**-oh-mee | |
| tomography | toh-**MOG**-rah-fee | |
| tonsillitis | **ton**-sih-**LYE**-tis | |
| tracheotomy | **tray**-kee-**OT**-toh-mee | |
| venous | **VEE**-nus | |
| visceromegaly | **VIS**-er-oh-**meg**-ah-lee | |

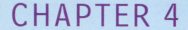

# CHAPTER 4
# Common Prefixes

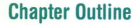

## Chapter Outline

## Learning Objectives

*After studying this chapter and completing the exercises, you should be able to do the following:*

1. State the meaning of prefixes found in this chapter.
2. Pronounce, spell, define, and write medical terms that use prefixes in this chapter.
3. Identify prefixes that have the same meaning.
4. Identify prefixes that have the opposite meaning.

## Introduction

This chapter introduces you to the most common prefixes. It starts by listing new roots and suffixes used in this chapter. The next section displays the prefix and its meaning first, followed by words using the prefix.

## 4.1 New Roots and Suffixes

Use these additional roots and suffixes when studying the medical terms in this chapter.

| ROOT | MEANING |
|------|---------|
| cellul/o | cell |
| cis/o | to cut |
| cost/o | rib |
| duct/o | to draw |
| later/o | side |
| sect/o | to cut |
| son/o | sound |
| versi/o | turning; tilting; tipping |

| SUFFIX | MEANING |
|--------|---------|
| -drome | run |
| -genous | produced by |
| -iasis | abnormal condition |
| -ion | process |
| -mortem | death |
| -opsy | to view |
| -partum | delivery |
| -plasia; -plasm | development; formation |
| -pnea | breathing |
| -tic | pertaining to |
| -um | structure |
| -uria | urination; urine |
| -y | condition; process |

## 4.2   Learning the Terms

Use the following suggestions for learning medical terms:

1. Pronounce the term repeatedly until it is easy for you.
2. Write it down. Ensure the spelling is correct.
3. Also write the definition. If possible, relate the word to a word, thought, or picture that will help you remember it.
4. Analyze the term with the method taught in this text.

| PREFIX<br>a(n)- | | MEANING<br>no; not |
|---|---|---|
| *Term* | *Term Analysis* | *Definition* |
| **apnea**<br>(**AP**-nee-ah) | -pnea = breathing | not breathing |
| **anuria**<br>(ah-**NOO**-ree-ah) | -uria = urine; urination | no urine (being formed in the kidney) |

**Helping You Remember**   The prefix "a-" changes to "an-" in the word "anuria" because the suffix begins with a vowel.

| PREFIX<br>ab- | | MEANING<br>away from |
|---|---|---|
| *Term* | *Term Analysis* | *Definition* |
| **abduction**<br>(ab-**DUCK**-shun) | -ion = process<br>duct/o = to draw | process of drawing away from the midline |

| PREFIX<br>ad- | | MEANING<br>toward |
|---|---|---|
| *Term* | *Term Analysis* | *Definition* |
| **adduction**<br>(ah-**DUCK**-shun) | -ion = process<br>duct/o = to draw | process of drawing toward the midline |

| PREFIX ana- | | MEANING up; apart |
| --- | --- | --- |
| Term | Term Analysis | Definition |
| **anatomy** (ah-**NAT**-oh-mee) | -tomy = process of cutting | the study of the structure or parts of the body |

| PREFIX ante- | | MEANING before |
| --- | --- | --- |
| Term | Term Analysis | Definition |
| **antenatal** (**an**-tee-**NAY**-tal) | -al = pertaining to nat/o = birth | pertaining to before birth, referring to the fetus; prenatal |
| **Note:** Fetus is the name given to the unborn infant. | | |
| **antepartum** (**an**-tee-**PAR**-tum) | -partum = delivery, labor, childbirth | before childbirth, referring to the mother |

| PREFIX anti- | | MEANING against |
| --- | --- | --- |
| Term | Term Analysis | Definition |
| **antibiotic** (**an**-tih-bye-**OT**-ick) | -tic = pertaining to bi/o = life | drugs used against bacteria that have infected the body |

**Helping You Remember**

The prefix *anti-* means "against." Note that both the prefix and its meaning contain the letter "i."
The prefix *ante-* means "before." Both the prefix and its meaning contain the letter "e."

| PREFIX auto- | | MEANING self |
| --- | --- | --- |
| Term | Term Analysis | Definition |
| **autopsy** (**AW**-top-see) | -opsy = to view | internal and external examination of the body after death to determine the cause of death. Also called a **necropsy** (**NECK**-rop-see) or postmortem examination |

| PREFIX<br>bi- (see di-) | | MEANING<br>two |
| --- | --- | --- |
| Term | Term Analysis | Definition |
| **bilateral**<br>(bye-**LAT**-er-al) | -al = pertaining to<br>later/o = side | pertaining to two sides |

| Helping You Remember | A bicycle has two wheels. |
| --- | --- |

| PREFIX<br>circum- | | MEANING<br>around |
| --- | --- | --- |
| Term | Term Analysis | Definition |
| **circumduction**<br>(**ser**-kum-**DUCK**-shun) | -ion = process<br>duct/o = to draw | process of moving a limb in<br>a circular motion |

| PREFIX<br>contra- | | MEANING<br>against |
| --- | --- | --- |
| Term | Term Analysis | Definition |
| **contraindication**<br>(**kon**-trah-**in**-dih-**KAY**-shun) | indication = a sign or<br>symptom that serves to<br>reveal a disease or<br>condition exists | a medical reason that indicates a specific<br>treatment, i.e., medications, procedure,<br>or surgery, should not be performed<br>because it may harm the patient.<br><br>*Example: Drugs used to treat acne are<br>contraindicated in pregnancy because of<br>possible harmful effects to the fetus.* |
| **contralateral**<br>(**kon**-trah-**LAT**-er-ahl) | -al = pertaining to<br>later/o = side | pertaining to the opposite side |

| PREFIX<br>di- | | MEANING<br>two |
| --- | --- | --- |
| Term | Term Analysis | Definition |
| **dissection**<br>(dye-**SECK**-shun) | -ion = process<br>sect/o = to cut | the process of cutting and separating<br>parts of the body |

| PREFIX dys- | | MEANING bad; difficult; painful; abnormal |
|---|---|---|
| Term | Term Analysis | Definition |
| **dysplasia** (dis-**PLAY**-zha) | -plasia = development; formation | abnormal development |
| **dyspnea** (**DISP**-nee-ah) | -pnea = breathing | difficult breathing |
| **dysuria** (dis-**YOO**-ree-ah) | -uria = urine; urination | painful urination |
| **dystrophy** (**DIS**-troh-fee) | -trophy = nourishment; growth; development | abnormal development. *Example: muscular dystrophy* |

| PREFIX endo- | | MEANING within |
|---|---|---|
| Term | Term Analysis | Definition |
| **endogenous** (en-**DOJ**-eh-nus) | -genous = produced by | produced from within the body; disease that originates from within the body. *Example: adult chicken pox (shingles) is the reactivation of the virus that caused childhood chicken pox. The virus has stayed inactive within the body for years.* |

| PREFIX epi- | | MEANING upon; above |
|---|---|---|
| Term | Term Analysis | Definition |
| **epicardium** (ep-ih-**KAR**-dee-um) | -um = structure cardi/o = heart | outer wall of the heart |

| PREFIX ex- (see also exo-) | | MEANING out |
|---|---|---|
| Term | Term Analysis | Definition |
| **excision** (eck-**SIH**-zhun) | -ion = process cis/o = to cut | process of cutting out; the surgical removal of tissue from the body |

| PREFIX<br>exo-; ecto- | | MEANING<br>out |
| --- | --- | --- |
| Term | Term Analysis | Definition |
| **exogenous**<br>(eck-**SOJ**-eh-nus) | -genous = produced by | produced outside the body; also known as **ectogenous** (eck-**TOJ**-eh-nus) |

| PREFIX<br>hyper- | | MEANING<br>above; excessive |
| --- | --- | --- |
| Term | Term Analysis | Definition |
| **hyperplasia**<br>(**high**-per-**PLAY**-zha) | -plasia = development; formation | excessive formation of cells; abnormal increase in the **number** of normal cells in normal tissue. May indicate a precancerous condition. Do not confuse with hypertrophy, which is enlargement of an organ due to an increase in the **size** of cells. |

| PREFIX<br>hypo- | | MEANING<br>below; deficient |
| --- | --- | --- |
| Term | Term Analysis | Definition |
| **hypogastric**<br>(**high**-poh-**GAS**-trick) | -ic = pertaining to<br>gastr/o = stomach | pertaining to below the stomach |
| **hypochondriasis**<br>(**high**-poh-kon-**DRY**-ah-sis) | -iasis = abnormal condition<br>chondr/o = cartilage | mental illness characterized by persistent thoughts that one has a serious illness despite complete medical evaluation and reassurance that there is no such illness |

| PREFIX<br>in- | | MEANING<br>in; into |
| --- | --- | --- |
| Term | Term Analysis | Definition |
| **incision**<br>(in-**SIH**-zhun) | -ion = process<br>cis/o = to cut | process of cutting |
| **inversion**<br>(in-**VER**-zhun) | -ion = process<br>versi/o = turning; tilting; tipping | turning inward, as in the turning of the sole of the foot inward. The opposite is **eversion** (ee-**VER**-zhun), turning outward. |

| PREFIX infra- | | MEANING below |
| --- | --- | --- |
| Term | Term Analysis | Definition |
| infracostal (in-frah-**KOS**-tal) | -al = pertaining to cost/o = rib | pertaining to below the rib |

| PREFIX inter- | | MEANING between |
| --- | --- | --- |
| Term | Term Analysis | Definition |
| intercellular (in-ter-**SEL**-yoo-lar) | -ar = pertaining to cellul/o = cell | pertaining to between the cells |
| intercostal (in-ter-**KOS**-tal) | -al = pertaining to cost/o = rib | pertaining to between the ribs |

| PREFIX intra- | | MEANING within |
| --- | --- | --- |
| Term | Term Analysis | Definition |
| intracranial (in-trah-**KRAY**-nee-al) | -al = pertaining to crani/o = head | pertaining to within the head |
| intramuscular (in-trah-**MUS**-kyoo-lar) | -ar = pertaining to muscul/o = muscle | pertaining to within a muscle |
| intravenous (in-trah-**VEE**-nus) | -ous = pertaining to ven/o = vein | pertaining to within a vein |

**In Brief**

infra- = below
inter- = between
intra- = within

| PREFIX macro- | | MEANING large |
| --- | --- | --- |
| Term | Term Analysis | Definition |
| macrocephaly (mack-roh-**SEF**-eh-lee) | -y = condition; process cephal/o = head | abnormally large head |

| PREFIX **meta-** | | MEANING **beyond** |
|---|---|---|
| *Term* | *Term Analysis* | *Definition* |
| **metaplasia** (**met**-ah-**PLAY**-zha) | **-plasia** = formation; development | change in formation |
| **metastasis** (meh-**TAS**-tah-sis) | **-stasis** = stopping; controlling | the uncontrolled spread of cancerous cells from one organ to another |

| PREFIX **micro-** | | MEANING **small** |
|---|---|---|
| *Term* | *Term Analysis* | *Definition* |
| **microscope** (**MY-**kroh-skohp) | -scope = instrument used to visually examine | an instrument used to view objects too small to be seen with the naked eye |

| PREFIX **neo-** | | MEANING **new** |
|---|---|---|
| *Term* | *Term Analysis* | *Definition* |
| **neoplasm** (**NEE-**oh-plazm) | -plasm = development; formation | new growth of tissue; a tumor. The tumor can be **benign** (bee-**NIGHN**), meaning harmless, or **malignant** (mah-**LIG**-nant), meaning harmful. |

| PREFIX **pan-** | | MEANING **all** |
|---|---|---|
| *Term* | *Term Analysis* | *Definition* |
| **panhysterectomy** (**pan**-hiss-ter-**ECK**-toh-mee) | -ectomy = excision; surgical removal hyster/o = uterus | surgical removal of the entire uterus |

| PREFIX **para-** | | MEANING **beside; near** |
|---|---|---|
| *Term* | *Term Analysis* | *Definition* |
| **parenteral drugs** (pah-**REN**-ter-al) | -al = pertaining to enter/o = small intestine | therapeutic drugs placed in the body in ways other than through the digestive tract. Parenteral drugs are given by injection into several sites, including the skin, muscle, vein, or spine. |

| PREFIX per- | | MEANING through |
|---|---|---|
| Term | Term Analysis | Definition |
| **percutaneous** (**per**-kyou-**TAY**-nee-us) | -ous = pertaining to cutane/o = skin | pertaining to through the skin |

**In Brief**

**pan-** = all
**pre-** = before
**pro-** = before
**per-** = through

| PREFIX peri- | | MEANING around |
|---|---|---|
| Term | Term Analysis | Definition |
| **perineuritis** (**per**-ih-nyoo-**RYE**-tis) | -itis = inflammation neur/o = nerve | inflammation around the nerve |

| PREFIX post- | | MEANING after |
|---|---|---|
| Term | Term Analysis | Definition |
| **postmortem** (pohst-**MOR**-tehm) **examination** | -mortem = death examination = to look at; to inspect | inspection of the body after death; autopsy |
| **postpartum** (pohst-**PAR**-tum) | -partum = delivery; labor; childbirth | after childbirth, with reference to the mother |

| PREFIX pre- | | MEANING before |
|---|---|---|
| Term | Term Analysis | Definition |
| **prenatal** (pree-**NAY**-tal) | -al = pertaining to nat/o = birth | pertaining to before birth, referring to the fetus |

| PREFIX pro- | | MEANING before |
| --- | --- | --- |
| Term | Term Analysis | Definition |
| **prodrome** (**PROH-**drohm) | -drome = run | symptom or symptoms occurring before the onset of disease. *Example: chest pain, tiredness, and shortness of breath are prodromal symptoms of a heart attack.* |

| PREFIX retro- | | MEANING back |
| --- | --- | --- |
| Term | Term Analysis | Definition |
| **retroversion** (**ret**-roh-**VER**-zhun) | -ion = process versi/o = turning; tipping; tilting | backward turning or tipping of an organ |

| PREFIX sub- | | MEANING under; below |
| --- | --- | --- |
| Term | Term Analysis | Definition |
| **subcutaneous** (**sub**-kyoo-**TAY**-nee-us) | -ous = pertaining to cutane/o = skin | pertaining to under the skin (Figure 4-1) |

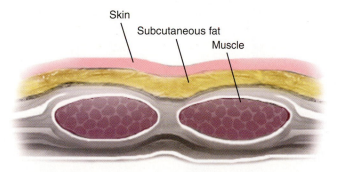

Skin
Subcutaneous fat
Muscle

**Figure 4-1** Skin and subcutaneous fat.

| **sublingual** (sub-**LING**-gwal) | -al = pertaining to lingu/o = tongue | pertaining to under the tongue |
| --- | --- | --- |

| PREFIX supra- | | MEANING above |
|---|---|---|
| Term | Term Analysis | Definition |
| **suprarenal** (**soo**-prah-**REE**-nal) | -al = pertaining ren/o = kidney | pertaining to above the kidney |

| PREFIX trans- | | MEANING through; across |
|---|---|---|
| Term | Term Analysis | Definition |
| **transection** (tran-**SECK**-shun) | -ion = process sect/o = cut | process of cutting across (Figure 4-2) |

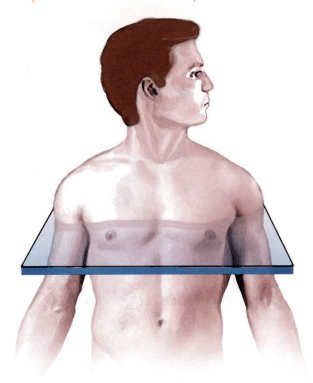

**Figure 4-2** Transection (the process of cutting across the body or an organ).

| PREFIX<br>ultra- | | MEANING<br>beyond |
|---|---|---|
| *Term* | *Term Analysis* | *Definition* |
| **ultrasonography**<br>(**ul**-trah-son-**OG**-<br>rah-fee) | -graphy = process of recording<br>son/o = sound | process of recording an image of<br>internal structures by using high<br>frequency sound waves (Figure 4-3).<br>Also known as ultrasound or<br>**sonogram** (**SOHN**-oh-gram) |

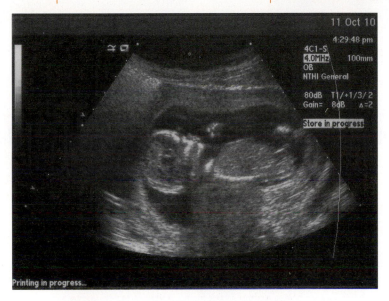

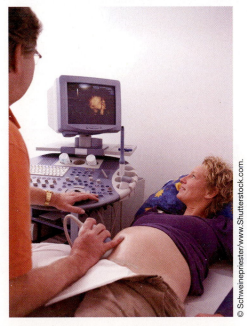

**Figure 4-3**  A. Image of fetal ultrasound at about 15 weeks. B. Ultrasonography is a noninvasive procedure that monitors fetal development during pregnancy.

## 4.3  Summary of Prefixes That Have the Same Meaning

| PREFIX | MEANING |
|---|---|
| epi-; hyper-; supra- | above |
| ante-; pre-; pro- | before |
| hypo-; infra-; sub- | below |
| meta-; ultra- | beyond |
| endo-; intra- | within |
| ex-; exo-; ecto- | out |

## 4.4  Summary of Prefixes That Have the Opposite Meaning

| PREFIX | MEANING |
|---|---|
| hyper-<br>hypo- | excessive<br>deficient |
| post-<br>ante-; pre-; pro- | after<br>before |
| epi-; hyper-; supra-<br>hypo-; infra-; sub- | above<br>below |
| in-<br>ex-; exo-; ecto- | in; into<br>out |

## 4.5  Review Exercises

### EXERCISE 4-1  Matching Word Elements with Meaning

*Match the word element in Column A with its meaning in Column B.*

| | Column A | Column B |
|---|---|---|
| _____ | **1.** trans- | A. before |
| _____ | **2.** anti- | B. difficult |
| _____ | **3.** endo- | C. below |
| _____ | **4.** para- | D. across |

|            | Column A       | Column B       |
| ---------- | -------------- | -------------- |
| _____ | **5.** ante-   | E. excessive   |
| _____ | **6.** infra-  | F. after       |
| _____ | **7.** hyper-  | G. against     |
| _____ | **8.** post-   | H. beside      |
| _____ | **9.** dys-    | I. around      |
| _____ | **10.** peri-  | J. within      |

## EXERCISE 4-2 **Definitions**

*Write the meaning of the prefix in the space provided.*

**a. sub-** _____

**b. dys-** _____

**c. ex-** _____

**d. bi-** _____

**e. post-** _____

**f. anti-** _____

**g. intra-** _____

**h. ante-** _____

**i. hypo-** _____

**j. a(n)-** _____

**k. hyper-** _____

**l. endo-** _____

**m. pre-** _____

**n. peri-** _____

**o. ab-** _____

**p. ad-** _____

**q. contra-** _____

**r. di-** _____

**s. pan-** _____

**t. para-** _____

u. **meta-** _____

v. **per-** _____

w. **retro-** _____

x. **supra-** _____

y. **auto-** _____

z. **micro-** _____

## EXERCISE 4-3  Identifying and Defining Word Parts

_In the words listed below, separate the medical term into its word parts with a slash. Then, define the term in the space provided. The first question is answered for you._

a. **pre/nat/al** pertaining to before birth _____

b. **postmortem** _____

c. **perineuritis** _____

d. **apnea** _____

e. **dysuria** _____

f. **antenatal** _____

g. **subcutaneous** _____

h. **hypogastric** _____

i. **bilateral** _____

j. **intramuscular** _____

k. **dyspnea** _____

l. **infracostal** _____

m. **hyperplasia** _____

n. **endogenous** _____

o. **adduct** _____

p. **contralateral** _____

q. **dissection** _____

r. **parenteral** _____

s. **macrocephaly** _____

t. **inversion** _____

**EXERCISE 4-4** **Word Building and Sentence Completion**

*Build a known medical word by matching one of the prefixes from the left-hand column with the correct root or suffix in the right-hand column. Then, complete the following sentences using the correct medical word.*

| PREFIX | ROOT OR SUFFIX |
|--------|----------------|
| anti- | -cutaneous |
| a- | -gnosis |
| infra- | -pnea |
| sub- | -biotics |
| pro- | -costal |

1. I have an infection. The physician gave me a prescription for _____.

2. Salina broke her arm. The physician said her bone would repair itself quickly. He said that the _____ was good.

3. Miguel received an injection under his skin. It is called a(n) _____ injection.

4. Sometimes when I am sleeping I stop breathing. The physician says I have sleep _____.

5. The pain is located below the ribs. The physician said this was _____ pain.

**EXERCISE 4-5** **Spelling**

*Circle the word that is correctly spelled in each group below.*

1. antenatal            antinatal            antenatul
2. antebiotic           antibyotic           antibiotic
3. bylateral            bilateral            billateral
4. dispnea              dyspnea              dysneea
5. dysuria              dysurea              disuria
6. exsision             eccision             excision
7. intracranal          intracranial         intracraneal
8. perineuritis         perenuritis          perineuritus
9. postmortum           postmortem           postmoretem
10. subqutaneus         subcutaneus          subcutaneous

## 4.6   Pronunciation and Spelling

1. Listen to each word on the audio file provided on the Student Companion Website.

2. Pronounce each word carefully.

3. Spell each word in the space provided.

| Word | Pronunciation | Spelling |
|------|---------------|----------|
| antenatal | **an**-tee-**NAY**-tal | |
| antepartum | **an**-tee-**PAR**-tum | |
| antibiotic | **an**-tih-bye-**OT**-ick | |
| anuria | ah-**NOO**-ree-ah | |
| apnea | **AP**-nee-ah | |
| autopsy | **AW**-top-see | |
| bilateral | bye-**LAT**-er-al | |
| circumduction | **ser**-kum-**DUCK**-shun | |
| contraindication | **kon**-trah-**in**-dih-**KAY**-shun | |
| contralateral | **kon**-trah-**LAT**-er-ahl | |
| dissection | dye-**SECK**-shun | |
| dysplasia | dis-**PLAY**-see-ah | |
| dyspnea | **DISP**-nee-ah | |
| dysuria | dis-**YOO**-ree-ah | |
| endogenous | en-**DOJ**-eh-nus | |
| epicardium | **ep**-ih-**KAR**-dee-um | |
| excision | eck-**SIH**-zhun | |
| exogenous | eck-**SOJ**-eh-nus | |
| hyperplasia | **high**-per-**PLAY**-see-ah | |
| hypochondriasis | **high**-poh-kon-**DRY**-ah-sis | |
| hypogastric | **high**-poh-**GAS**-trick | |
| incision | in-**SIH**-zhun | |
| inversion | in-**VER**-zhun | |
| infracostal | **in**-frah-**KOS**-tal | |

| Word | Pronunciation | Spelling |
|---|---|---|
| intracranial | **in**-trah-**KRAY**-nee-al | |
| intramuscular | **in**-trah-**MUS**-kyoo-lar | |
| macrocephaly | **mack**-roh-**SEF**-eh-lee | |
| metaplasia | **met**-ah-**PLAY**-zha | |
| metastasis | meh-**TAS**-tah-sis | |
| microscope | **MY**-kroh-skohp | |
| panhysterectomy | **pan**-hiss-ter-**ECK**-toh-mee | |
| parenteral | pah-**REN**-ter-al | |
| percutaneous | **per**-kyou-**TAY**-nee-us | |
| perineuritis | **per**-ih-nyoo-**RYE**-tis | |
| postmortem | pohst-**MOR**-tehm | |
| postpartum | pohst-**PAR**-tum | |
| prenatal | pre-**NAY**-tal | |
| retroversion | **ret**-roh-**VER**-zhun | |
| subcutaneous | **sub**-kyoo-**TAY**-nee-us | |
| sublingual | sub-**LING**-gwal | |
| suprarenal | **soo**-prah-**REE**-nal | |
| transection | tran-**SECK**-shun | |
| ultrasonography | **ul**-trah-son-**OG**-rah-fee | |

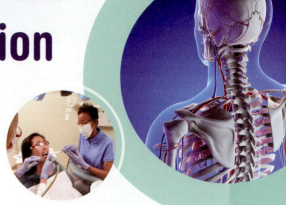

# Body Organization

## Chapter Outline

## Learning Objectives

*After studying this chapter and completing the exercises, you should be able to do the following:*

1. Name the cavities of the body and their related organs.
2. Define the anatomical position.
3. Define common terms used for directions.
4. Name and locate the abdominopelvic regions.
5. Name and locate the abdominopelvic quadrants.
6. Pronounce, spell, define, and write medical terms common to the body as a whole.
7. Listen, read, and study, so you can speak and write.

## Introduction

This chapter will teach you common terminology relating to the organization of the body. You will also learn the terms used to describe the position of the body and the placement of various body parts.

## 5.1  Body Cavities

**PRACTICE FOR LEARNING: Body Cavities**

Write the words below in the correct spaces on Figure 5-1. To help you, the number beside the word tells you where it goes on the figure. Be sure to pronounce each word as you write it. Repeat the pronunciation several times if you find the word hard to say.

1. dorsal cavity (**DOR**-sal **KAH**-vih-tee)
2. ventral cavity (**VEN**-tral)
3. cranial cavity (**KRAY**-nee-al)
4. vertebral cavity (**VER**-teh-bral)
5. abdominal cavity (ab-**DOM**-ih-nal)
6. pelvic cavity (**PEL**-vick)
7. thoracic cavity (thoh-**RAS**-ick)

When you study the body cavities, think of a backpack. The backpack has empty spaces called pouches. Some are big, some are small. The body has empty spaces inside it as well. But they are not called pouches. They are called cavities.

The body has two main cavities: the dorsal and the ventral. The dorsal cavity is also called the posterior cavity, because it is at the back of the body. Posterior refers to the

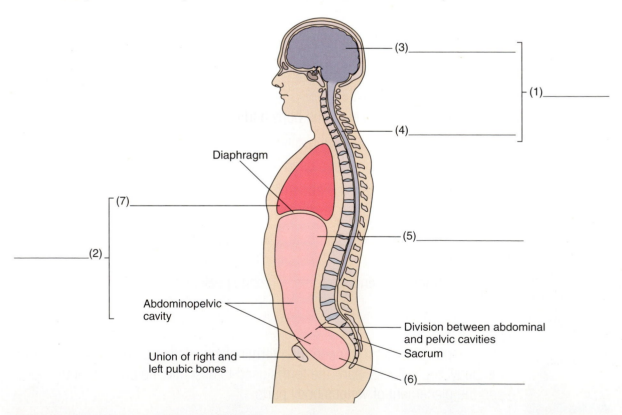

**Figure 5-1** Major body cavities and subdivisions

back. The ventral cavity is also called the anterior cavity, because it is at the front of the body. Anterior refers to the front. Each of these cavities has further subdivisions, which are shown in Figure 5-1.

## Dorsal Cavity

The dorsal cavity is subdivided into two parts: the cranial cavity and vertebral cavity. The cranial cavity is inside the skull. The brain is contained in the cranial cavity. The vertebral cavity is inside the vertebral column, or spine. The spinal cord (a group of nerves) is contained in the vertebral cavity.

## Ventral Cavity

The ventral cavity contains many internal organs including the heart, lungs, kidneys, digestive organs, and others. These internal organs are also called **viscera** (**VIS**-er-ah). A large muscle called the **diaphragm** (**DYE**-ah-fram) divides the ventral cavity into upper and lower cavities. The upper cavity is called the thoracic cavity. The lower cavity is the **abdominopelvic** (ab-**dom**-ih-noh-**PEL**-vick) cavity.

The thoracic cavity contains the heart and lungs. The abdominopelvic cavity is divided into two smaller cavities: the abdominal cavity and the pelvic cavity. The abdominal cavity is above the pelvic cavity. It contains organs such as the liver, intestines, stomach, and kidneys. The pelvic cavity contains some reproductive organs, the urinary bladder, and parts of the intestine.

| In Brief | The **dorsal cavity** is subdivided into the cranial and vertebral cavities. The **ventral cavity** is subdivided into the thoracic and abdominopelvic cavities. |
| --- | --- |

## PRACTICE FOR LEARNING: Body Cavities

Fill in the blanks with the most appropriate answer.

1. Write the two major body cavities. _____ and _____

2. What body organ would you find in the cranial cavity? _____
   Vertebral cavity? _____

3. Name the two cavities contained in the ventral cavity. _____ and
   _____

4. The stomach and kidneys are found in which body cavity? _____

5. The urinary bladder is found in which body cavity? _____

Answers: 1. dorsal (posterior) and ventral (anterior). 2. brain; spinal cord.
3. thoracic; abdominopelvic. 4. abdominal. 5. pelvic.

## 5.2 Directional Terminology

### Anatomical Position

If you are going to tell someone how to get somewhere, you both need to understand what east, west, north, and south mean. These words are called directional terms because they tell direction.

In health care, we need directional terms that will accurately describe where particular body structures are located. The problem is that bodies can move. You can lie on your back, your front, or either side. You can stand or sit. A change in position would change the meaning of the directional terms.

There is a simple solution to this problem. Everyone using directional terminology in health care must think of the body in a standard position. This is known as the **anatomical position**. It is illustrated in Figure 5-2A. The body is standing erect, arms by the side, with head, palms, and feet facing forward. All directional terms assume that the body is in this position.

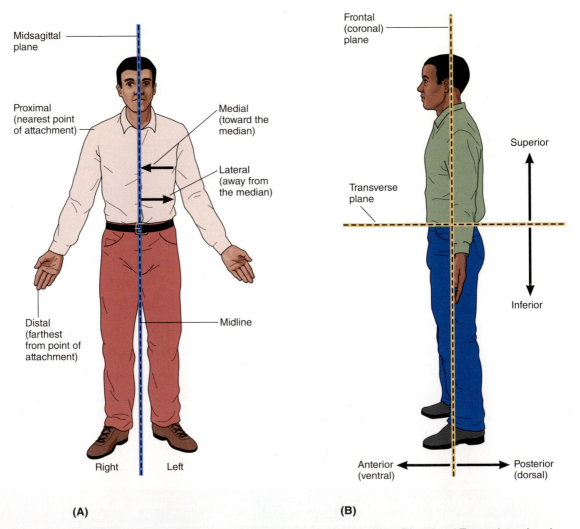

(A)                                                            (B)

**Figure 5-2** Anatomical position and directional terms A. Anatomical position. Directional Terms: lateral and medial; proximal and distal B. Superior and inferior; anterior and posterior.

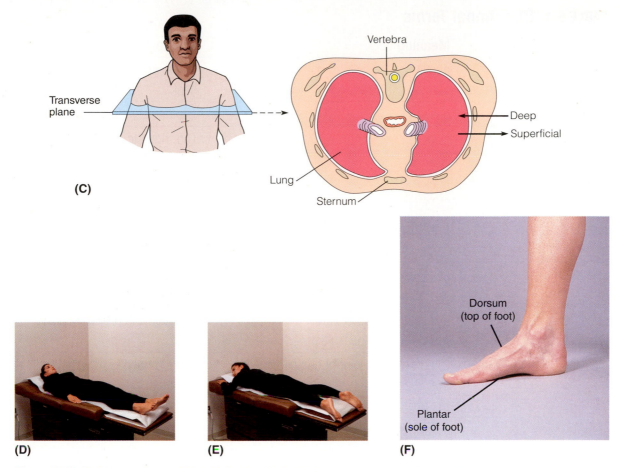

**Figure 5-2** C. Deep and superficial. D. Supine. E. Prone. F. Dorsum and plantar (continued).

> **In Brief**   **Anatomical position** is standing erect, arms by the side, head, palms, and feet facing forward.

## Directional Terms

As stated above, we need directional terms to describe the position of body parts, particularly in relation to each other. Directional terms are also useful in communicating the location of diseases when they appear in the body.

All of the directional terms are listed in Table 5-1. To help you remember them, they are grouped in opposite pairs. For example, the terms "superior" and "inferior" are grouped because they are opposites: superior means "above," and inferior means "below." Figures 5-2 A–F illustrate the use of the terms.

> **Helping You Remember**   To remember the meaning of supine, notice that supine has "up" as part of the word.

**TABLE 5-1  Directional Terms**

| Directional Term | Meaning | Example |
|---|---|---|
| superior | above | The head is superior to the neck. |
| inferior | below | The neck is inferior to the head. |
| ventral (anterior) | front | The thoracic cavity is anterior to the vertebral cavity. |
| dorsal (posterior) | back | The vertebral cavity is posterior to the thoracic cavity. |
| medial | toward the midline of the body | The big toe is medial to the small toe. |
| lateral | away from the midline of the body | The small toe is lateral to the big toe. |
| proximal | 1. nearest to the point of attachment to the trunk | The elbow is proximal to the wrist. |
| | 2. nearest the point of origin (In the digestive tract, the mouth is the point of origin.) | The stomach is proximal to the intestine. |
| distal | 1. farthest from the point of attachment to the trunk | The knee is distal to the hip. |
| | 2. farthest from the point of origin | The intestine is distal to the stomach. |
| superficial | near the surface of the body | The skin is superficial to muscle. |
| deep | away from the surface of the body | The muscle is deep to skin. |
| supine | lying on the back, face up | During an operation on the abdomen, the patient is placed in the supine position. |
| prone | lying on the abdomen | For a back operation, the patient is placed in the prone position. |
| plantar | bottom of the foot; sole of the foot | Plantar warts are on the sole of the foot. |
| dorsum | top of the foot | The dorsum of the foot is the top of the foot. |

## PRACTICE FOR LEARNING: Directional Terms

1. Write the opposite meaning of the following directional terms. The first one is done for you.

   **a.** anterior <u>posterior</u>

   **b.** lateral _____

   **c.** proximal _____

   **d.** deep _____

   **e.** prone _____

   **f.** dorsum _____

2. Choose the correct answer from the choices in parentheses.

   **g.** The neck is (inferior/superior) to the chin.

   **h.** Your mouth is (medial/lateral) to your ear.

   **i.** You have stepped on a sharp object. The bottom of your foot starts to bleed. You have cut the (plantar/dorsum) area of your foot.

   **j.** Jacque has a sunburn on the surface of his skin. The sunburn is said to be (superficial/deep).

   **k.** A patient is having an operation on her breast. The patient will be placed on the operating table in the (supine/prone) position.

   **l.** Ed has a rash on his chest and a bruise under his armpit. The bruise is (lateral/medial) to the rash.

   > Answers: a. posterior. b. medial. c. distal. d. superficial. e. supine. f. plantar.
   > g. inferior. h. medial. i. plantar. j. superficial. k. supine. l. lateral.

## 5.3 | Body Planes

Sections of the body are often referred to as anatomical planes (flat surfaces). Imagine cutting an organ, vertically or horizontally. Once this is done, a flat surface is exposed. This surface is called a **plane** (**PLAYN**). Because an organ can be cut in different ways, there are different kinds of planes. They are listed in Table 5-2 and illustrated in Figure 5-3.

> **Helping You Remember**
>
> To help you remember that sagittal separates a structure into right and left, think of the astrological sign of Sagittarius. With its bow and arrow, Sagittarius can hit a body structure, slicing it into right and left portions.

**TABLE 5-2  Planes of the Body**

| Plane | Definition |
| --- | --- |
| frontal; coronal (**KOR**-eh-nal) | separates a structure into anterior and posterior portions |
| sagittal (**SAJ**-ih-tal) | separates a structure into right and left portions. If the sagittal section divides the body into equal portions, it is called a **midsagittal** section. |
| transverse; horizontal | separates a structure into superior and inferior portions |

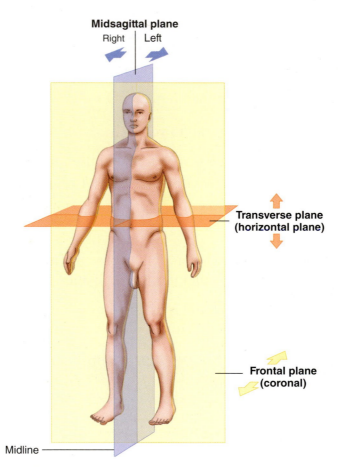

**Figure 5-3** Planes of the body.

## 5.4  Abdominopelvic Regions

PRACTICE FOR LEARNING: **Abdominopelvic Regions**

Write the words below in the correct spaces beside Figure 5-4. To help you, the number beside the word tells you where it goes on the figure. Be sure to pronounce each word as you write it. Repeat the pronunciation several times if you find the word hard to say.

1. right hypochondriac region (**high**-poh-**KON**-dree-ack)

2. epigastric region (**ep**-ih-**GAS**-trick)

3. left hypochondriac region (**high**-poh-**KON**-dree-ack)

4. right lumbar region (**LUM**-bar)

5. umbilical region (um-**BILL**-ih-cahl)

6. left lumbar region (**LUM**-bar)

7. right inguinal or iliac region (**ING**-gwih-nal or **ILL**-ee-ack)

8. hypogastric region (**high**-poh-**GAS**-trick)

9. left inguinal or iliac region (**ING**-gwih-nal or **ILL**-ee-ack)

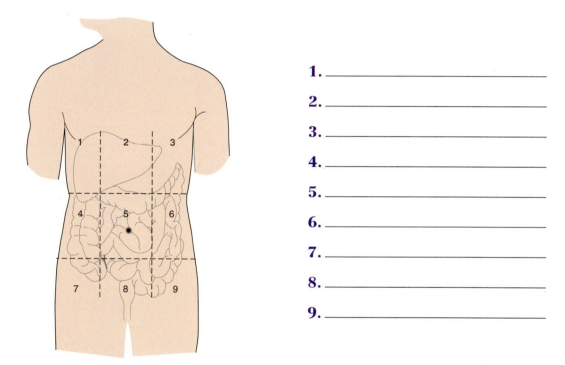

1. _____

2. _____

3. _____

4. _____

5. _____

6. _____

7. _____

8. _____

9. _____

**Figure 5-4**  Abdominopelvic regions.

Looking at the outside of the body, the abdominopelvic area can be divided into nine regions. As you can see in Figure 5-4, it looks like a tic-tac-toe board. Each region is given a name and each region contains specific organs.

When a patient has pain in the abdominopelvic area, the name of the region is used to communicate the exact location of the pain. For example, a physician may say, "The pain is in the right iliac region." This means the pain is located in the patient's right hip area.

When you are looking at illustrations, be careful to remember that the right and left abdominal regions refer to the patient's right or left, not yours.

## 5.5   Abdominopelvic Quadrants

**PRACTICE FOR LEARNING: Abdominopelvic Quadrants**

Write the words below in the correct spaces beside Figure 5-5. To help you, the number beside the word tells you where it goes on the figure. Be sure to pronounce each word as you write it. Repeat the pronunciation several times if you find the word hard to say.

1. right upper quadrant (RUQ)
2. left upper quadrant (LUQ)
3. right lower quadrant (RLQ)
4. left lower quadrant (LLQ)

The abdominopelvic area can also be divided into four areas called quadrants (Figure 5-5).

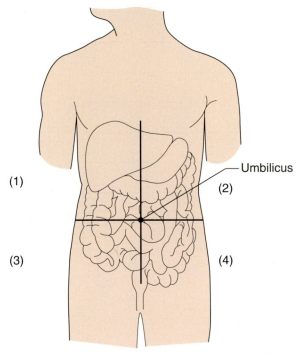

1. _____

2. _____

3. _____

4. _____

**Figure 5-5**  Abdominopelvic quadrants.

## 5.6 New Roots, Suffixes, and Prefixes

Use these additional roots when studying the medical terms of this chapter.

| ROOT | MEANING |
|---|---|
| anter/o | front |
| dors/o | back |
| ili/o | hip |
| infer/o | below; downward |
| inguin/o | groin |
| medi/o | middle |
| poster/o | back |
| proxim/o | near |
| super/o | above; toward the head |
| ventr/o | front |
| vertebr/o | vertebra (any of 33 bones making up the spine) |

## 5.7 Learning the Terms

Use the following suggestions for learning medical terms:

1. Pronounce the term repeatedly until it is easy for you.
2. Write it down. Ensure the spelling is correct.
3. Also write the definition. If possible, relate the word to a word, thought, or picture that will help you remember it.
4. Analyze the term with the method taught in this text.

### Suffixes

| SUFFIX<br>-ac | | MEANING<br>pertaining to |
|---|---|---|
| *Term* | *Term Analysis* | *Definition* |
| iliac<br>(ILL-ee-ack) | ili/o = hip | pertaining to the hip |

| SUFFIX -al | MEANING pertaining to | |
|---|---|---|
| Term | Term Analysis | Definition |
| **abdominal** (ab-**DOM**-ih-nal) | abdomin/o = abdomen (The abdomen is the portion of the body between the chest and pelvis) | pertaining to the abdomen |
| **cranial** (**KRAY**-nee-al) | crani/o = skull | pertaining to the skull |
| **dorsal** (**DOR**-sal) | dors/o = back | pertaining to the back of the body or organ; posterior (Figure 5-2B) |
| **inguinal** (**ING**-gwih-nal) | inguin/o = groin (the groin is the fold between the thigh and lower abdomen) | pertaining to the groin |
| **lateral** (**LAT**-er-al) | later/o = side | pertaining to the side (Figure 5-2A) |
| **medial** (**MEE**-dee-al) | medi/o = middle | pertaining to the middle (Figure 5-2A) |
| **proximal** (**PROCK**-sih-mal) | proxim/o = near; close to | pertaining to something being near a specific point (Figure 5-2A) |
| **spinal** (**SPYE**-nal) | spin/o = spine; vertebral column | pertaining to the spine |
| **ventral** (**VEN**-tral) | ventr/o = front | pertaining to the front; anterior (Figure 5-2B) |
| **vertebral** (**VER**-teh-bral) | vertebr/o = vertebra | pertaining to any one of the 33 bones making up the spine |
| **visceral** (**VIS**-er-al) | viscer/o = internal organs | pertaining to the internal organs |

**Helping You Remember**  The combining form is spelled abdom**in**/o. The word is spelled abdom**en**.

| SUFFIX -ic | | MEANING pertaining to |
|---|---|---|
| *Term* | *Term Analysis* | *Definition* |
| epigastric (**ep**-ih-**GAS**-trick) | epi- = above; upon gastr/o = stomach | pertaining to upon the stomach (Figure 5-4) |
| pelvic (**PEL**-vick) | pelv/o = pelvis | pertaining to the pelvis |
| thoracic (thoh-**RAS**-ick) | thorac/o = chest | pertaining to the chest |

| SUFFIX -ior | | MEANING pertaining to |
|---|---|---|
| *Term* | *Term Analysis* | *Definition* |
| anterior (an-**TEER**-ee-or) | anter/o = front | pertaining to the front (Figure 5-2B) |
| inferior (in-**FEER**-ee-or) | infer/o = below; downward | pertaining to below or in a downward position; a structure below another structure (Figure 5-2B) |
| posterior (pos-**TEER**-ee-or) | poster/o = back | pertaining to the back of the body or an organ (Figure 5-2B) |
| superior (soo-**PEER**-ee-or) | super/o = above; toward the head | pertaining to above or toward the head (Figure 5-2B) |

## 5.8 Review Exercises

### EXERCISE 5-1 Matching Word Parts with Meaning

*Match the meaning in Column A with the word part in Column B.*

| | Column A | Column B |
|---|---|---|
| _____ | **1.** hip | A. gastr/o |
| _____ | **2.** back | B. thorac/o |
| _____ | **3.** near | C. anter/o |
| _____ | **4.** above; upon | D. -ic |
| _____ | **5.** stomach | E. ili/o |

|  | Column A | Column B |
|---|---|---|
| _____ | **6.** below | F. epi- |
| _____ | **7.** front | G. crani/o |
| _____ | **8.** pertaining to | H. dors/o |
| _____ | **9.** chest | I. infer/o |
| _____ | **10.** skull | J. proxim/o |

## EXERCISE 5-2  Directional Terms

*Match each directional term in Column A with its meaning in Column B.*

|  | Column A | Column B |
|---|---|---|
| _____ | **1.** superior | A. pertaining to the skull |
| _____ | **2.** anterior | B. pertaining to the hip |
| _____ | **3.** thoracic | C. above; toward the head |
| _____ | **4.** visceral | D. pertaining to the front |
| _____ | **5.** epigastric | E. pertaining to below the stomach |
| _____ | **6.** iliac | F. pertaining to upon the stomach |
| _____ | **7.** cranial | G. pertaining to the chest |
| _____ | **8.** hypogastric | H. pertaining to internal organs |

## EXERCISE 5-3  Defining Directional Terms

*Underline the root and then define the medical word. The first question is answered for you.*

1. **<u>hypogastr</u>ic** pertaining to below the stomach _____

2. **iliac** _____

3. **dorsal** _____

4. **inguinal** _____

5. **visceral** _____

6. **cranial** _____

7. **anterior** _____

8. **superior** _____

## EXERCISE 5-4  True/False

*Circle True if the statement is correct. Circle False if the statement is not correct.*

1. The liver is located in the pelvic cavity.                              True    False

2. The abdominal cavity is superior to the thoracic cavity.                True    False

3. The small toe is medial to the big toe.                                 True    False

4. The wrist is proximal to the elbow.                                     True    False

5. Prone is lying on the abdomen.                                          True    False

6. The right iliac region is in the right upper quadrant.                  True    False

7. Dorsum refers to the back of a structure                               True    False

8. The right hypochondriac region of the abdomen is in the RUQ.            True    False

## EXERCISE 5-5  Spelling

*Circle the words that are spelled incorrectly in the list below. Then correct the spelling in the space provided.*

1. epigastric _____

2. abdomenal _____

3. inquinal _____

4. thorasic _____

5. vicseral _____

6. anterior _____

7. medial _____

## Animation

Watch a video on Body Planes.

## 5.9  Pronunciation and Spelling

1. Listen to each word on the audio file provided on the Student Companion Website.

2. Pronounce each word carefully.

3. Spell each word in the space provided.

| Word | Pronunciation | Spelling |
|------|---------------|----------|
| epigastric | **ep**-ih-**GAS**-trick | |
| hypogastric | **high**-poh-**GAS**-trick | |
| iliac | **ILL**-ee-ack | |
| abdominal | ab-**DOM**-ih-nal | |
| cranial | **KRAY**-nee-al | |
| dorsal | **DOR**-sal | |
| inguinal | **ING**-gwih-nal | |
| medial | **MEE**-dee-al | |
| proximal | **PROCK**-sih-mal | |
| spinal | **SPYE**-nal | |
| ventral | **VEN**-tral | |
| visceral | **VIS**-er-al | |
| pelvic | **PEL**-vick | |
| thoracic | thoh-**RAS**-ick | |
| inferior | in-**FEER**-ee-or | |
| posterior | pos-**TEER**-ee-or | |
| superior | soo-**PEER**-ee-or | |

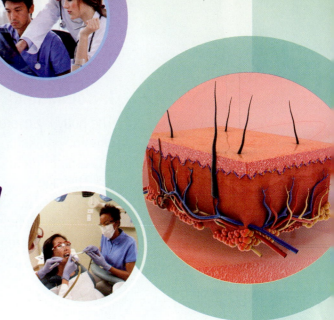

## CHAPTER 6

# Skin: The Integumentary System

## Chapter Outline

## Learning Objectives

*After studying this chapter and completing the exercises, you should be able to do the following:*

1. Identify the cells, tissues, and accessory structures of the system.
2. Identify the layers of the skin and describe the structures found in these layers.
3. List the functions of the skin.
4. Pronounce, spell, define, and write medical terms common to this system.
5. Describe common diseases of the system.
6. Listen, read, and study, so you can speak and write.

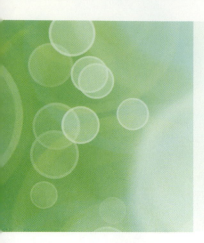

## Introduction

The body is covered with skin, nails, and hair. Together with glands found in the skin they make up the integumentary (in-**teg**-yoo-**MEN**-tar-ee) system. It gets its name from the Latin word *integumentum* meaning "covering."

The skin is an organ, just like the heart and lungs. It is the largest organ in the body. The skin has two layers. The outer layer (epidermis) helps prevent harmful substances from entering the body. The inner layer (dermis) contains glands that secrete important substances, nerves that carry electrical impulses, and blood vessels that help keep the body at the right temperature.

## 6.1 | Skin and Subcutaneous Tissue

**PRACTICE FOR LEARNING: Layers of the Skin and Subcutaneous Tissue**

Write the words below in the correct spaces on Figure 6-1. To help you, the number beside the word tells you where it goes on the figure. Be sure to pronounce each word as you write it. Repeat the pronunciation several times if you find the word hard to say. Only numbers 1–3 will be labeled here.

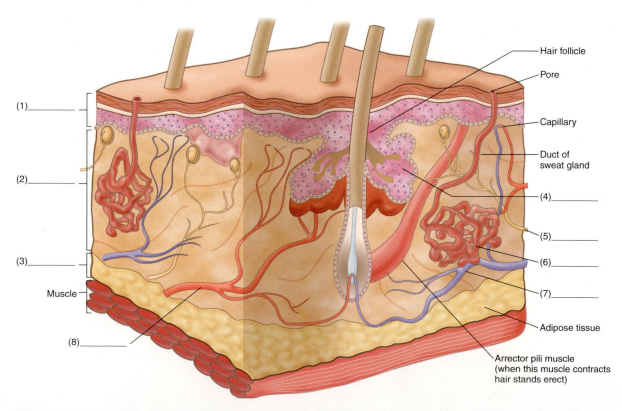

**Figure 6-1** Layers of the skin and subcutaneous tissue. Structures associated with the dermis.

1. epidermis (**ep**-ih-**DER**-mis)

2. dermis (**DER**-mis)

3. subcutaneous tissue (**sub**-kyoo-**TAY**-nee-us **TISH**-yoo)

Figure 6-1 shows you the layers of tissue. The outer layer is part of the skin and is called the epidermis. Underneath it is another layer of skin called the dermis. Underneath the dermis is a fatty layer called subcutaneous tissue. It is not part of the skin. The subcutaneous tissue attaches the skin to muscles close to the surface.

> **In Brief**
>
> The **epidermis** is the outer layer of skin.
> The **dermis** is under the epidermis.
> **Subcutaneous** tissue is under the dermis.

## Epidermis

In Chapter 2, you learned that organs are made of tissues and tissues are made of cells. The epidermis is an organ made of tissue called **epithelium** (**ep**-ih-**THEE**-lee-um). The cells are called **epithelial** (**ep**-ih-**THEE**-lee-al) cells. The epidermis is a protective covering over the entire body and lines body cavities and covers organs.

The epidermis protects us from the sun's rays by producing **melanin** (**MEL**-ah-nin). Melanin is produced by cells in the epidermis called **melanocytes** (meh-**LAN**-oh-sights). Darker skin has more melanocytes than lighter skin. Skin with more melanin has better protection from the sun.

Skin also protects by keeping infectious materials from entering the body and it waterproofs the body and prevents fluid loss.

> **In Brief**
>
> **Epidermis**
>
> Protects from sun, infection, and fluid loss

## Dermis

### PRACTICE FOR LEARNING: **Dermis**

Write the words below in the correct spaces in Figure 6-1. To help you, the number beside the word tells you where it goes on the figure. Be sure to pronounce each word as you write it. Repeat the pronunciation several times if you find the word hard to say.

4. sebaceous (seh-**BAY**-shus) gland

5. nerve (**NURV**)

**6.** sweat gland (**SWET GLAND**)

**7.** vein (**VAYN**)

**8.** artery (**AR**-ter-ee)

The dermis is made of connective tissue. A major component of connective tissue is **collagen** (**KOL**-ah-jen), which makes the skin flexible and strong.

If you look at Figure 6-1, you can see that the dermis contains blood vessels. If you are cut down to this layer, you will bleed. The blood vessels supply nutrients to the epidermis and dermis. They also help control body temperature.

The dermis also contains nerves. They give us sensations such as touch, pain, temperature, and pressure. Also in the dermis are glands and hair follicles. These parts are discussed below under the heading Accessory Structures.

> **In Brief**    The organs located in the **dermis** are: blood vessels, nerves, glands, and hair follicles.

## Subcutaneous Tissue

Subcutaneous tissue is deep to the dermis and is composed of mostly adipose (**AD**-ih-pohs) tissue. Its cells are called adipocytes. Besides storing fat, this layer loosely connects the skin to the underlying muscles and protects us from injury. It is also known as **superficial fascia** (**FASH**-ee-ah). Fascia is connective tissue that holds parts together. In this case, it holds the skin to the muscles. It is called superficial fascia because the subcutaneous tissue is closer to the surface of the body than the fascia surrounding the muscle.

### PRACTICE FOR LEARNING: Epidermis and Dermis

Choose the correct answer from the choices in parentheses.

**1.** The function of the epidermis is (protection/sensation).

**2.** The tissue making up the epidermis is (epithelial/connective) tissue.

**3.** The substance that gives the skin a darker color is (melanin/sebum).

**4.** The dermis is made of (epithelial/connective) tissue.

**5.** A function of the blood vessels in the dermis is (sensation/temperature regulation).

**6.** Collagen is most likely to be found in the (epithelial/connective/muscle) tissue.

7. Superficial fascia is also known as (epidermis/ dermis/ subcutaneous tissue).

8. Adipocytes are (skin/fat) cells commonly found in the (epidermis/dermis/ superficial fascia).

> Answers: 1. protection. 2. epithelial. 3. melanin. 4. connective. 5. temperature regulation. 6. connective. 7. subcutaneous tissue. 8. fat; superficial fascia

## 6.2   Accessory Structures

### Glands

There are glands in the dermis that secrete substances necessary for skin function. **Sebaceous** glands secrete oil called **sebum** (**SEE**-bum). It keeps the skin and the hair soft and pliable (flexible). **Sweat** glands help regulate temperature by secreting sweat onto the surface of the skin. When the sweat evaporates, the skin cools. Specialized glands in the ear named **ceruminous** (seh-**ROO**-min-us) glands secrete **cerumen** (seh-**ROO**-men), a waxy substance that helps prevent bacterial infection.

### Hair Follicles

There are also hair follicles in the dermis (Figure 6-1). They grow the hairs that cover our skin in certain places. When hair is lost on top of the head, the person is said to be bald. The medical word for bald is **alopecia** (**al**-oh-**PEE**-she-ah). The opposite, the presence of excessive body and facial hair, especially in women, is called **hirsutism** (**HER**-soot-iz-um).

### Nails

Nails are protective coverings on the ends of fingers and toes. Nails are epithelial cells that have been hardened. At the base of each nail is the white, half-moon shaped **lunula** (**LOO**-nuh-lah). The word "luna" means moon. It is from the lunula that the nail grows. Other anatomical structures are the **nail bed** and the cuticle or **eponychium** (**ep**-oh-**NICK**-ee-um).

---

**In Brief**

**Accessory Structures**

glands, hair, nails

**Glands**

sebaceous, sweat, ceruminous

**Nails**

includes lunula, nail bed, eponychium

## 6.3 | New Roots, Suffixes, and Prefixes

Use these additional roots, suffixes, and prefixes when studying the terms in this chapter.

| ROOT | MEANING |
| --- | --- |
| chem/o | drug |
| cry/o | cold |
| crypt/o | hidden |
| melan/o | black |
| myc/o | fungus |
| staphyl/o | resembling a bunch of grapes |
| strept/o | twisted |
| xer/o | dry |

| SUFFIX | MEANING |
| --- | --- |
| -cle | small |
| -edema | swelling |
| -ion | process |
| -ium | structure |
| -ose | pertaining to |
| -sis | condition |

| PREFIX | MEANING |
| --- | --- |
| tele- | distant |

## 6.4 | Learning the Terms

Use the following suggestions for learning medical terms.

1. Pronounce the term repeatedly until it is easy for you.
2. Write it down. Ensure the spelling is correct.
3. Also write the definition. If possible, relate the word to a word, thought, or picture that will help you remember it.
4. Analyze the term with the method taught in this text.

## Roots

| ROOT<br>adip/o (see also lip/o) | | MEANING<br>fat |
| --- | --- | --- |
| Term | Term Analysis | Definition |
| adipose<br>(AD-ih-pohs) | -ose = pertaining to | pertaining to fat |

| ROOT<br>bi/o | | MEANING<br>life |
| --- | --- | --- |
| Term | Term Analysis | Definition |
| biopsy<br>(BYE-op-see) | -opsy = to view | a procedure involving the removal of a piece of living tissue, which is then examined for any abnormalities |

| ROOT<br>cutane/o (see also derm/o and dermat/o) | | MEANING<br>skin |
| --- | --- | --- |
| Term | Term Analysis | Definition |
| subcutaneous<br>(sub-kyoo-TAY-nee-us) | sub- = under<br>-ous = pertaining to | pertaining to under the skin |

| ROOT<br>cyan/o | | MEANING<br>blue |
| --- | --- | --- |
| Term | Term Analysis | Definition |
| cyanosis<br>(sigh-ah-NOH-sis) | -sis = condition | bluish discoloration of skin (Figure 6-2) |

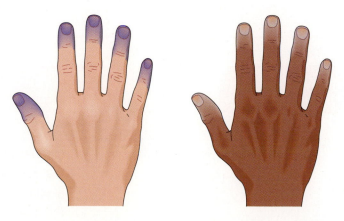

**Figure 6-2**  Cyanosis.

| ROOT derm/o; dermat/o | | MEANING skin |
| --- | --- | --- |
| Term | Term Analysis | Definition |
| dermatitis (der-mah-TYE-tis) | -itis = inflammation | inflammation of the skin |
| dermatologist (der-mah-TOL-oh-jist) | -logist = one who specializes in the study of | one who specializes in the study of the skin and its diseases |
| hypodermic (high-poh-DER-mick) | -ic = pertaining to hypo- = under; below | pertaining to under the skin |

**Note:** The prefixes hypo- and sub- cannot be interchanged with the roots meaning skin. Hypo- is used with the root **derm/o**, and sub- is used with the root **cutane/o**.

| ROOT erythem/o | | MEANING red |
| --- | --- | --- |
| Term | Term Analysis | Definition |
| erythema (er-ih-THEE-mah) | "-a" is a noun ending | red discoloration of the skin |
| erythematous (er-ih-THEM-ah-tus) | -ous = pertaining to | pertaining to redness of the skin |

| ROOT kerat/o | | MEANING hard; horn-like |
| --- | --- | --- |
| Term | Term Analysis | Definition |
| keratosis (ker-ah-TOH-sis) | -osis = abnormal condition | any skin growth, such as a wart or callus, in which there is overgrowth or thickness of the skin |

| ROOT lip/o | | MEANING fat |
| --- | --- | --- |
| Term | Term Analysis | Definition |
| lipedema (lip-eh-DEE-mah) | -edema = swelling | chronic abnormal condition that is characterized by the accumulation of fat and fluid in the tissues just under the skin of the hips and legs. |

| Term | Term Analysis | Definition |
|------|---------------|------------|
| lipoma<br>(lih-**POH**-mah) | -oma = tumor; mass | tumor or mass containing fat |
| liposuction<br>(**lip**-oh-**SUCK**-shun) | suction = process of aspirating or withdrawing | withdrawal of fat from the subcutaneous tissue |

| ROOT<br>necr/o | | MEANING<br>death |
|---------------|---|------------------|
| **Term** | **Term Analysis** | **Definition** |
| necrotic tissue<br>(neh-**KROT**-ick) | -tic = pertaining to | pertaining to the death of tissues. Example: decubitus ulcer (Figure 6-3) |

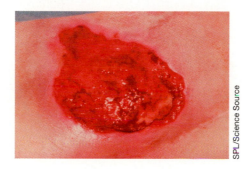

SPL/Science Source

**Figure 6-3** Decubitus ulcer (pressure sore, bedsore).

**Note:** Decubitus means lying down. A **decubitus** (deh-**KYOU**-bih-tus) ulcer is also known as a pressure sore or bedsore. It is caused by lying on a body part for too long. This puts constant pressure on the skin, especially over bony areas such as elbows. The pressure cuts off the circulation to the part. The skin becomes necrotic (dies) because of the lack of oxygen. When necrotic tissue is sloughed (falls off), it leaves an open sore (Figure 6-3). Figure 6-6c illustrates necrotic tissue before it is sloughed. In this case the necrosis is from a burn.

| ROOT<br>onych/o (see ungu/o) | | MEANING<br>nail |
|------------------------------|---|-----------------|
| **Term** | **Term Analysis** | **Definition** |
| eponychium<br>(**ep**-oh-**NICK**-ee-um) | -ium = structure<br>epi- = upon | structure upon the nail; cuticle |
| onychocryptosis<br>(**on**-ih-koh-krip-**TOH**-sis) | -osis = abnormal condition<br>crypt/o = hidden | in-grown toenail |
| onychomycosis<br>(**on**-ih-koh-my-**KOH**-sis) | -osis = abnormal condition<br>myc/o = fungus | **fungal** infection of the nail; also known as tinea unguium (**TIN**-ee-ah **UNG**-gwim) |

| ROOT **pedicul/o** | | MEANING **lice** |
|---|---|---|
| Term | Term Analysis | Definition |
| **pediculosis** (peh-**dick**-yoo-**LOH**-sis) | -osis = abnormal condition | infestation with lice |

| ROOT **ras/o** | | MEANING **scrape** |
|---|---|---|
| Term | Term Analysis | Definition |
| **abrasion** (ab-**RAY**-zhun) | -ion = process ab- = away from | scraping away of the superficial layers of injured skin; for example, scraping your skin on the cement results in an abrasion. Also known as an **excoriation** (**ecks**-kor-ee-**AY**-shun) |

| ROOT **ungu/o** | | MEANING **nail** |
|---|---|---|
| Term | Term Analysis | Definition |
| **subungual** (sub-**UNG**-gwal) | -al = pertaining to sub- = under | pertaining to under the nail |

| ROOT **vesic/o** | | MEANING **small sac; bladder** |
|---|---|---|
| Term | Term Analysis | Definition |
| **vesicle** (**VES**-ih-kul) | -cle = small | a blister; a small elevation on the skin filled with clear fluid |

## Suffixes

| SUFFIX **-coccus** | | MEANING **berry-shape** |
|---|---|---|
| Term | Term Analysis | Definition |
| **staphylococcus** (staf-ih-loh-**KOCK**-us) | staphyl/o = resembling a bunch of grapes | berry-shaped bacteria growing in small clusters, like grapes |
| **streptococcus** (strep-toh-**KOCK**-us) | strept/o = resembling twisted chains | berry-shaped bacteria growing in twisted chains |

| SUFFIX -cyte | | MEANING cell |
| --- | --- | --- |
| Term | Term Analysis | Definition |
| melanocyte (meh-**LAN**-oh-sight) | melan/o = black | cells producing melanin |

| SUFFIX -derma | | MEANING Skin |
| --- | --- | --- |
| Term | Term Analysis | Definition |
| scleroderma (**skler**-oh-**DER**-mah) | scler/o = hard | skin becomes hard and swollen because the connective tissues become thick and hard |
| xeroderma (**zer**-oh-**DER**-mah) | xer/o = dry | extreme dryness of the skin |

| SUFFIX -therapy | | MEANING Treatment |
| --- | --- | --- |
| Term | Term Analysis | Definition |
| chemotherapy (**kee**-moh-**THER**-ah-**pee**) | chem/o = drugs | treatment with drugs. Usually refers to the use of drugs on cancer patients. |
| cryotherapy (**krye**-oh-**THER**-ah-**pee**) | cry/o = cold | destruction of unwanted tissue, such as warts, by freezing with liquid nitrogen. The freezing destroys the tissue (Figure 6-4). |

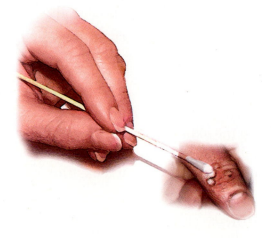

**Figure 6-4**  Cryotherapy.

| Term | Term Analysis | Definition |
|---|---|---|
| **laser therapy** (**LAY**-zer **THER**-ah-pee) | laser = intense beam of light | removal of skin lesions such as birthmarks or tattoos using an intense beam of light called a laser. Lasers are also used in cosmetic surgeries. |

**Note:** In this example, therapy is used as a word rather than a suffix.

| Term | Term Analysis | Definition |
|---|---|---|
| **radiotherapy** (**ray**-dee-oh-**THER**-ah-pee) | radi/o = x-rays | the use of radiation to treat disease, usually cancer. Radiotherapy is not used to diagnose disease. |
| **teletherapy** (**tel**-eh-**THER**-ah-pee) | tele- = distant | radiation treatment applied to a tumor at a distance from the body |

## 6.5    Pathology

### Burns

A burn is an injury to the skin caused by heat, chemicals, electricity, or radiation. Burns can be described by how deep the burn is and by the area of skin burned. Look at Figures 6-5 and 6-6 as you read the descriptions below:

- **First-degree burn (superficial burn)** is a burn to the epidermis only. There is redness but no vesicles (blisters). An example is a sunburn.

- **Second-degree burn (partial-thickness burn)** involves the epidermis and upper portion of the dermis. The skin is red. There are vesicles (blisters).

- **Third-degree burn (full-thickness burn)** involves the epidermis and all of the dermis. The subcutaneous tissue may be damaged.

- **Fourth-degree burn** involves the epidermis, dermis, subcutaneous tissue, and muscle.

### Bruises

A bruise is a discoloration to the skin from a ruptured blood vessel. The skin is not broken and blood accumulates in the tissue spaces. A bruise, is also known as a **contusion** (kon-**TOO**-zhun). Bruises can take on different looks each with a different name. These are listed below:

- **Ecchymosis** (**ek**-ih-**MOH**-sis) (plural ecchymos**es**) is a large, irregular area of purplish discoloration (Figure 6-7A).

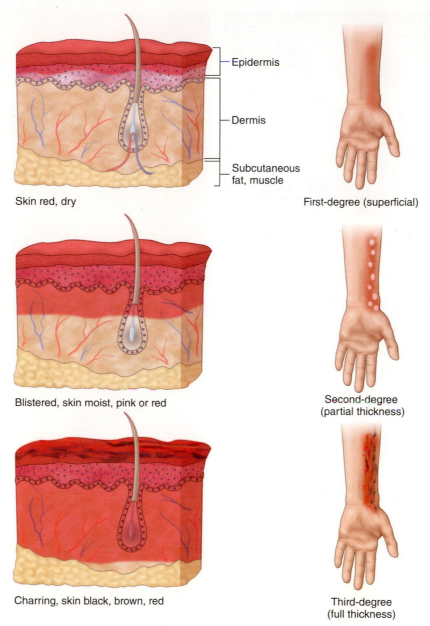

**Figure 6-5** Superficial (first degree), partial thickness (second degree), and full thickness (third degree). The degree of the burn is determined by the layers of skin involved.

- **Hematoma** is a mass or collection of blood causing a swelling under the skin. Hematomas are often named after their location. For example, **subungual hematoma**.

- **Petechiae** (peh-**TEE**-kee-ee) are small pinpoint hemorrhages under the skin (Figure 6-7B).

- **Purpura** (**PER**-per-ah) is a broad term that includes a number of conditions characterized by bleeding into the skin such as ecchymoses and petechiae. Purpura means purple, the color of the bruise (Figure 6-7C).

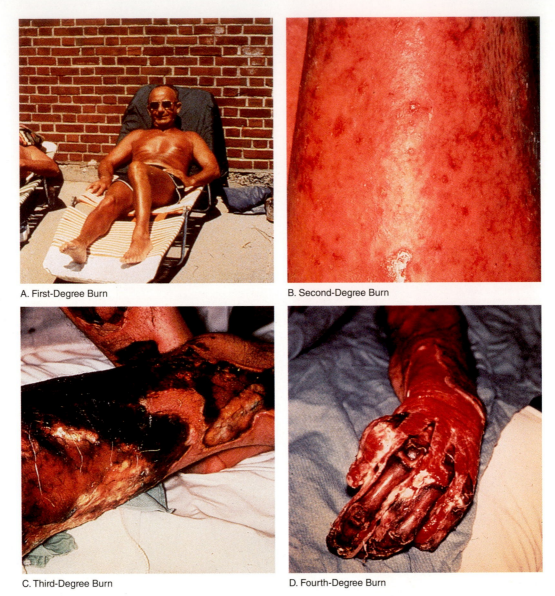

A. First-Degree Burn

B. Second-Degree Burn

C. Third-Degree Burn

D. Fourth-Degree Burn

**Figure 6-6**  Burns. A. First-degree burn. B. Second-degree burn. C. Third-degree burn. D. Fourth-degree burn.
(All photographs courtesy of the Phoenix Society for Burn Survivors, Inc.)

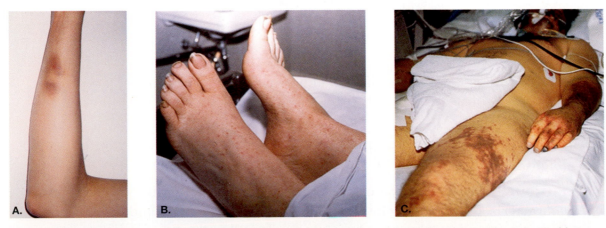

A.

B.

C.

**Figure 6-7**  A. Ecchymoses. B. Petechiae. C. Purpura: Purple discoloration of skin. Ecchymosis and petechiae are examples of purpura.

## Cutaneous Lesions (LEE-zhunz)

A skin lesion is any abnormality caused by disease or injury (trauma). Any deviation from the normal appearance of the skin can be called a lesion. Distinguishing the various kinds of skin lesions is important, since they characterize specific diseases. (Figure 6-8A–G)

- **Cicatrix** (**sick**-ah-**TRICKS**) is normal scar tissue resulting from the normal healing of a wound.
- **Cyst** (**SIST**) is a small closed sac or cavity filled with fluid or semifluid. Example: ovarian cyst (Figure 6-8A)
- **Fissure** is a crack-like sore. Often seen on the heels and between the toes when the skin is very dry (Figure 6-8B).
- **Macule** (**MACK**-yool) is a discolored, unelevated area of skin. Example: birthmarks (Figure 6-8C)
- **Papule** (**PAP**-yool) is a solid, elevated area of skin. Example: acne (Figure 6-8D)
- **Pustule** (**PUS**-tyool) is a small, elevated area of skin that contains pus. Example: acne, abscess (Figure 6-8E)
- **Vesicle** is an elevated area of skin containing clear fluid. Example: blister (Figure 6-8F). A blister larger than 0.5 cm is called a **bulla** (**BOO**-lah).

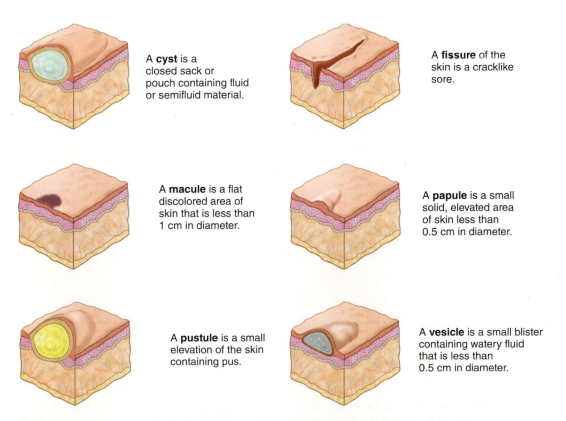

A **cyst** is a closed sack or pouch containing fluid or semifluid material.

A **fissure** of the skin is a cracklike sore.

A **macule** is a flat discolored area of skin that is less than 1 cm in diameter.

A **papule** is a small solid, elevated area of skin less than 0.5 cm in diameter.

A **pustule** is a small elevation of the skin containing pus.

A **vesicle** is a small blister containing watery fluid that is less than 0.5 cm in diameter.

**Figure 6-8**  Cutaneous Lesions. A. Cyst. B. Fissure. C. Macule. D. Papule. E. Pustule. F. Vesicle.

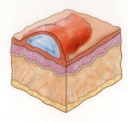

A **wheal** is a raised circular area of skin usually pale in center, surrounded by redness.

**Figure 6-8** G. Wheal (continued).

- **Wheal** (**WHEEL**) is a raised, circular area of skin usually pale in the center, surrounded by redness. Example: mosquito bite and hives (also known as **urticaria**) (yoo-tih-**KEHR**-ee-ah) (Figure 6-8G).

## Exanthem

**Exanthem** (egg-**ZAN**-thum) is a widespread rash.

## Infections

### Bacterial Infections

- **Furuncle** (**FYOO**-run-kul) are also known as boils. They are large, tender, swollen areas around hair follicles or sebaceous glands. A cluster of boils is called a **carbuncle** (**KAR**-bun-kul). Boils are caused by a staphylococcus infection.
- **Cellulitis** (**sell**-yoo-**LYE**-tis) is an inflammation of the connective tissue underlying the epidermis caused by staphylococcus or streptococcus.
- **Impetigo** (**im**-peh-**TYE**-goh) is a superficial but highly contagious skin infection that usually affects infants and children. Characteristic red sores appear on the face.
- **Necrotizing fascitis** (**NEK**-roh-tye-zing fah-**SIGH**-tis) is a severe infection caused by streptococcus bacteria causing inflammation of the fascia and resulting in tissue death. If left untreated, the infected body tissue becomes necrotic. Can be fatal. Also known as flesh-eating disease.

### Fungal Infections

- **Candidiasis** (**kan**-dih-**DYE**-ah-sis) is a yeast infection occurring on the skin and mucous membrane. Also known as **moniliasis** (**mon**-ih-**LYE**-eh-sis). If the fungus appears in the oral cavity, the condition is called **thrush**. The mucous membrane of the vagina can also be affected, resulting in an inflamed vagina.
- **Tinea** (**TIN**-ee-ah) is a fungal infection that can grow on skin, hair, and nails.

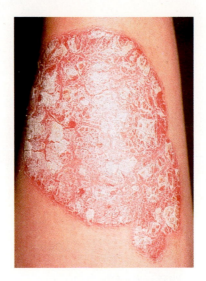

**Figure 6-9**  Psoriasis. (Courtesy of Robert A. Silverman, MD, Pediatric Dermatology, Georgetown University.)

## Viral Infection

- **Verrucae** (veh-**ROO**-see) are small, hard skin lesions caused by the human papillomavirus. Verrucae is commonly known as warts.

## Psoriasis (sor-EYE-ah-sis)

Psoriasis is a chronic inflammation of the skin (Figure 6-9). The skin appears erythematous (red), with silvery scales. Symptoms include xeroderma and pruritus (proo-**EYE**-tus). Pruritus means itchy. Psoriasis is not infectious.

## Tumors, Neoplasms

An abnormal growth of tissue cells. Tumors can be **benign** or **malignant**. Benign tumors are noncancerous, usually harmless, and do not spread from one location to another. Malignant tumors are cancerous and harmful and usually spread or **metastasize** (meh-**TAS**-tah-size). Common benign and malignant tumors are listed below. Treatment involves removal of the tumor by surgery, laser, radiation, and/or chemotherapy.

### Benign Tumors

- **Papilloma** (**pap**-ih-**LOH**-mah) a benign nipple-like growth projecting from epithelial tissue (papill/o = nipple). Example: a wart.
- **Lipoma** (lih-**POH**-mah) is a benign tumor of fatty tissue.

### Malignant Tumors

- **Carcinoma** (**kar**-sih-**NOH**-mah) is a malignant tumor of epithelial cells. Two types are basal (**BAY**-sal) cell and squamous (**SKWAY**-mus) cell carcinomas.

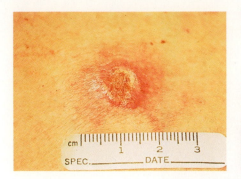
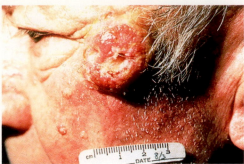

**Figure 6-10**  Carcinoma of the skin. A. Basal cell carcinoma. B. Squamous cell carcinoma.
(Courtesy of Robert A. Silverman, MD, Pediatric Dermatology, Georgetown University.)

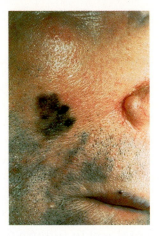

**Figure 6-11**  Melanoma. (Courtesy of Robert A. Silverman, MD, Pediatric Dermatology, Georgetown University.)

- **Basal cell carcinoma** is a malignant tumor of the epidermis. Unlike other malignant skin cancers, it rarely spreads to other locations (Figure 6-10A).
- **Squamous cell carcinoma** is also a malignant tumor of the epidermis. It has a tendency to spread to other organs (Figure 6-10B).
- **Melanoma** (**mel**-ah-**NOH**-mah) is a malignant tumor arising from the melanocytes in the epidermis (Figure 6-11).
- **Sarcoma** (sar-**KOH**-mah) is a malignant tumor arising from connective tissues of the skin. One example is Kaposi sarcoma, a type of skin cancer that is a typical complication of AIDS.

Basal cell carcinoma, squamous cell carcinoma, and some types of melanomas are most commonly treated by Mohs (**MOHZ**) surgery. This type of surgery removes cancerous tissues in layers. This limits the loss of normal tissue and provides the highest cure rate.

**Helping You Remember**  Mohs surgery is an eponym. A disease named for the person who discovered or described it first. Eponyms can also apply to structures, operations, and procedures.

## 6.6   Look-Alike and Sound-Alike Words

*Below is a list of look-alike and sound-alike words. Study the definitions of each set of words. Questions will follow in the Review Exercises.*

### TABLE 6-1  Look-Alike and Sound-Alike Words

| | |
|---|---|
| ablation | treatment that involves the excision of body tissue or the destruction of its function through surgery, hormones, drugs, heat, chemicals, or electricity |
| abrasion | an injury caused by scraping |
| glands | organs that secrete chemicals |
| glans | the tip of the penis (glans penis) |
| patience | showing self-control |
| patients | persons under medical care |
| vesical | pertaining to the bladder |
| vesicle | blister |
| plantar | the sole of the foot |
| planter | container for a plant |
| cirrhosis | any chronic disease of the liver |
| psoriasis | skin condition characterized by silvery scales |
| Mohs | surgery for melanoma |
| mow | to mow (cut) the lawn with a lawnmower |
| wheal | a raised, circular area of skin, usually pale in the center, and surrounded by redness |
| wheel | round object that turns, such as the wheel on a bicycle |

## 6.7   Review Exercises

### EXERCISE 6-1  Look-Alike and Sound-Alike Words

*Read the sentences carefully and circle the word in parentheses that correctly completes the meaning. Use Table 6-1 if it helps you.*

**1.** Genital warts are sexually transmitted. They often appear on the (**glands/glans**) penis.

**2.** After swallowing the medication, the patient broke out in (**vesicals/vesicles**).

3. Cryotherapy was used to treat the (**plantar/planter**) warts on the bottom of the foot.

4. All of the (**patients/patience**) showed up at the medical clinic at the same time. It took a lot of (**patients/patience**) to look after them.

5. The patient has been given a cream to treat his (**cirrhosis/psoriasis**).

6. After he (**mohs/mows**) the lawn, Juan will travel to the hospital for treatment of his melanoma. (**Mohs/Mows**) surgery will be performed.

7. During the bike race, rider number 82 fell off the bike and slid on the pavement. There was a large (**abrasion/ablation**) extending the length of the thigh.

8. Following antibiotic treatment for a urinary tract infection, Georgia broke out in (**wheals/wheels**) on 80 percent of her body.

## EXERCISE 6-2  Matching Word Parts with Meanings

*Match the word part in Column A with its meaning in Column B.*

| | Column A | Column B |
|---|---|---|
| _____ | **1.** adip/o | A. blue |
| _____ | **2.** cry/o | B. scrape |
| _____ | **3.** bi/o | C. nail |
| _____ | **4.** cyan/o | D. life |
| _____ | **5.** necr/o | E. tumor |
| _____ | **6.** erythem/o | F. fungus |
| _____ | **7.** radi/o | G. fat |
| _____ | **8.** myc/o | H. pertaining to |
| _____ | **9.** ras/o | I. away from |
| _____ | **10.** -opsy | J. skin |
| _____ | **11.** -tic | K. cold |
| _____ | **12.** ab- | L. death |
| _____ | **13.** onych/o | M. x-rays |
| _____ | **14.** derm/o | N. red |
| _____ | **15.** -oma | O. to view |

## EXERCISE 6-3  Matching Medical Words with Definitions

*Match the term in Column A with its definition in Column B.*

| | Column A | Column B |
|---|---|---|
| _____ | **1.** epidermis | A. tissue making up the dermis |
| _____ | **2.** sebum | B. bald |

| | Column A | Column B |
|---|---|---|
| _____ | **3.** alopecia | C. pertaining to fat |
| _____ | **4.** epithelium | D. treatment with drugs |
| _____ | **5.** adipose | E. top layer of skin |
| _____ | **6.** erythema | F. scraping away of skin |
| _____ | **7.** connective | G. keeps hair soft |
| _____ | **8.** chemotherapy | H. death of tissue |
| _____ | **9.** abrasion | I. red discoloration |
| _____ | **10.** necrotic | J. tissue making up the epidermis |

## EXERCISE 6-4 Word Completion

*Complete the medical word by adding the most appropriate word element. The first question is completed for you.*

1. A specialist in the study of the skin is a dermato**logist**.

2. Pertaining to fat is _____ ose.

3. Under the skin is _____ cutaneous.

4. Under the skin is _____ dermic.

5. Pertaining to the death of tissues is _____ tic.

6. A tumor or mass containing fat is _____ oma.

7. Cell producing melanin is called melano _____.

8. Treatment with drugs _____ therapy.

## EXERCISE 6-5 Spelling

*Circle any misspelled words in the list below and correctly spell them in the space provided.*

1. **subqutaneous** _____

2. **sebaceous** _____

3. **malanin** _____

4. **sweet glands** _____

5. **epithelial** _____

6. **airythemia** _____

    **7. soriasis** _____

    **8. metastasize** _____

    **9. subungwal** _____

  **10. ecchymosis** _____

## EXERCISE 6-6 Pathology

*Choose the correct answer and write it in the space provided.*

  **1.** A term describing a group of boils is _____

     carbuncle    ecchymoses    furuncle    petechiae

  **2.** A contusion is another name for _____

     boil    bruise    crushed    furuncle

  **3.** A partial-thickness burn is a _____ burn

     first-degree    second-degree    third-degree

  **4.** A chronic skin condition characterized by redness and silvery scales is

    _____

     cellulitis    impetigo    psoriasis    xeroderma

  **5.** The term used to describe the spreading of a tumor from one location to another
    is _____

     abrasion    cyanosis    metastasis    necrosis

  **6.** A malignant tumor of connective tissue is called a _____

     carcinoma    hematoma    papilloma    sarcoma

  **7.** Staphylococci are

     bacteria    fungus    parasite    virus

  **8.** Tumors that are noncancerous are said to be _____

     benign    malignant    metastatic

  **9.** A wart is an example of a(n) _____

     adipoma    carcinoma    lipoma    papilloma

 **10.** A melanoma is generally considered a _____ tumor

     benign    malignant

**11.** The term *excoriation* is also known as _____

abrasion     erythema     keratosis     pruritus

**12.** A patient complains of red and itchy skin. The medical term for itchy is

_____

abrasive     erythematous     necrotic     pruritus

**13.** A discolored, unelevated area of skin is a _____

vesicle     macule     papule     wheal

**14.** A blister is also known as a _____

vesicle     macule     papule     wheal

**15.** A raised, circular area of skin usually pale in the center, surrounded by redness is
a _____

vesicle     macule     papule     wheal

## Animations

Visit the companion website to watch a video on **burns**.

## 6.8  Pronunciation and Spelling

*Listen, read, and study, so you can speak and write.*

**1.** Listen to each word on the audio file provided on the Student Companion Website.

**2.** Pronounce each word carefully.

**3.** Spell each word in the space provided.

| Word | Pronunciation | Spelling |
|------|---------------|----------|
| **abrasion** | ab-**RAY**-zhun | |
| **adipose** | **AD**-ih-pohs | |
| **biopsy** | **BYE**-op-see | |
| **carcinoma** | kar-sih-**NOH**-mah | |
| **cryotherapy** | **krye**-oh-**THER**-ah-pee | |
| **cyanosis** | **sigh**-ah-**NOH**-sis | |
| **dermatitis** | der-mah-**TYE**-tis | |

| Word | Pronunciation | Spelling |
|------|---------------|----------|
| dermatologist | der-mah-TOL-oh-jist | |
| dermis | DER-mis | |
| epidermis | ep-ih-DER-mis | |
| epithelial | ep-ih-THEE-lee-al | |
| epithelium | ep-ih-THEE-lee-um | |
| eponychium | ep-oh-NICK-ee-um | |
| erythematous | er-ih-THEM-ah-tus | |
| hypodermic | high-poh-DER-mick | |
| keratosis | ker-ah-TOH-sis | |
| laser therapy | LAY-zer THER-ah-pee | |
| lipedema | lip-eh-DEE-mah | |
| lipoma | lih-POH-mah | |
| liposuction | lip-oh-SUCK-shun | |
| melanin | MEL-ah-nin | |
| melanocytes | meh-LAN-oh-sights | |
| melanoma | mel-ah-NOH-mah | |
| necrotic | neh-KROT-ick | |
| onychocryptosis | on-ih-koh-krip-TOH-sis | |
| onychomycosis | on-ih-koh-my-KOH-sis | |
| papilloma | pap-ih-LOH-mah | |
| pruritus | proo-EYE-tus | |
| psoriasis | sor-EYE-ah-sis | |
| sebaceous | seh-BAY-shus | |
| staphylococcus | staf-ih-loh-KOCK-us | |
| streptococcus | strep-toh-KOCK-us | |
| subcutaneous | sub-kyoo-TAY-nee-us | |
| subungual | sub-UNG-gwal | |
| vesicle | VES-ih-kul | |
| xeroderma | zer-oh-DER-mah | |

# CHAPTER 7

# Skeletal System

## Chapter Outline

## Learning Objectives

*After studying this chapter and completing the review exercises, you should be able to do the following:*

1. Name and locate the major bones of the body.
2. Describe the structure and functions of bones and joints.
3. Pronounce, spell, and define the medical terms related to the skeletal system.
4. Describe the common diseases related to the skeletal system.
5. Listen, read, and study so you can speak and write.

## Introduction

The skeletal system is made up of 206 bones. They are attached to each other at joints. In this chapter you will learn about the location of the major bones, the structure of bones, and how bones contribute to body function. You will also learn about the structure of joints and how they function to produce movement.

## 7.1   Major Bones of the Body

**PRACTICE FOR LEARNING: Major Bones of the Body**

Write the words below in the correct spaces on Figure 7-1. To help you, the number beside the word tells you where it goes on the figure. Be sure to pronounce each word as you write it. Repeat the pronunciation several times if you find the word hard to say. The common names and adjectival forms are listed in Table 7-1.

1. cranium (**KRAY**-nee-um)
2. facial bones (**FAY**-shal)
3. thorax (**THOR**-acks)
4. carpals (**KAR**-palz)
5. metacarpals (**met**-ah-**KAR**-palz)
6. phalanges (fah-**LAN**-jeez)
7. tarsals (**TAR**-salz)
8. metatarsals (**met**-ah-**TAR**-salz)
9. phalanges (fah-**LAN**-jeez)
10. fibula (**FIB**-yoo-lah)
11. tibia (**TIB**-ee-ah)
12. patella (pah-**TEL**-ah)
13. femur (**FEE**-mur)
14. pelvis (**PEL**-vis)
15. ulna (**ULL**-nah)
16. radius (**RAY**-dee-us)
17. humerus (**HEW**-mer-us)
18. vertebra (**VER**-teh-brah)
19. scapula (**SKAP**-yoo-lah)
20. clavicle (**KLAV**-ih-kul)

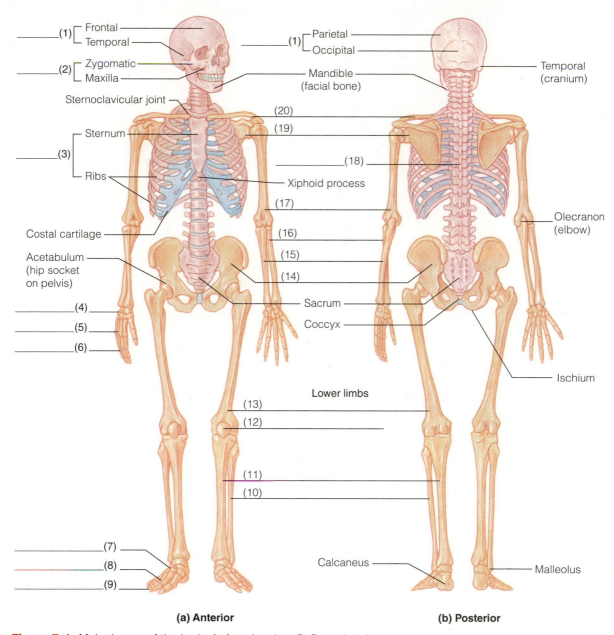

**Figure 7-1**  Major bones of the body. A. Anterior view. B. Posterior view.

## PRACTICE FOR LEARNING: **Bones and Other Structures of the Skull**

Write the words below in the correct spaces on Figure 7-2. To help you, the number beside the word tells you where it goes on the figure. Be sure to pronounce each word as you write it. Repeat the pronunciation several times if you find the word hard to say.

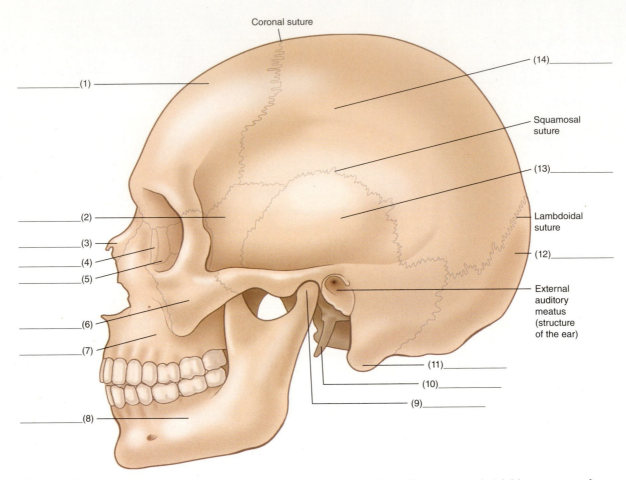

**Figure 7-2** Lateral view of the skull. Sutures are immovable joints. Mastoid process and styloid process are for muscle attachment.

1. frontal (**FRUN**-tal) bone
2. sphenoid (**SFEE**-noyd) bone
3. nasal (**NAY**-zal) bone
4. lacrimal (**LACK**-rih-mal) bone
5. ethmoid (**ETH**-moyd) bone
6. zygoma (zye-**GOH**-mah)
7. maxilla (**MACK**-sil-ah)
8. mandible (**MAN**-dih-bull)
9. temporomandibular (**tem**-por-oh-man-**DIB**-you-lar) joint
10. styloid (**STIGH**-loyd) process
11. mastoid (**MASS**-toyd) process
12. occipital (ock-**SIP**-ih-tal) bone
13. temporal (**TEM**-por-al) bone
14. parietal (pah-**RYE**-eh-tal) bone

### TABLE 7-1  Major Bones, their Common Names, and Adjectival Forms

| Bone | Common Name | Adjectival Form |
| --- | --- | --- |
| calcaneus | heel | calcaneal |
| carpus | wrist | carpal |
| clavicle | collarbone | clavicular |
| coccyx | tailbone | coccygeal |
| cranium | skull | cranial |
| femur | thigh bone | femoral |
| humerus | upper arm | humeral |
| ilium | hip or pelvis | iliac |
| mandible | lower jaw | mandibular |
| maxilla | upper jaw | maxillary |
| metacarpus | bones of hand | metacarpals |
| metatarsus | bones of foot | metatarsals |
| olecranon | elbow | olecranal |
| patella | kneecap | patellar |
| phalanges | fingers or toes | phalangeal |
| scapula | shoulder blade | scapular |
| sternum | breastbone | sternal |
| tarsus | ankle bones | tarsals |
| thorax | chest | thoracic |
| tibia | shin | tibial |
| vertebra | backbone | vertebral |
| zygoma | cheek | zygomatic |

## PRACTICE FOR LEARNING: Major Bones of the Body

**I.** Using Figure 7-1 answer the following questions;

   **a.** The parietal and temporal bones are bones of the _____.

   **b.** The tibia is also known as the _____.

   **c.** Where is the occipital bone located on the cranium? _____

   **d.** Where is the parietal bone located on the cranium? _____

   **e.** Name two bones of the thorax. _____

**f.** On which bone is the acetabulum located? _____

**g.** Name two bones making up the forearm. _____

**h.** Name two bones making up the lower leg. _____

**II.** Study Table 7-1 and then write the medical name for the following:

| Common Name | Medical Name |
|---|---|
| a. kneecap | |
| b. fingers or toes | |
| c. cheek bone | |
| d. elbow | |
| e. hip or pelvis | |
| f. breastbone | |
| g. collarbone | |
| h. shoulder blade | |
| i. wrist | |
| j. tailbone | |

Answers: 1. a. cranium or skull. b. shin. c. back of cranium. d. crown or top of cranium. e. sternum and ribs. f. ilium or pelvic bone. g. radius; ulna. h. tibia; fibula. 2. a. patella. b. phalanges. c. zygomatic bone or zygoma. d. olecranon. e. ilium. f. sternum. g. clavicle. h. scapula. i. carpals. j. coccyx.

## 7.2  Bone Structure and Function

### Bone Structure

#### Cells and Minerals

Just like other organs, bones are made up of cells and tissues. Bones grow and renew themselves. Immature bone cells are called **osteoblasts** (**OS**-tee-oh-blasts). They grow into mature cells called **osteocytes** (**OS**-tee-oh-sights). Osteocytes form bone tissue called **osseous** (**OS**-ee-us) tissue.

**In Brief**

**Osteoblasts** are immature bone cells.

**Osteocytes** are mature bone cells.

Osteocytes form **osseous** tissue.

**Calcium** and **phosphorus** are minerals that make bone hard.

For bones to properly form and become hard and strong, we need to eat food that contains two minerals: **calcium** (**KAL**-see-um) and **phosphorus** (**FOS**-for-us). We also need plenty of vitamin D to help us absorb the calcium.

Cartilage is similar to bone but it is soft because it lacks the calcium deposits that make bone hard. Cartilage is found in all joints, the spinal column, and the rib cage.

## Bone Function

Bones have many functions. They provide protection and support, and allow movement to happen because they provide a rigid structure for the muscles to pull on. They also act as a storehouse for calcium and phosphorus, and release these minerals into the bloodstream when required. The inner part of the bone is called bone marrow. It produces blood cells that are necessary for life. This blood-forming process is called **hematopoiesis** (**he**-mah-toh-poy-**EE**-sis).

**PRACTICE FOR LEARNING: Bone Structure and Function**

Circle True if the statement is correct. Circle False if the statement is not correct.

1. Calcium is a mineral found in bone.            True or False

2. Bone marrow produces blood cells.            True or False

3. Osseous is a type of bone cell.            True or False

4. Osteoblasts are a type of bone cell.            True or False

> Answers: 1. True. 2. True. 3. False. 4. True.

## 7.3   Vertebral Column

**PRACTICE FOR LEARNING: Vertebral Column**

Write the bones of the vertebral column in the correct space on Figure 7-3. To help you, the number beside the bone tells you where it goes on the figure. Be sure to pronounce each word as you write it. Repeat the pronunciation several times if you find the word hard to say.

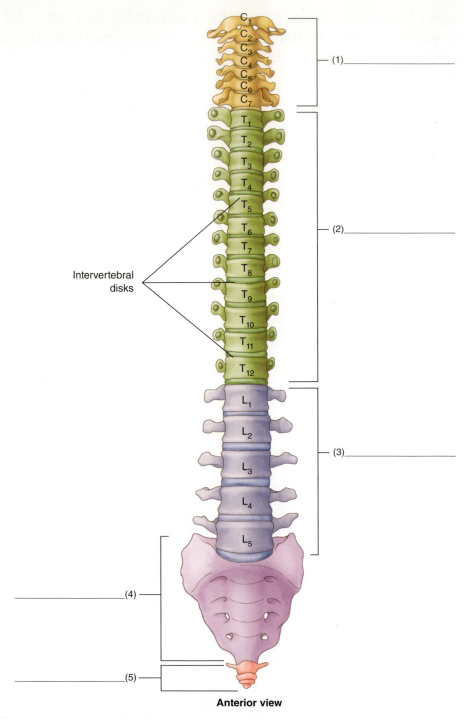

Intervertebral disks

Anterior view

**Figure 7-3**  Vertebral column, anterior view.

1. cervical vertebrae (**SER**-vih-kal **VER**-teh-bree)

2. thoracic (thoh-**RAS**-ick)

3. lumbar (**LUM**-bar)

4. sacrum (**SAY**-krum)

5. coccyx (**KOCK**-sicks)

The bones of the **vertebral** (**VER**-teh-brahl) **column** are organized into five groups. They are illustrated in Figure 7-3. The vertebral column is also called the spinal column, spine, or backbone.

The vertebral column consists of 33 bones arranged in a column that extends from the base of the skull to the lower back. Each bone is called a **vertebra** (**VER**-teh-brah) (plural vertebrae [**VER**-teh-bree]). There are 7 **cervical** vertebrae (C1 to C7), 12 **thoracic** vertebrae (T1 to T12), 5 **lumbar** vertebrae (L1 to L5), 5 fused bones called the **sacrum** (S1 to S5), and 4 fused bones called the coccyx or tailbone. Each vertebra has a round hole in the middle. The holes line up to form a canal. The spinal cord lies within this canal. The vertebrae protect the spinal cord, which is made up of nerves.

---

**In Brief**

The **vertebral column** is also known as the spinal column, spine, or backbone.

The **vertebral column** is made up of bone.

The **spinal cord** is made up of nerves.

---

In Figure 7-3 there is a diagram of a cushion of cartilage called the **intervertebral** (**in**-ter-**VER**-teh-bral) disc, which lies between each vertebrae. These discs allow the vertebrae to glide over each other, making movement smooth and painless.

---

**Helping You Remember**

Think of the vertebral column as a stack of doughnuts with the spinal cord passing through the holes. The intervertebral discs would be like thick wax paper placed between the doughnuts to prevent sticking.

---

## 7.4 Joints

A joint is where two bones come together. Movement occurs at joints. A joint is usually named after the bones that it joins. For example, the sternoclavicular (**ster**-noh-klah-**VICK**-yoo-lar) joint is the union between the sternum (stern/o) and clavicle (clavicul/o) (Figure 7-1).

For joints to work properly and without pain, it is important that the two bones glide smoothly over each other (Figure 7-4). This is accomplished by **articular** (ar-**TIK**-yoo-lar) **cartilage** and **synovial** (sih-**NOH**-vee-al) fluid inside the joint. The synovial fluid is produced by **synovial membrane** lining the joint.

Although most of the joints in the body are movable, there are a few immovable joints in the skull. These immovable joints are called **sutures**.

Also at joints (but not inside) are **tendons** (**TEN**-donz), **ligaments** (**LIG**-ah-ments), and **bursae** (**BUR**-see) (Figure 7-5). Tendons attach muscle to bone. Ligaments attach bone to bone. Bursae are tiny, purse-like sacs lined with synovial membrane and filled with

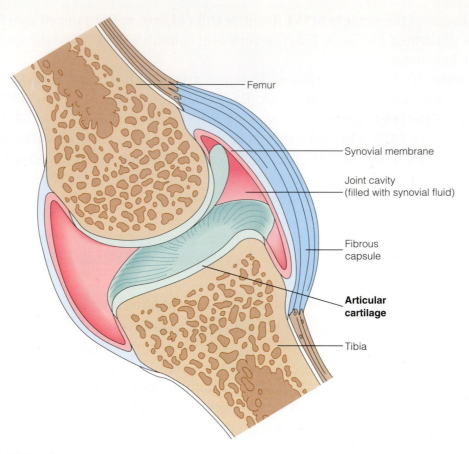

**Figure 7-4**   A joint cavity.

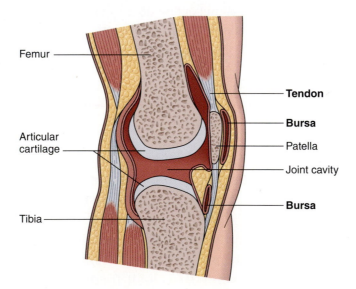

**Figure 7-5**   Bursae around a joint.

synovial fluid. Each **bursa** (**BUR**-sah) prevents friction between two structures that need to glide past each other when they move. The bursa can become inflamed through overuse, resulting in a condition called **bursitis** (bur-**SIGH**-tis). Baseball pitchers will sometimes develop bursitis at the shoulder, while tennis players often develop it in the elbow.

**PRACTICE FOR LEARNING: Vertebral Column and Joints**

Write the correct answers on the space provided:

1. Name the bones of the vertebral column. Write the number of bones in each segment.

   _____

   _____

2. Define a joint. _____

3. Where is articular cartilage located? _____

> Answers: 1. 7 cervical; 12 thoracic; 5 lumbar; 5 fused sacral bones; 4 fused coccygeal bones. 2. A joint is where two bones come together. 3. Covering ends of bone in joints.

## 7.5 New Roots, Suffixes, and Prefixes

Use these additional roots and suffixes when studying the terms in this chapter.

| ROOT | MEANING |
| --- | --- |
| ankyl/o | fusion of parts; stiffening |
| faci/o | face |
| kyph/o | humpback |
| lord/o | swayback |
| ped/o | child |
| sacr/o | sacrum |
| sarc/o | flesh |
| scoli/o | crooked |

| SUFFIX | MEANING |
| --- | --- |
| -desis | surgical fusion |
| -immune | immunity; safe (The immune system protects the body against disease.) |
| -listhesis | slipping |
| -luxation | dislocation |
| -malacia | softening |

## 7.6    Learning the Terms

Following these steps will make it easier for you to learn medical terms:

1. Pronounce the term repeatedly until it is easy for you.
2. Write it down. Ensure the spelling is correct.
3. Also write the definition. If possible, relate the word to a word, thought, or picture that will help you remember it.
4. Analyze the term with the method taught in this text.

### Roots

| ROOT<br>acetabul/o | | MEANING<br>acetabulum; hip socket |
|---|---|---|
| Term | Term Analysis | Definition |
| acetabular<br>(ass-eh-**TAB**-yoo-lar) | -ar = pertaining to | pertaining to the hip socket; the hip socket is a dent (depression) on the pelvic bone (ilium) |

| ROOT<br>arthr/o | | MEANING<br>joint |
|---|---|---|
| Term | Term Analysis | Definition |
| arthralgia<br>(ar-**THRAL**-jah) | -algia = pain | joint pain |
| arthritis<br>(ar-**THRIGH**-tis) | -itis = inflammation | inflammation of a joint. See Section 7.7 for more details. |
| arthrocentesis<br>(**ar**-throh-sen-**TEE**-sis) | -centesis = surgical puncture | surgical puncture to remove fluid from the joint cavity |
| arthrodesis<br>(**ar**-throh-**DEE**-sis) | -desis = surgical fusion | surgical fusion of a joint |
| arthropathy<br>(ar-**THROP**-ah-thee) | -pathy = disease | diseased joint |
| arthroplasty<br>(**AR**-throh-**plas**-tee) | -plasty = surgical repair or reconstruction | surgical repair of a joint. (Figures 7-6A and B) |

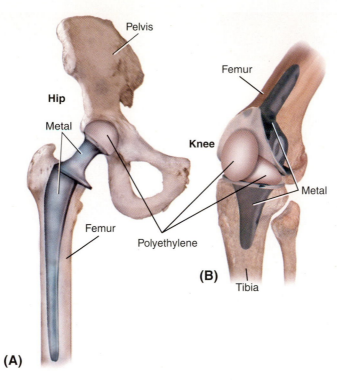

**Figure 7-6** Arthroplasty. A. Total hip replacement. B. Total knee replacement.

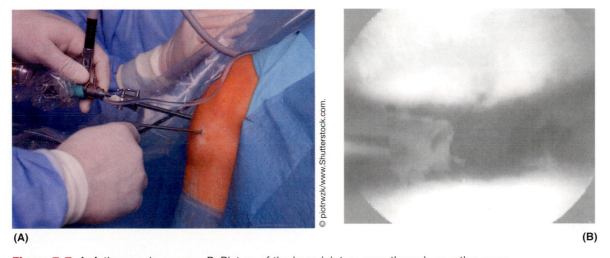

**Figure 7-7** A. Arthroscopic surgery. B. Picture of the knee joint as seen through an arthroscope.

| arthroscopy (ar-**THROS**-koh-pee) | -scopy = process of visual examination | process of visually examining the joint cavity by using an arthroscope (Figures 7-7A and B). |
|---|---|---|

| ROOT brachi/o | | MEANING arm |
|---|---|---|
| Term | Term Analysis | Definition |
| brachiocephalic (bray-kee-oh-seh-FAL-ik) | -ic = pertaining to cephal/o = head | pertaining to the arm and head |

| ROOT calcane/o | | MEANING heel |
|---|---|---|
| Term | Term Analysis | Definition |
| calcaneal (kal-KAY-nee-al) | -eal = pertaining to | pertaining to the heel |

| ROOT cervic/o | | MEANING neck |
|---|---|---|
| Term | Term Analysis | Definition |
| cervical (SER-vih-kal) | -al = pertaining to | pertaining to the neck |

| ROOT chondr/o | | MEANING cartilage |
|---|---|---|
| Term | Term Analysis | Definition |
| chondromalacia (kon-dro-mah-LAY-she-ah) | -malacia = soft | softening of cartilage |
| chondrocyte (KON-droh-sight) | -cyte = cell | cartilage cell |

| ROOT clavicul/o | | MEANING clavicle; collarbone |
|---|---|---|
| Term | Term Analysis | Definition |
| infraclavicular (in-frah-klah-VICK-yoo-lar) | -ar = pertaining to infra- = below; under | pertaining to below the collarbone. Also known as subclavicular and subclavian. |

| ROOT coccyg/o | | MEANING coccyx; tailbone |
|---|---|---|
| Term | Term Analysis | Definition |
| coccygeal (kock-**SIJ**-ee-al) | -eal = pertaining to | pertaining to the tailbone |

| ROOT cost/o | | MEANING rib |
|---|---|---|
| Term | Term Analysis | Definition |
| costal (**KOS**-tal) | -al = pertaining to | pertaining to the ribs |
| subcostal (sub-**KOS**-tal) | -al = pertaining to<br>sub- = under | pertaining to under the ribs |
| costochondritis (**kos**-toh-kon-**DRY**-tis) | -itis = inflammation<br>chondr/o = cartilage | inflammation of ribs and cartilage |
| costovertebral (**kos**-toh-**VER**-teh-bral) | -al = pertaining to<br>vertebr/o = vertebra | pertaining to ribs and vertebra |

| ROOT crani/o | | MEANING skull |
|---|---|---|
| Term | Term Analysis | Definition |
| craniofacial (**kray**-nee-oh-**FAY**-shal) | -al = pertaining to<br>faci/o = face | pertaining to the skull and face |
| craniotomy (**kray**-nee-**OT**-ah-mee) | -tomy = to cut; incision | incision into the skull |

| ROOT femor/o | | MEANING femur; thigh bone |
|---|---|---|
| Term | Term Analysis | Definition |
| femoral (**FEM**-or-al) | -al = pertaining to | pertaining to the femur |

| ROOT ili/o | | MEANING hip |
|---|---|---|
| *Term* | *Term Analysis* | *Definition* |
| iliac (**ILL**-ee-ack) | -ac = pertaining to | pertaining to the hip |
| iliosacral joint (**ill**-ee-oh-**SAY**-kral) | -al = pertaining to<br>sacr/o = sacrum | pertaining to the joint between the hip and sacrum; also known as the sacroiliac (**say**-kroh-**ILL**-ee-ack) joint |

| ROOT lumb/o | | MEANING lower back; loins |
|---|---|---|
| *Term* | *Term Analysis* | *Definition* |
| lumbodynia (**lum**-boh-**DIN**-yah) | -dynia = pain | pain in the lower back; lumbago |

| ROOT mandibul/o | | MEANING mandible; lower jaw |
|---|---|---|
| *Term* | *Term Analysis* | *Definition* |
| mandibular (man-**DIB**-yoo-lar) | -ar = pertaining to | pertaining to the mandible |

| ROOT maxill/o | | MEANING upper jaw |
|---|---|---|
| *Term* | *Term Analysis* | *Definition* |
| maxillary (**MACK**-sih-**lar**-ee) | -ary = pertaining to | pertaining to the upper jaw |

| ROOT myel/o | | MEANING bone marrow |
|---|---|---|
| *Term* | *Term Analysis* | *Definition* |
| myelogenous (**my**-eh-**LOJ**-en-us) | -genous = produced by | produced by the bone marrow |

| ROOT olecran/o | | MEANING elbow |
|---|---|---|
| *Term* | *Term Analysis* | *Definition* |
| olecranal (oh-**LECK**-ran-al) | -al = pertaining to | pertaining to the elbow |

| ROOT patell/o | | MEANING patella; kneecap |
|---|---|---|
| *Term* | *Term Analysis* | *Definition* |
| suprapatellar (**soo**-prah-pah-**TEL**-ar) | -ar = pertaining to<br>supra- = above | pertaining to above the kneecap |

| ROOT oste/o | | MEANING bone |
|---|---|---|
| *Term* | *Term Analysis* | *Definition* |
| osteitis (**os**-tee-**EYE**-tis) | -itis = inflammation | inflammation of the bone |
| osteomalacia (**os**-tee-oh-mah-**LAY**-shee-ah) | -malacia = softening | softening of bone |
| osteomyelitis (**os**-tee-oh-**my**-eh-**LYE**-tis) | -itis = inflammation<br>myel/o = bone marrow | inflammation of bone and bone marrow |
| osteonecrosis (**os**-tee-oh-neh-**KRO**-sis) | -sis = condition<br>necr/o = death | death of bone tissue due to the lack of blood supply |

| ROOT phalang/o | | MEANING phalanx; one of the bones making up the fingers or toes |
|---|---|---|
| *Term* | *Term Analysis* | *Definition* |
| interphalangeal joint (**in**-ter-fah-**LAN**-jee-al) | -al = pertaining to<br>inter- = between | pertaining to joints between the phalanges |

| ROOT radi/o | | MEANING radius (one of the bones of the lower arm) | |
| --- | --- | --- | --- |
| Term | Term Analysis | Definition | |
| radiocarpal joint (**ray**-dee-oh-**KAR**-pal) | -al = pertaining to  carp/o = wrist | pertaining to the joint between the radius and wrist | |

| ROOT scapul/o | | MEANING scapula; shoulder blade | |
| --- | --- | --- | --- |
| Term | Term Analysis | Definition | |
| subscapular (sub-**SKAP**-yoo-lar) | -ar = pertaining to  sub- = under; below | pertaining to under the shoulder blade; infrascapular | |

| ROOT spondyl/o | | MEANING vertebra | |
| --- | --- | --- | --- |
| Term | Term Analysis | Definition | |
| spondylolisthesis (**spon**-dih-loh-lis-**THEE**-sis) | -listhesis = slipping | forward slipping of one vertebra over another. Usually the fifth lumbar vertebra over the sacrum. | |

| ROOT synovi/o | | MEANING synovial membrane | |
| --- | --- | --- | --- |
| Term | Term Analysis | Definition | |
| synovectomy (**sin**-oh-**VECK**-toh-me) | -ectomy = excision | surgical removal of the synovial membrane | |

| ROOT thorac/o | | MEANING chest | |
| --- | --- | --- | --- |
| Term | Term Analysis | Definition | |
| thoracolumbar (thoh-**rack**-oh-**LUM**-bar) | -ar = pertaining to  lumb/o = lower back; loins | pertaining to the chest and lower back | |

| ROOT uln/o | | MEANING ulna (one of the bones of the lower arm) |
|---|---|---|
| Term | Term Analysis | Definition |
| ulnar (**ULL**-nar) | -ar = pertaining to | pertaining to the ulna |

## Suffixes

| SUFFIX -luxation | | MEANING displacement; dislocation |
|---|---|---|
| Term | Term Analysis | Definition |
| subluxation (**sub**-leck-**SAY**-shun) | sub- = under; below | partial displacement or dislocation of a bone from its joint |

| SUFFIX -oma | | MEANING tumor; mass |
|---|---|---|
| Term | Term Analysis | Definition |
| carcinoma (**kar**-sih-**NOH**-mah) | carcin/o = cancer | malignant tumor of epithelial cells |
| chondroma (kon-**DROH**-mah) | chondr/o = cartilage | benign tumor of cartilage |
| chondrosarcoma (**kon**-droh-sar-**KOH**-mah) | -sarcoma = malignant tumor of connective tissue. | malignant tumor of cartilage. Cartilage is a type of connective tissue. |
| osteoma (**os**-tee-**OH**-mah) | oste/o = bone | benign tumor of bone |
| osteosarcoma (**os**-tee-oh-sar-**KOH**-mah) | -sarcoma = malignant tumor of connective tissue | malignant tumor of bone. Bone is a type of connective tissue. |
| sarcoma (sar-**KOH**-mah) | sarc/o = flesh | sarcoma can also be used as a word on its own to mean a malignant tumor of connective tissue |

| SUFFIX -osis | | MEANING abnormal condition |
|---|---|---|
| Term | Term Analysis | Definition |
| kyphosis (kye-**FOH**-sis) | kyph/o = humpback | abnormal increase in the outward curvature of the thoracic spine (Figure 7-8A) |
| lordosis (lor-**DOH**-sis) | lord/o = swayback | abnormal increase in the forward curvature of the lumbar spine (Figure 7-8B) |
| scoliosis (**skoh**-lee-**OH**-sis) | scoli/o = crooked | abnormal lateral curvature of the spine (Figure 7-8C) |

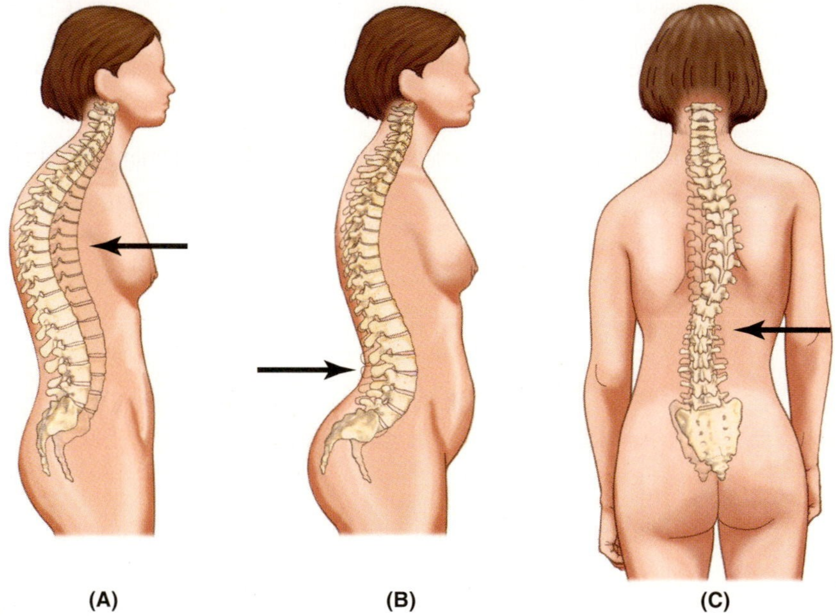

(A)                    (B)                    (C)

**Figure 7-8**  Abnormal Curvatures of the spine. (A) Kyphosis. (B) Lordosis. (C) Scoliosis

# Prefixes

| PREFIX auto- | | MEANING self |
|---|---|---|
| Term | Term Analysis | Definition |
| autoimmune disease (**aw**-toh-ih-**MYOON**) | -immune = immunity; safe | immune response to one's own body tissue; destruction of one's own cells by one's own immune system. An example of an autoimmune disease is rheumatoid arthritis. (See under pathology for more detail on rheumatoid arthritis.) |

**Note:** The immune system helps protect the body against harmful substances.

| PREFIX ortho- | | MEANING straight |
|---|---|---|
| *Term* | *Term Analysis* | *Definition* |
| **orthopedics** (**or**-thoh-**PEE**-dicks) | -ic = pertaining to ped/o = child | surgical specialty dealing with the correction of deformities and dysfunctions of the skeletal system. |

## 7.7 Pathology

### Fractures

A fracture is a break or crack in a bone.

### Types of Fractures

- **Greenstick** fracture means a bone is partially broken on one side and bent on the other (Figure 7-9A).

- **Closed fracture**, also known as a simple fracture, means a bone is broken but there is no open cut in the skin (Figure 7-9B).

- **Open fracture**, also known as a compound fracture, means a bone is broken and there is an open cut in the skin (Figure 7-9C).

- **Comminuted** (**kom**-ih-**NOOT**-id) fracture means the bone has been splintered (Figure 7-9D).

- **Colles** (**KOHL**-eez) fracture is of the distal radius near the wrist (Figure 7-9E).

- **Pathological** fracture means the bone breaks because it is weak from disease.

### Treatment

The treatment of fractures involves reduction and immobilization. Reduction means placing the bones back together. Immobilization results from placing a cast over the broken bone to prevent movement.

If an incision in the skin is not necessary to place the bones back together, the procedure is called **closed reduction** (Figure 7-9F). If it is necessary to incise (cut) the skin in order to see how to place the bones back together, the procedure is called **open reduction**. When the fracture is severe, screws, nails, or pins may be needed to hold the bones in place. This procedure is called **open reduction internal fixation** (**ORIF**) (Figure 7-9G).

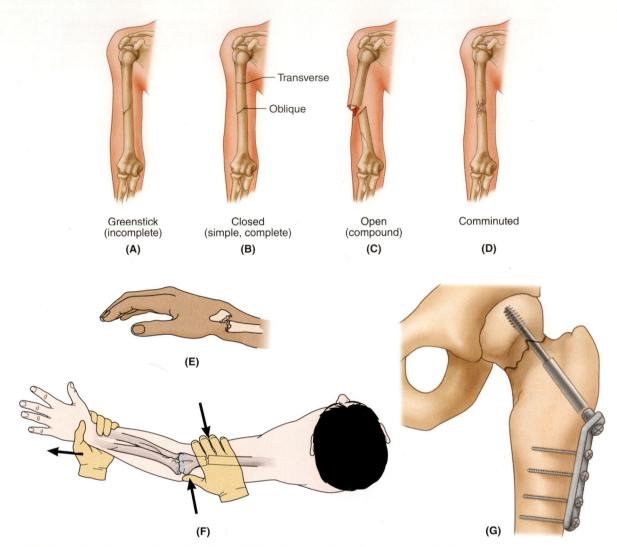

Transverse

Oblique

| Greenstick (incomplete) | Closed (simple, complete) | Open (compound) | Comminuted |
|:---:|:---:|:---:|:---:|
| (A) | (B) | (C) | (D) |

(E)

(F)

(G)

**Figure 7-9** Fractures: A. Greenstick (incomplete). B. Closed (simple, complete). C. Open (compound). D. Comminuted. E. Colles. F. Closed reduction. G. Open reduction internal fixation.

## Herniated Intervertebral Disc; Slipped Disc

A portion of the intervertebral disc moves out of place (herniates). The result is that a nerve may be pinched, causing pain (Figure 7-10). Although herniation can occur at any point along the vertebral column, the lumbar vertebrae are most often affected because of the weight they bear.

## Osteoarthritis (os-tee-oh-ar-**THRIGH**-tis) (OA)

Chronic progressive degeneration of the articular cartilage. It is the most common form of arthritis (Figure 7-11). The exact cause is unknown, but joint injury and cartilage degeneration may leave the ends of bone without cartilage and without protection from opposing bony surfaces. Movement is painful because bone rubs on bone without protection from the articular cartilage.

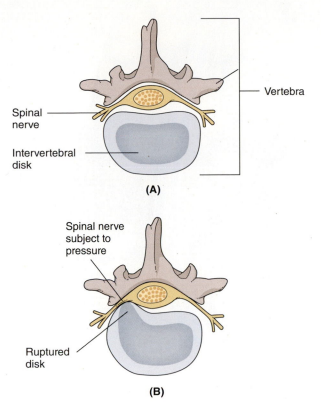

Vertebra

Spinal nerve

Intervertebral disk

**(A)**

Spinal nerve subject to pressure

Ruptured disk

**(B)**

**Figure 7-10** A. Normal intervertebral disc. B. Herniated intervertebral disc places pressure on spinal cord.

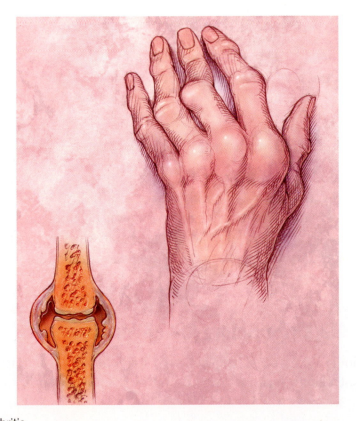

**Figure 7-11** Osteoarthritis.

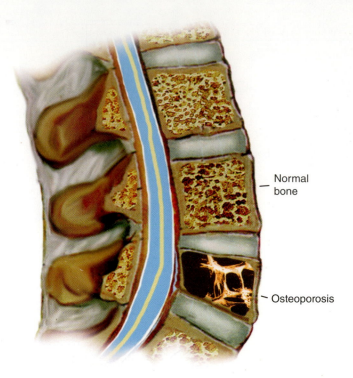

Normal
bone

Osteoporosis

**Figure 7-12**  Osteoporosis.

## Osteoporosis (os-tee-oh-pah-ROH-sis)

Loss of bone mass (density of bone), especially in the thoracic vertebrae (Figure 7-12). The bone becomes thin, porous, and weak. Pathological fractures are common because of the weak bone.

## Rheumatoid Arthritis (ROO-mah-toyd) (RA)

A chronic autoimmune disease that first attacks joints. It can progress to other body organs including skin, blood vessels, and lungs. An autoimmune disease occurs when the body's immune system fails to recognize its own cells as normal and attacks the body's tissues as if they were foreign invaders. In rheumatoid arthritis, the synovial membranes at the joint are attacked, making movement difficult.

## 7.8  Look-Alike and Sound Alike Words

Below is a list of look-alike and sound-alike words. Study the spelling and definitions of each set of words. Questions will follow in the Review Exercises.

### TABLE 7-2 Look-Alike and Sound-Alike Words

| | |
|---|---|
| **hypercalcemia** | increased amounts of calcium in the blood |
| **hyperkalemia** | increased amounts of potassium in the blood |
| **humeral** | pertaining to the humerus |
| **humoral** | pertaining to body fluids |
| **humerus** | the arm bone |
| **humorous** | funny |
| **ilium** | hip bone |
| **ileum** | third portion of the small intestine |
| **malleolus** | bony bump on the distal end of the tibia and fibula |
| **malleus** | bone of the middle ear |
| **sprain** | stretching or tearing of a ligament |
| **strain** | stretching or tearing of a tendon or muscle |

## 7.9    Review Exercises

### EXERCISE 7-1 Look-Alike and Sound-Alike Words

*Read the sentences carefully and circle the word in parentheses that correctly completes the meaning. Use Table 7-2 if it helps you.*

1. In (**humoral/humeral**) immunity, antibodies are released into the blood.

2. While bouncing on the bed, Julio fell off and broke his (**humorous/humerus**). This was not (**humorous/humerus**).

3. José slipped on the rocks and broke the distal tibia at the (**malleus/malleolus**).

4. Jack had a difficult time hearing. The MRI showed degeneration of the (**malleolus/malleus**).

5. While skiing, Anastasia tore her shoulder ligaments. The diagnosis was a (**sprain/strain**) of the shoulder.

6. (**Hypercalcemia/Hyperkalemia**) is due to kidney dysfunction resulting in abnormal potassium levels.

## EXERCISE 7-2  Matching Word Parts with Meanings

*Match the word part in Column A with its meaning in Column B.*

| Column A | Column B |
|---|---|
| _____ **1.** arthr/o | A. cartilage |
| _____ **2.** -pathy | B. inflammation |
| _____ **3.** -plasty | C. softening |
| _____ **4.** -scopy | D. tumor |
| _____ **5.** chondr/o | E. under |
| _____ **6.** cost/o | F. joint |
| _____ **7.** oste/o | G. rib |
| _____ **8.** myel/o | H. straight |
| _____ **9.** -itis | I. malignant tumor of |
| _____ **10.** orth/o | connective tissue |
| _____ **11.** -malacia | J. self |
| _____ **12.** -cyte | K. child |
| _____ **13.** -oma | L. safe |
| _____ **14.** -al | M. disease |
| _____ **15.** sub- | N. bone |
| _____ **16.** -sarcoma | O. cell |
| _____ **17.** -centesis | P. process of viewing |
| _____ **18.** auto- | Q. bone marrow |
| _____ **19.** -immune | R. surgical puncture |
| _____ **20.** ped/o | S. pertaining to |
|  | T. surgical reconstruction |

## EXERCISE 7-3  Short Answer—Anatomy

*Answer the following in the space provided.*

**1.** Name two cells found in osseous tissue. _____
_____

**2.** Bones come together to form _____.

**3.** How are joints named? _____

**4.** Name two mineral substances found in bone.
_____

**5.** The tailbone is also known as the _____.

6. The bones of the skull are called the _____. The bones of the chest are called the _____.

7. Tendons attach _____. Ligaments attach

_____.

8. What type of tissue is the spinal column made up of? What type of tissue is the spinal cord made up of? _____

9. Name the five divisions of the vertebral column. State the number of bones in each division.

_____

_____

_____

10. Name five functions of bone. _____

## EXERCISE 7-4  Location of Bones

*Match each bone with its location. The location may be used more than once.*

## Locations

arm _____

cranium _____

face _____

foot _____

hand _____

leg _____

pelvis _____

thorax _____

vertebral column _____

wrist _____

## Bones

1. calcaneus _____

2. fibula _____

**3.** carpals _____

**4.** sternum _____

**5.** metatarsals _____

**6.** olecranon _____

**7.** radius _____

**8.** occipital _____

**9.** zygomatic _____

**10.** maxilla _____

**11.** parietal _____

**12.** metacarpals _____

**13.** coccyx _____

**14.** ilium _____

**15.** sacrum _____

**16.** femur _____

**17.** humerus _____

**18.** ulna _____

**19.** patella _____

**20.** mandible _____

## EXERCISE 7-5 **Naming Bones**

*Write the common name of the following bones.*

**1.** cranium _____

**2.** zygomatic _____

**3.** mandible _____

**4.** maxilla _____

**5.** sternum _____

**6.** coccyx _____

**7.** humerus _____

**8.** olecranon _____

**9.** carpals _____

**10.** metacarpals _____

**11.** phalanges _____

**12.** ilium _____

**13.** femur _____

**14.** tibia _____

**15.** patella _____

## EXERCISE 7-6  Matching—Pathology

*I. Match the term in Column A with its description in Column B.*

|  | Column A | Column B |
|---|---|---|
| _____ | **1.** rheumatoid arthritis | A. loss of bone mass |
| _____ | **2.** reduction and immobilization | B. treatment for osteoarthritis |
|  |  | C. autoimmune disease |
| _____ | **3.** osteoarthritis | D. treatment for fractures |
| _____ | **4.** osteoporosis | E. degeneration of articular cartilage |
| _____ | **5.** arthroplasty |  |

*II. Match the term in Column A with its description in Column B.*

|  | Column A | Column B |
|---|---|---|
| _____ | **6.** kyphosis | F. inflammation causing fusion of joints between vertebrae |
| _____ | **7.** lordosis | G. partial dislocation |
| _____ | **8.** ankylosing spondylitis | H. increased forward curvature of lumbar spine |
| _____ | **9.** subluxation | I. forward slipping of one vertebrae over another |
| _____ | **10.** spondylolisthesis | J. increased outward curvature of thoracic spine |

*III. Match the term in Column A with its description in Column B.*

|  | Column A | Column B |
|---|---|---|
| _____ | **11.** open fracture | K. fracture of distal radius |
| _____ | **12.** closed fracture | L. bone is splintered |
| _____ | **13.** Colles | M. fractured bone with broken skin |
| _____ | **14.** comminuted fracture | N. bone is partially broken on one side and bent on the other |
| _____ | **15.** greenstick | O. fractured bone with no broken skin |

## EXERCISE 7-7 Definitions—Learning the Terms

*Give the meanings of the following terms.*

**1.** arthralgia _____

**2.** chondromalacia _____

**3.** subcostal _____

**4.** osteitis _____

**5.** osteosarcoma _____

**6.** osteomyelitis _____

**7.** orthopedics _____

**8.** myelogenous _____

**9.** arthropathy _____

**10.** osteomalacia _____

**11.** spondylolisthesis _____

**12.** subluxation _____

**13.** open/compound fracture _____

**14.** scoliosis _____

**15.** herniated intervertebral disc _____

## EXERCISE 7-8 Definitions in Context

*Define the bolded terms in context. Use your dictionary if necessary.*

**1.** Severe **arthropathy** in the back involves the **sacroiliac joint**.

    **a.** arthropathy _____

    **b.** sacroiliac joint _____

**2.** **Reduction** and **immobilization** have been performed on a previously noted **Colles fracture**.

    **c.** reduction and immobilization _____

    **d.** Colles fracture _____

**3.** It was felt he would benefit from **arthroscopy** and repair of the **articular cartilage**.

    **e.** arthroscopy _____

    **f.** articular cartilage _____

**4.** The patient's x-ray showed a **comminuted** fracture of the right **femur** and **greenstick** fracture of the left **humerus**. He was admitted for **open reduction and internal fixation** of right femur.

**g.** comminuted _____

**h.** femur _____

**i.** greenstick _____

**j.** humerus _____

**k.** open reduction and internal fixation _____

## EXERCISE 7-9  Word Building

*I. Use the root arthr/o to build medical words for the following definitions:*

**a.** joint pain _____

**b.** inflammation of a joint _____

**c.** surgical puncture to remove fluid from the joint cavity _____

**d.** diseased joint _____

**e.** surgical reconstruction of a joint _____

**f.** process of visually examining a joint cavity _____

*II. Use the root chondr/o to build medical words for the following definitions:*

**a.** softening of cartilage _____

**b.** benign tumor of cartilage _____

**c.** cartilaginous cell _____

*III. Use the root oste/o to build medical words for the following definitions:*

**a.** inflammation of bone _____

**b.** benign tumor of bone _____

**c.** softening of bone _____

**d.** inflammation of bone and bone marrow _____

**e.** malignant tumor of bone _____

*IV. Use the suffix -osis to build medical words for the following definitions*

**a.** Increase in the outward curvature of the thoracic spine _____

**b.** Increase in the forward curvature of the lumbar spine _____

**c.** Abnormal lateral curvature of the spine _____

*V. Use the suffix -al to build medical words for the following definitions:*

    **a.** pertaining to the head and face _____

    **b.** pertaining to the lower jaw _____

    **c.** pertaining to the neck _____

    **d.** pertaining to under the collarbone _____

    **e.** pertaining to the elbow _____

## EXERCISE 7-10  Spelling

*Circle any words that are spelled incorrectly in the list below. Then correct the spelling in the space provided.*

    **1.** calcaneus _____

    **2.** osseous _____

    **3.** mylogenus _____

    **4.** cocyxx _____

    **5.** humeral _____

    **6.** vertabral _____

    **7.** phalanges _____

    **8.** reumatoid _____

    **9.** imobilization _____

  **10.** cartalage _____

## EXERCISE 7-11  Labeling—Bones

Using the body structures listed below, label Figure 7-13. Write your answer on the numbered space provided below, or if you prefer, on the diagram.

| | | |
|---|---|---|
| carpals | humerus | scapula |
| clavicle | metacarpals | tarsals |
| cranium | metatarsals | thorax |
| facial bones | patella | tibia |
| femur | phalanges | ulna |
| fibula | radius | vertebra |
| hip bones | | |

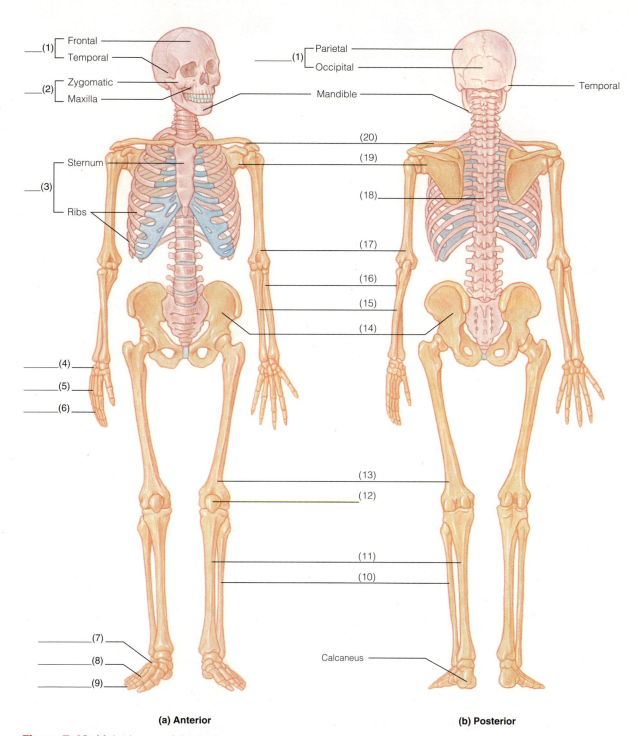

Frontal
Temporal
Zygomatic
Maxilla
Sternum
Ribs
Parietal
Occipital
Temporal
Mandible
Calcaneus

(a) Anterior                                    (b) Posterior

**Figure 7-13**  Major bones of the body.

Example:

1. **cranium** _____

2. _____

3. _____

4. _____

5. _____

6. _____

7. _____

8. _____

9. _____

10. _____

11. _____

12. _____

13. _____

14. _____

15. _____

16. _____

17. _____

18. _____

19. _____

20. _____

## Animations

Visit the companion website to view the video on **kyphosis**, **lordosis**, and **scoliosis**.

Also watch the following videos: **Osteorheumatoid Arthritis**; **Arthroscopy**; **Internal Fixation of a Fracture**.

## 7.10   Pronunciation and Spelling

**1.** Listen to each word on the audio file provided on the Student Companion Website.

**2.** Pronounce each word carefully.

**3.** Spell each word in the space provided.

| Word | Pronunciation | Spelling |
|------|---------------|----------|
| acetabular | **ass**-eh-**TAB**-yoo-lar | _____ |
| arthralgia | ar-**THRAL**-jee-ah | _____ |
| arthritis | ar-**THRIGH**-tis | _____ |

| Word | Pronunciation | Spelling |
|------|---------------|----------|
| arthrocentesis | **ar**-throh-sen-**TEE**-sis | |
| arthrodesis | **ar**-throh-**DEE**-sis | |
| arthroplasty | **AR**-throh-**plas**-tee | |
| arthroscopy | ar-**THROS**-koh-pee | |
| carpals | **KAR**-palz | |
| chondrocyte | **KON**-droh-sight | |
| chondroma | kon-**DROH**-mah | |
| chondromalacia | **kon**-droh-mah-**LAY**-she-ah | |
| chondrosarcoma | **kon**-droh-sar-**KOH**-mah | |
| clavicle | **KLAV**-ih-kul | |
| coccyx | **KOCK**-sicks | |
| cranium | **KRAY**-nee-um | |
| ethmoid | **ETH**-moyd | |
| facial | **FAY**-shal | |
| femur | **FEE**-mur | |
| fibula | **FIB**-yoo-lah | |
| frontal | **FRUN**-tal | |
| humerus | **HEW**-mer-us | |
| kyphosis | kye-**FOH**-sis | |
| lacrimal | **LACK**-rih-mal | |
| lordosis | lor-**DOH**-sis | |
| mandible | **MAN**-dih-bull | |
| maxilla | **MACK**-sil-ah | |
| metacarpals | **met**-ah-**KAR**-palz | |
| metatarsals | **met**-ah-**TAHR**-salz | |
| myelogenous | **my**-eh-**LOJ**-en-us | |
| occipital | ock-**SIP**-ih-tal | |
| orthopedics | **or**-thoh-**PEE**-dicks | |
| osseous | **OS**-ee-us | |

| Word | Pronunciation | Spelling |
|------|---------------|----------|
| osteitis | os-tee-EYE-tis | |
| osteoma | os-tee-OH-ma | |
| osteomalacia | os-tee-oh-mah-LAY-shee-ah | |
| osteomyelitis | os-tee-oh-my-eh-LYE-tis | |
| osteoporosis | os-tee-oh-por-OH-sis | |
| osteosarcoma | os-tee-oh-sar-KOH-mah | |
| patella | pah-TEL-ah | |
| phalanges | fah-LAN-jeez | |
| radius | RAY-dee-us | |
| sacrum | SAY-krum | |
| scapula | SKAP-yoo-lah | |
| scoliosis | skoh-lee-OH-sis | |
| sphenoid | SFEE-noyd | |
| sternum | STER-num | |
| subcostal | sub-KOS-tal | |
| tarsals | TAHR-salz | |
| temporal | TEM-por-al | |
| temporomandibular | tem-por-oh-man-DIB-you-lar | |
| thorax | THOR-acks | |
| tibia | TIB-ee-ah | |
| ulna | ULL-nah | |
| vertebral column | VER-teh-bral KOL-um | |
| zygomatic | zye-goh-MAT-ick | |

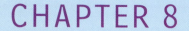

# CHAPTER 8

# Muscular System

## Chapter Outline

## Learning Objectives

*After studying this chapter and completing the review exercises, you should be able to:*

1. Name three types of muscle tissue and state the location of each.
2. Name and define types of muscular movement.
3. Name, locate, and state the function of common skeletal muscles.
4. Pronounce, spell, define, and write the medical terms related to the muscular system.
5. Describe common diseases related to the muscular system.
6. Listen, read, and study so you can speak and write.

## Introduction

All bodily movement is performed by muscle. Bend your arm and move your hand toward your shoulder. The muscles in your forearm and upper arm have made this happen. They are called **voluntary** muscles because you can make them move when you want them to. At the same time you were doing this, your heart kept beating even though you were not thinking about it. The heart is an example of **involuntary** muscle. It does its job without being told.

## 8.1  Major Muscles of the Body

PRACTICE FOR LEARNING: **Major Muscles of the Body**

Write the muscles listed below in the correct spaces in Figure 8-1A and B. To help you, the number beside the muscle tells you where it goes on the figure. Be sure to pronounce each word as you write it. Repeat the pronunciation several times if you find the word hard to say.

### Anterior View

1. facial muscles (**FAY**-shul **MUSS**-elz)
2. sternocleidomastoid (**stern**-oh-**kleye**-doh-**MASS**-toyd)
3. pectoralis major (**peck**-tor-**AL**-iss **MAY**-jor)
4. serratus anterior (seh-**RAY**-tuss an-**TEER**-ee-or)
5. abdominal muscles (ab-**DOM**-ih-nul)
6. adductors of thigh (ah-**DUCK**-terz)
7. sartorius (sar-**TOR**-ee-us)
8. quadriceps femoris (**KWAH**-drih-seps **FEM**-or-iss)
9. biceps brachii (**BYE**-seps **BRAY**-kee)

### Posterior View

10. trapezius (trah-**PEE**-zee-us)
11. triceps brachii (**TRIGH**-seps **BRAY**-kee)
12. latissimus dorsi (lah-**TIS**-ih-mus)
13. gluteus maximus (**GLOO**-tee-us **MAX**-ih-muss)
14. gastrocnemius (**gas**-troh-**NEE**-mee-us)
15. Achilles tendon (ah-**KILL**-eez **TEN**-don)
16. hamstrings (**HAM**-stringz)
17. deltoid (**DEL**-toyd)

| Helping You Remember | The words "biceps" and "triceps" always end in "s," whether they are referring to one muscle or more than one. |

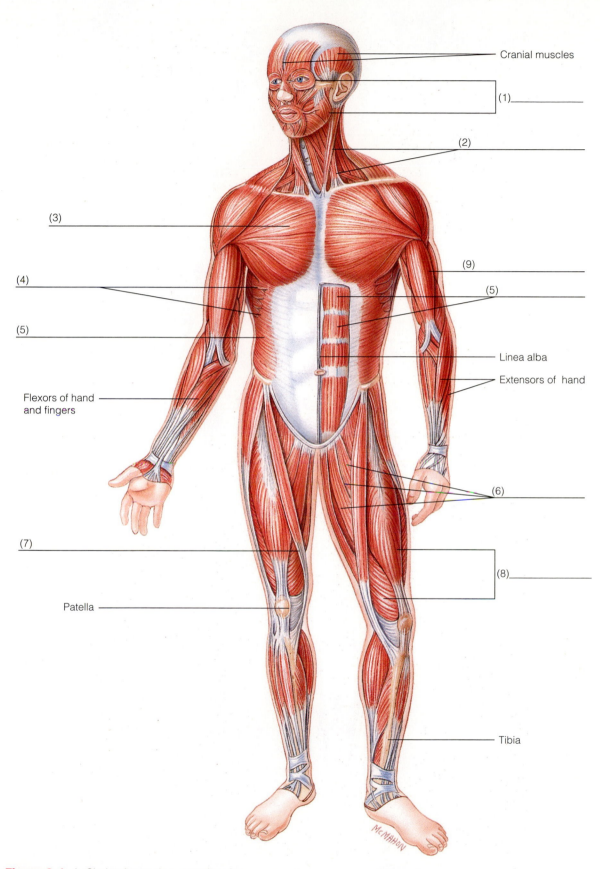

Cranial muscles

(1)_____

(2)

(3)

(9)

(4)

(5)

(5)

Linea alba

Extensors of hand

Flexors of hand
and fingers

(6)

(7)

(8)_____

Patella

Tibia

**Figure 8-1**  A. Skeletal muscles, anterior view.

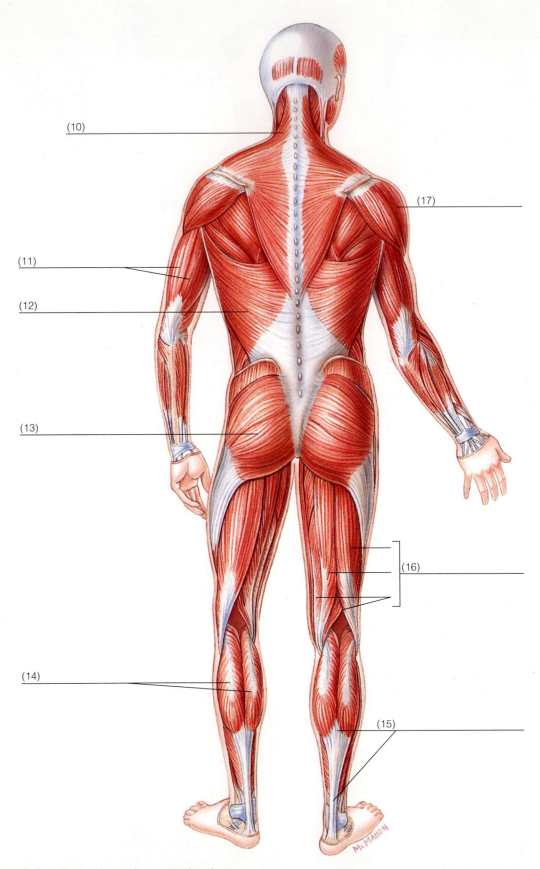

(10)

(17)

(11)

(12)

(13)

(16)

(14)

(15)

**Figure 8-1** B. Skeletal muscles, posterior view.

## 8.2 Types of Muscle Tissue

The cells found in muscle are called muscle fibers. They are long, slender, and thread-like. They can **contract** (kon-**TRAKT**), which means they can shorten their length. This makes movement possible. Muscle fibers form three types of muscle tissue: **cardiac** (**KAR**-dee-ack), **visceral** (**VISS**-er-al), and **skeletal** (**SKEL**-eh-tal). Cardiac muscle is located in the heart and functions to pump blood. Visceral muscles move internal organs such as the respiratory tract, digestive tract, and blood vessels. Skeletal muscles are located on top of bone. They move bone by pulling on it.

**In Brief**

There are three types of muscle tissue:

**cardiac**

**visceral**

**skeletal**

All muscle is wrapped in a band of connective tissue called **fascia** (**FASH**-ee-ah), as illustrated in Figure 8-2. This is called deep fascia.

In this chapter you will learn only about the skeletal muscles.

**PRACTICE FOR LEARNING: Muscle Types**

Fill in the blanks with the correct answer.

1. Muscle cells are also called _____.

2. Name three types of muscle tissue: _____, _____, and _____.

3. What is the main function of muscle tissue? _____

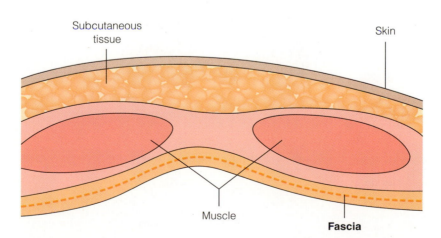

**Figure 8-2** Fascia wraps around muscle.

**4.** Where are visceral muscles located? _____

**5.** Where are skeletal muscles located? _____

**6.** Define deep fascia. _____

> Answers: 1. muscle fibers. 2. cardiac, skeletal, and visceral. 3. movement; contraction. 4. internal organs. 5. on top of bones. 6. band of connective tissue around the muscle

## 8.3  Movements of Skeletal Muscles

All skeletal muscles are connected to two bones. This makes movement possible. When the muscle contracts, one of the two bones it is connected to moves because the muscle pulls on the bone. This is illustrated in Figure 8-3.

The muscles are connected to bones by bands of connective tissue. Some of these tissues are thin and cordlike. They are called tendons (Figure 8-3). Broader bands of connective tissues are called **aponeuroses** (**ah**-poh-new-**ROH**-seez).

### Types of Muscle Movements

Muscles move bone in different ways. The common movements are listed below and are illustrated in Figures 8-4 to 8-8.

- **Flexion** means decreasing the angle between two bones, such as bending the neck forward or bending a limb.

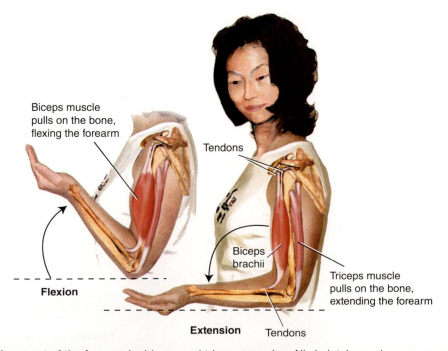

Biceps muscle pulls on the bone, flexing the forearm

Tendons

Flexion

Biceps brachii

Triceps muscle pulls on the bone, extending the forearm

Extension          Tendons

**Figure 8-3**  Movement of the forearm by biceps and triceps muscles. All skeletal muscles are connected to bones by tendons. Bone movement occurs when the muscle pulls on the bone.

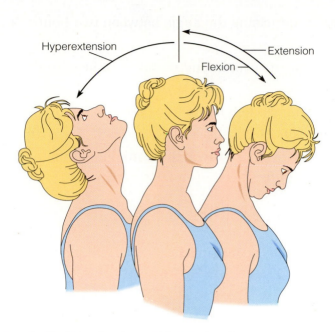

**Figure 8-4** Muscle movements: flexion, extension, and hyperextension.

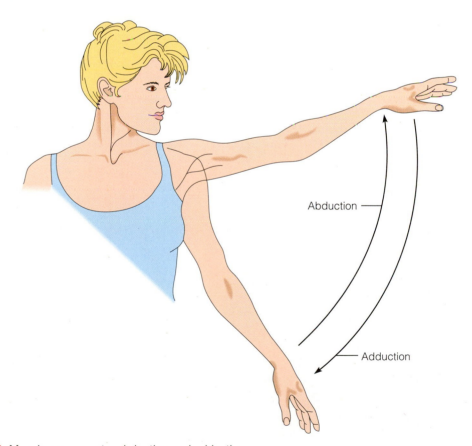

**Figure 8-5** Muscle movements: abduction and adduction.

- **Extension** means increasing the angle between two bones; it is a return from flexion.
- **Hyperextension** means overextending the joint beyond straight (beyond the anatomical position).
- **Abduction** means movement **away** from the midline of the body, usually involving the upper or lower limbs.
- **Adduction** means movement **toward** the midline of the body, usually involving the upper or lower limbs.

> **Helping You Remember**  Notice that adduction has the word "add" in it, meaning "to bring things together."

- **Pronation** means turning the palm down or backward.
- **Supination** means turning the palm up or toward the front.
- **Eversion** means movement of the sole of the foot outward, away from the midline.
- **Inversion** means movement of the sole of the foot inward, toward the midline.

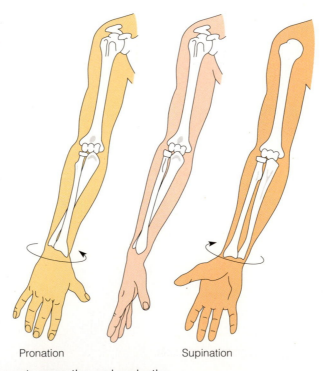

Pronation                   Supination

**Figure 8-6**  Muscle movements: pronation and supination.

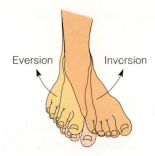

**Figure 8-7** Muscle movements: eversion and inversion.

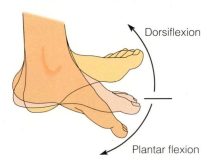

**Figure 8-8** Muscle movements: dorsiflexion and plantar flexion.

- **Dorsiflexion** means flexion at the ankle moving the foot upward.
- **Plantar flexion** means flexion at the ankle pointing the toes toward the ground.

## PRACTICE FOR LEARNING: Muscle Movements

Fill in the blanks with the correct muscle movement:

1. Overextending the joint beyond the anatomical position.
   _____

2. Movement of the sole inward toward the midline.
   _____

3. Turning the palm down or backward.
   _____

4. Movement toward the midline of the body.
   _____

5. Decreasing the angle between two bones.
   _____

6. Turning the palm up or toward the front.
   _____

**7.** Flexion at the ankle pointing the toes toward the ground.

_____

**8.** Movement away from the midline of the body.

_____

> Answers: 1. hyperextension. 2. inversion. 3. pronation. 4. adduction. 5. flexion.
> 6. supination. 7. plantar flexion. 8. abduction.

## 8.4   New Roots, Suffixes, and Prefixes

Use these additional roots, suffixes, and prefixes when studying the terms in this chapter.

| ROOT | MEANING |
|------|---------|
| fibr/o | fiber |
| skelet/o | skeleton |

| SUFFIX | MEANING |
|--------|---------|
| -asthenia | no strength |
| -cele | hernia; protrusion or displacement of an organ through a structure that normally contains it |
| -clonus | violent action; turmoil |
| -ia | condition |

| PREFIX | MEANING |
|--------|---------|
| brady- | slow |
| hemi- | half |
| para- | abnormal; beside; near |
| quadri-; tetra- | four |

## 8.5   Learning the Terms

Following these steps will make it easier for you to learn medical terms:

**1.** Pronounce the term repeatedly until it is easy for you.

**2.** Write it down. Ensure the spelling is correct.

3. Also write the definition. If possible, relate the word to a word, thought, or picture that will help you remember it.

4. Analyze the term with the method taught in this text.

## Roots

| ROOT | | MEANING |
| --- | --- | --- |
| **condyl/o** | | **a small rounded bony process or projection like the elbow; condyle (KON-dil)** |
| *Term* | *Term Analysis* | *Definition* |
| **epicondylitis** (**ep**-ih-**kon**-dih-**LYE**-tis) | epi- above; on; upon<br>-itis = inflammation | inflammation of tissue surrounding the elbow |

| ROOT | | MEANING |
| --- | --- | --- |
| **fasci/o** | | **fascia (band of connective tissue surrounding the muscle)** |
| *Term* | *Term Analysis* | *Definition* |
| **fascial** (**FASH**-ee-al) | -al = pertaining to | pertaining to fascia |
| **fascitis** (fah-**SIGH**-tis). Also, **fasciitis** (fas-ee-**EYE**-tis) | -itis = inflammation | inflammation of the fascia |

| ROOT | | MEANING |
| --- | --- | --- |
| **kinesi/o** | | **movement** |
| *Term* | *Term Analysis* | *Definition* |
| **kinesiology** (kih-**nee**-see-**OL**-oh-jee) | -logy = study of | study of movement |

| ROOT | | MEANING |
| --- | --- | --- |
| **muscul/o (see also my/o)** | | **muscle** |
| *Term* | *Term Analysis* | *Definition* |
| **muscular** (**MUS**-kyoo-lar) | -ar = pertaining to | pertaining to muscle |
| **musculoskeletal** (**mus**-kyoo-loh-**SKEL**-eh-tal) | -al = pertaining to<br>skelet/o = skeleton | pertaining to the muscles and skeleton |

| ROOT my/o | | MEANING muscle |
|---|---|---|
| *Term* | *Term Analysis* | *Definition* |
| **electromyography** (ee-**leck**-troh-my-**OG**-rah-fee) | -graphy = process of recording electr/o = electricity | process of recording the electrical activity of a muscle |
| **fibromyalgia** (**figh**-broh-my-**AL**-jee-ah) | -algia = pain fibr/o = fiber | chronic muscle pain |
| **myasthenia gravis (MG)** (**mye**-as-**THEE**-nee-ah **GRAH**-vis) | -asthenia = no strength; muscle weakness gravis = grave or severe | weakening and fatigue of the skeletal muscles. The disease is caused by abnormalities at the neuromuscular junction. |
| **myocele** (**MY**-oh-seel) | -cele = hernia; protrusion or displacement of an organ through a structure that normally contains it | hernia of muscle; protrusion of muscle through its fascia |
| **myoclonus** (**my**-oh-**KLOH**-nus) | -clonus = violent action; turmoil | sudden involuntary jerking of a muscle or group of muscles |

| ROOT tendin/o; ten/o | | MEANING tendon |
|---|---|---|
| *Term* | *Term Analysis* | *Definition* |
| **tendinitis** (**ten**-dih-**NIGH**-tis) | -itis = inflammation | inflammation of a tendon |
| **tendinous** (**TEN**-dih-nus) | -ous = pertaining to | pertaining to a tendon |
| **tenotomy** (teh-**NOT**-eh-me) | -tomy = to cut | cutting of a tendon |

| ROOT ton/o | | MEANING tone; tension |
|---|---|---|
| *Term* | *Term Analysis* | *Definition* |
| **atonic** (ah-**TON**-ick) | -ic = pertaining to a- = no; not; lack of | pertaining to no tone or tension |
| **dystonia** (dis-**TOH**-nee-ah) | -ia = condition dys- = abnormal; bad; difficult; painful | abnormal muscle tone |

| Term | Term Analysis | Definition |
|------|---------------|------------|
| **myotonia**<br>(**my**-oh-**TOH**-nee-ah) | -ia = condition<br>my/o = muscle | muscle is unable to relax; a type of dystonia |
| **tonic**<br>(**TON**-ick) | -ic = pertaining to | pertaining to tone |

## Suffixes

| SUFFIX<br>-kinesia; -kinesis | | MEANING<br>movement |
|------|------|------|
| Term | Term Analysis | Definition |
| **bradykinesia**<br>(**brad**-ee-kih-**NEE**-zee-ah) | brady- = slow | slow movement |
| **dyskinesia**<br>(**dis**-kih-**NEE**-zee-ah) | dys- = poor; bad; difficult; painful; abnormal | poor muscle movement |
| **hyperkinesis**<br>(**high**-per-kih-**NEE**-sis) | hyper- = excessive; above normal | excessive movement; hyperactivity |

| SUFFIX<br>-paresis | | MEANING<br>weakness or incomplete paralysis |
|------|------|------|
| Term | Term Analysis | Definition |
| **hemiparesis**<br>(**hem**-ee-pah-**REE**-sis) | hemi- = half | weakness or partial paralysis affecting either the right or left side of the body |
| **myoparesis**<br>(**my**-oh-pah-**REE**-sis) | my/o = muscle | weak or slight muscular paralysis |

| SUFFIX<br>-plegia | | MEANING<br>paralysis |
|------|------|------|
| Term | Term Analysis | Definition |
| **paraplegia**<br>(**par**-ah-**PLEE**-jee-ah) | para- = abnormal | paralysis of the lower trunk and legs. The trunk refers to the body, not including the head and extremities. |
| **quadriplegia**<br>(**kwad**-rih-**PLEE**-jee-ah) | quadri- = four | paralysis of all four extremities. Also known as tetraplegia. |

| SUFFIX -penia | | MEANING decrease; deficiency |
| --- | --- | --- |
| Term | Term Analysis | Definition |
| sarcopenia (**sar**-koh-**PEE**-nee-ah) | sarc/o = flesh | loss of muscle mass, strength, and function that comes with aging |

| SUFFIX -taxia | | MEANING order |
| --- | --- | --- |
| Term | Term Analysis | Definition |
| ataxia (ah-**TACKS**-ee-ah) | a- = no; not; lack of | no muscular coordination |

## 8.6  Pathology

### Carpal Tunnel Syndrome (CTS)

A syndrome is a group of signs and symptoms that indicates a specific disease. A sign is something that the physician can observe, such as swelling. A symptom is something that the patient experiences, such as pain.

The carpal tunnel (Figure 8-9) is a small passageway in the wrist on the palmar side (the palm side) of the forearm. This passageway is made of ligaments. It protects the median nerve and tendons on the palmar side of the wrist. When the tendons and ligaments in this area are overused, they become inflamed, putting pressure on the median nerve. This causes numbness, pain, and weakness.

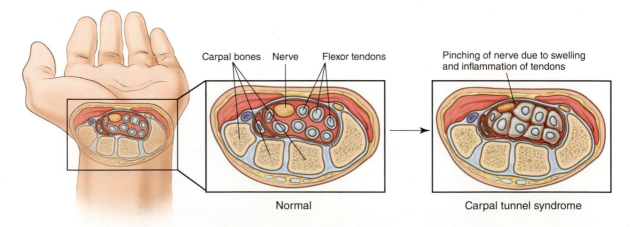

**Figure 8-9** Carpal Tunnel Syndrome The carpal tunnel is located at the wrist. Tendons pass through this tunnel. When the tendons become inflamed, pressure is placed on the median nerve causing pain, numbness, and weakness.

## Muscular Dystrophy (MD)

"Muscular dystrophy" is a broad term that includes a number of inherited disorders of the skeletal muscles. The main features are muscular weakness and degeneration of muscle tissue. The most common type is **Duchenne** (doo-**SHEN**) muscular dystrophy. There is no cure for the disease.

## Rotator Cuff Tendinitis

The rotator cuff is a group of tendons. The tendons hold the shoulder joint in place (Figure 8-10A). Rotator cuff tendinitis is the inflammation of these tendons (Figure 8-10B). The major cause is overuse. Swimmers, tennis players, and baseball pitchers are particularly prone to rotator cuff tendinitis.

## Strain

A strain results from overstretching or tearing a muscle. It is commonly called a pulled muscle. Do not confuse a strain with a **sprain**. A sprain is a tearing of a ligament.

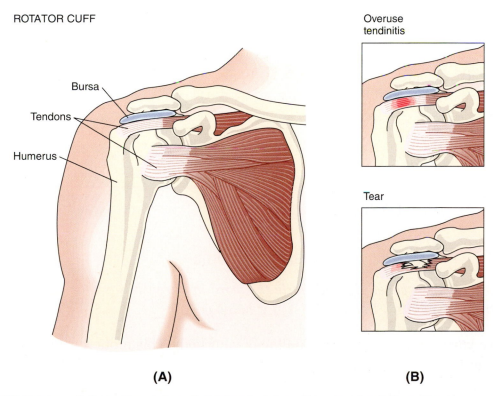

**Figure 8-10** Rotator cuff. A. Healthy rotator cuff. B. Injured rotator cuff (overuse tendinitis and tear).

## 8.7   Look-Alike and Sound-Alike Words

Below is a list of look-alike and sound-alike words. Study the spelling and definitions of each set of words. Questions will follow in the Review Exercises.

### TABLE 8-1   Look-Alike and Sound-Alike Words

| | |
|---|---|
| **abduction** | to draw away from the midline of the body |
| **adduction** | to draw toward the midline of the body |
| **myelography** | process of recording the spinal cord |
| **myography** | process of recording a muscle |
| **fascial** | pertaining to the fascia |
| **facial** | pertaining to the face |
| **flexor** | a muscle that flexes a joint |
| **flexure** | a portion of a structure that is bent |
| **peroneal** | pertaining to the muscles over the fibula. Term of the muscular system |
| **peritoneal** | pertaining to the peritoneum. The peritoneum is a membrane lining the abdominopelvic cavity. Term of the digestive system |
| **perineal** | pertaining to the perineum. The perineum is the area between the vagina and anus in the female. In the male, it is the area between the scrotum and anus. Term of the reproductive system. |

## 8.8   Review Exercises

### EXERCISE 8-1   Look-Alike and Sound-Alike Words

*Read the sentences carefully and circle the word in parentheses that correctly completes the meaning. Use Table 8-1 if it helps you.*

1. Move your leg away from the midline of your body. This motion is (**abduction/ adduction**).

2. Muscle disease may be assessed by (**myelography/myography**).

3. Plantar (**fascial/facial**) pain can be caused by flat feet.

4. The (**fascial/facial**) muscles can wrinkle the forehead and pucker the lips.

**5.** Bob cannot bend his wrist because the (**flexor/flexure**) muscles were damaged in a motorcycle accident.

**6.** Debra tore the (**peroneal/peritoneal/perineal**) area when she delivered her baby.

**7.** The (**peroneal/peritoneal/perineal**) cavity in the abdomen was filled with fluid.

**8.** The (**peroneal/peritoneal/perineal**) muscle is responsible for abduction of the foot.

## EXERCISE 8-2 Match Word Parts with Meanings

*Match the word part in Column A with its meaning in Column B:*

| | Column A | Column B |
|---|---|---|
| _____ | **1.** fasci/o | A. order |
| _____ | **2.** -ia | B. pertaining to |
| _____ | **3.** kinesi/o | C. pain |
| _____ | **4.** my/o | D. to cut |
| _____ | **5.** -taxia | E. tendon |
| _____ | **6.** -ous | F. muscle |
| _____ | **7.** -tomy | G. band of tissue surrounding muscle |
| _____ | **8.** -algia | H. tension |
| _____ | **9.** ton/o | I. movement |
| _____ | **10.** ten/o | J. condition |

## EXERCISE 8-3 Short Answer—Anatomy and Physiology

*Answer the following in the space provided.*

**1.** Name three types of muscle tissue.

_____

_____

**2.** What is the primary function of muscle?

_____

**3.** State the difference between:

**a.** pronation and supination _____

**b.** dorsiflexion and plantar flexion _____

**c.** hyperextension and extension _____

## EXERCISE 8-4 Location of Muscles

*Match the muscle with its location using the locations listed below:*

arm _____

back _____

chest _____

leg _____

neck _____

shoulder _____

trunk _____

**1.** quadriceps _____

**2.** serratus anterior _____

**3.** pectoralis major _____

**4.** adductors _____

**5.** gastrocnemius _____

**6.** triceps brachii _____

**7.** hamstrings _____

**8.** Achilles tendon _____

**9.** biceps brachii _____

**10.** trapezius _____

**11.** latissimus dorsi _____

**12.** deltoid _____

**13.** sartorius _____

**14.** sternocleidomastoid _____

## EXERCISE 8-5  Definitions—Anatomy, Physiology, Pathology

*Give the meaning of the following*:

**1. muscle fibers** _____

**2. tendons** _____

**3. fascia** _____

**4. adduction** _____

**5. eversion** _____

**6. ataxia** _____

**7. rotator cuff tendinitis** _____

**8. fibromyalgia** _____

**9. dystonia** _____

**10. tenotomy** _____

## EXERCISE 8-6  Definitions in Context

*Define the bolded terms in context in the space below. Use your dictionary if necessary.*

### Discharge Summary

HISTORY OF PRESENT ILLNESS: The patient is a seven-year-old boy who showed signs of muscular weakness at age three to four years. The diagnosis of **muscular dystrophy** was made when a muscle **biopsy** confirmed **degeneration** of muscle fibers. He is still walking and was started on drug **therapy** four months ago.

PHYSICAL EXAMINATION: On examination, the patient is a pleasant young fellow. He has **proximal** muscle weakness. He has **hypertrophy** and some shortening of the **Achilles tendon**. General physical examination is within normal limits.

COURSE IN HOSPITAL: While in the hospital, an **intravenous** line was started, and blood samples were taken for tests during a 24-hour period. The course in hospital was uneventful.

Most Responsible Diagnosis: Muscular Dystrophy

    **a.** muscular dystrophy _____

    **b.** biopsy _____

    **c.** degeneration _____

**d.** therapy _____

**e.** proximal _____

**f.** hypertrophy _____

**g.** Achilles tendons _____

**h.** intravenous _____

## EXERCISE 8-7  Word Building

*I. Use the root ton/o to build terms for the following definitions.*

    **a.** pertaining to no tone or tension _____

    **b.** abnormal muscle tone _____

    **c.** muscle is unable to relax _____

    **d.** pertaining to tone _____

*II. Use the suffix -kinesia to build terms for the following definitions.*

    **a.** slow movement _____

    **b.** impaired movement _____

    **c.** excessive movement _____

*III. Use the correct suffix, -plegia or -paresis, to build terms for the following definitions.*

    **a.** slight muscular paralysis _____
    _____

    **b.** paralysis of both legs and the lower part of the body
    _____

    **c.** paralysis of all four extremities _____

    **d.** slight paralysis or weakness affecting half of the body _____

## EXERCISE 8-8  Spelling

*Circle any misspelled words in the list below and correctly spell them in the space provided.*

    **1.** quadraceps _____

    **2.** sternocliedomastoid _____

    **3.** serratus _____

**4.** adducter muscles _____

**5.** plantar _____

**6.** trapezious _____

**7.** latisimus dorsi _____

**8.** gastrocnemius _____

**9.** Achilles _____

**10.** biceps brachii _____

## EXERCISE 8-9  Labeling

*I. Skeletal Muscles, Anterior View*

*Using the body structures listed below, label Figures 8-11. Write your answers in the numbered space provided below, or if you prefer, on the diagram.*

abdominal muscles

adductors

biceps brachii

facial muscles

pectoralis major

quadriceps femoris

sartorius

serratus major

sternocleidomastoid

**1.** _____

**2.** _____

**3.** _____

**4.** _____

**5.** _____

**6.** _____

**7.** _____

**8.** _____

**9.** _____

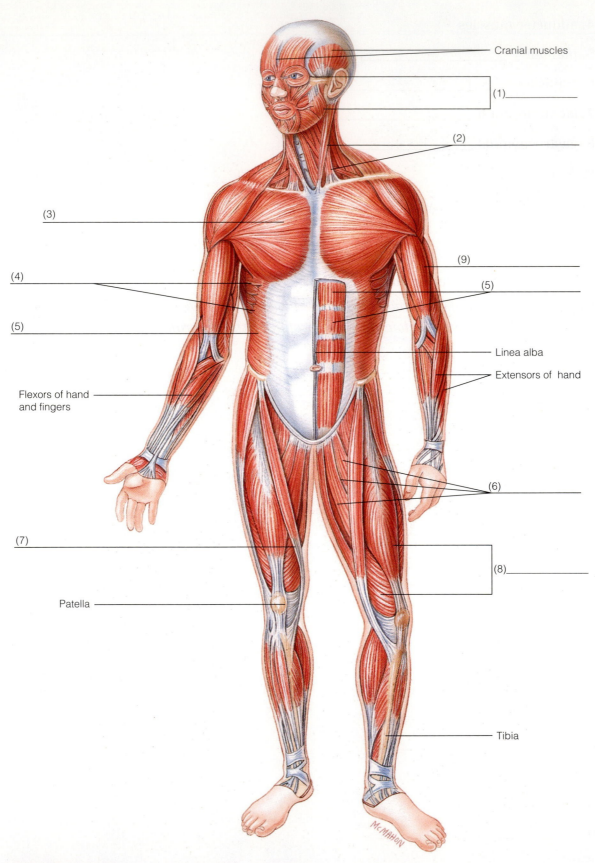

Cranial muscles

(1)_____

(2)

(3)

(4)

(9)

(5)

(5)

Linea alba

Extensors of hand

Flexors of hand
and fingers

(6)

(7)

(8)_____

Patella

Tibia

**Figure 8-11** Skeletal muscles, anterior view.

*II. Skeletal Muscles, Posterior View*

*Using the body structures listed below, label Figure 8-12. Write your answers in the numbered space provided.*

Achilles tendon

deltoid

gastrocnemius

gluteus maximus

hamstrings

latissimus dorsi

trapezius

triceps brachii

**10.** _____

**11.** _____

**12.** _____

**13.** _____

**14.** _____

**15.** _____

**16.** _____

**17.** _____

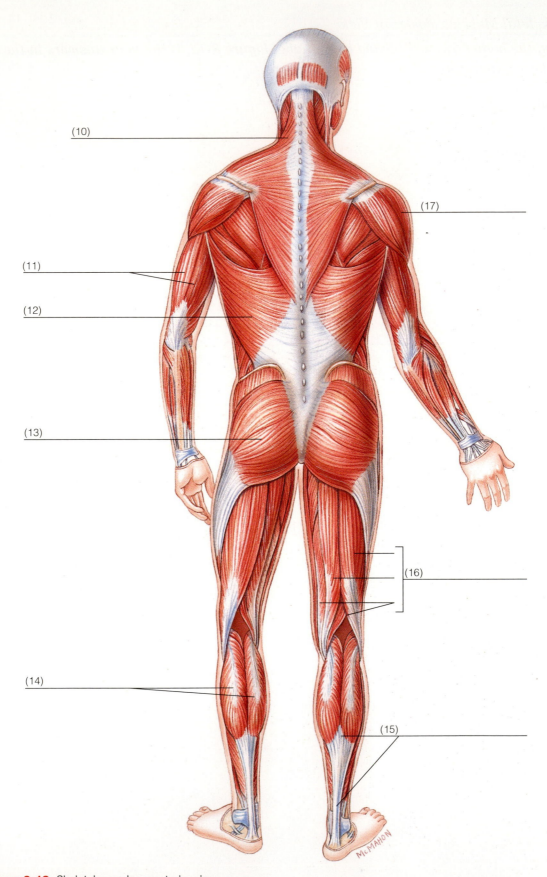

**Figure 8-12** Skeletal muscles, posterior view.

## 8.9 Pronunciation and Spelling

*Listen, read, and study, so you can speak and write effectively.*

1. Listen to each word on the audio file provided on the Student Companion Website.

2. Pronounce each word carefully.

3. Spell each word in the space provided.

| Word | Pronunciation | Spelling |
|------|---------------|----------|
| atonic | ah-**TON**-ick | |
| biceps brachii | **BYE**-seps **BRAY**-kee | |
| deltoid | **DEL**-toyd | |
| dorsiflexion | **dor**-sih-**FLECK**-shun | |
| dyskinesia | **dis**-kih-**NEE**-zee-ah | |
| dystonia | dis-**TOH**-nee-ah | |
| electromyography | ee-**leck**-troh-my-**OG**-rah-fee | |
| fascia | **FASH**-ee-ah | |
| fascitis | fah-**SIGH**-tis | |
| fibromyalgia | **figh**-broh-my-**AL**-jee-ah | |
| gastrocnemius | **gas**-troh-**NEE**-mee-us | |
| hemiparesis | **hem**-ee-pah-**REE**-sis | |
| inversion | in-**VER**-zhun | |
| kinesiology | kih-**nee**-see-**OL**-oh-jee | |
| latissimus dorsi | lah-**TISS**-ih-mus **DOR**-see | |
| muscular | **MUS**-kyoo-lar | |
| muscular dystrophy | **MUS**-kyoo-lar **DISS**-troh-fee | |
| musculoskeletal | **mus**-kyoo-loh-**SKEL**-eh-tal | |
| myasthenia gravis | (**mye**-as-**THEE**-nee-ah **GRAH**-vis) | |
| myocele | **MY**-oh-seel | |
| myoclonus | **my**-oh-**KLOH**-nus | |
| myoparesis | **my**-oh-pah-**REE**-sis | |

| Word | Pronunciation | Spelling |
|------|---------------|----------|
| myopathy | my-**OP**-ah-thee | |
| paraplegia | **par**-ah-**PLEE**-jee-ah | |
| pectoralis major | **peck**-tor-**AL**-iss **MAY**-jor | |
| plantar flexion | **PLAN**-tar **FLECK**-shun | |
| pronation | proh-**NAY**-shun | |
| quadriplegia | **kwad**-rih-**PLEE**-jee-ah | |
| sarcopenia | **sar**-koh-**PEE**-nee-ah | |
| serratus anterior | seh-**RAY**-tuss an-**TEER**-ee-or | |
| sternocleidomastoid | **stern**-oh-**kleye**-doh-**MASS**-toyd | |
| supination | **soo**-pih-**NAY**-shun | |
| tendinous | **TEN**-dih-nus | |
| tenotomy | teh-**NOT**-oh-me | |
| trapezius | trah-**PEE**-zee-us | |
| triceps brachii | **TRIGH**-seps **BRAY**-kee | |

## CHAPTER 9

# Nervous System

## Chapter Outline

## Learning Objectives

*After studying this chapter and completing the review exercises, you should be able to:*

1. Name and describe the divisions of the nervous system.
2. State the function of nerve cells.
3. Name, locate, and describe the structures and functions of the brain and spinal cord.
4. Describe the peripheral nervous system.
5. Pronounce, spell, define, and write the medical terms related to the nervous system.
6. Describe common diseases related to the nervous system.
7. Listen, read, and study so you can speak and write.

## Introduction

The nervous system helps your body adjust to what is happening to it. If you touch something hot, the nervous system sends signals to the brain that make you quickly pull away. If the light around you grows stronger, the nervous system tells your eyes to adjust. If your body needs water, the nervous system makes you thirsty. The organs that carry the messages are called **nerves** (**NERVZ**). This chapter will teach you the terms you need to know about this very complicated system.

## 9.1  Major Organs of the Nervous System

**PRACTICE FOR LEARNING: Major Organs and Divisions**

Write the words below in the correct space in Figure 9-1. To help you, the number beside the word tells you where it goes on the figure. Be sure to pronounce each word as you write it. Repeat the pronunciation several times if you find the word hard to say.

1. brain (**BRAYN**)
2. spinal cord (**SPYE**-nal **KORD**)
3. central nervous system (CNS) (**SEN**-tral **NERV**-us **SIS**-tem)
4. peripheral nerves (per-**IF**-er-al **NERVZ**)
5. peripheral nervous system (PNS)

## 9.2  Divisions of the Nervous System

Figure 9-1 shows you the two main divisions of the nervous system. They are the central nervous system (CNS) and the peripheral nervous system (PNS).

The CNS consists of the brain and the spinal cord.

The PNS consists mostly of nerves. There are 12 pairs of **cranial** nerves. They extend from the brain. There are also 31 pairs of spinal nerves. They extend from the spinal cord. These nerves transmit electrical impulses to different parts of the body from the CNS. The nerves also transmit electrical impulses from all parts of the body back to the CNS.

## 9.3  Nerve Cells and Nerves

**Neurons** (**NOO**-ronz) are nerve cells. They are very tiny, long, and slender (Figure 9-2). They make up organs called nerves. Neurons carry electrical impulses (messages) to and from the brain and spinal cord. They vary in size (some are as long as 3 feet or 91 centimeters).

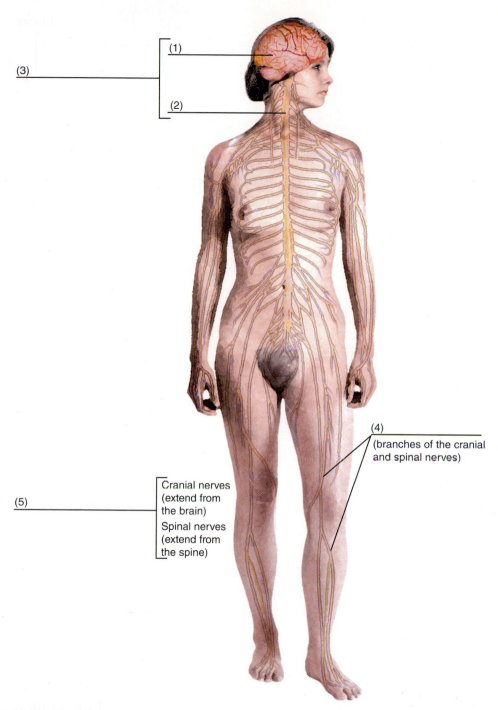

(1)

(3)

(2)

(4)
(branches of the cranial
and spinal nerves)

Cranial nerves
(extend from
the brain)

(5)

Spinal nerves
(extend from
the spine)

**Figure 9-1** Nervous system generalized.

Some neurons are covered with a white fatty substance called a **myelin sheath** (**MY**-eh-lin **SHEETH**). The myelin sheath acts as an insulator, keeping the impulse traveling from neuron to neuron until its destination is reached (Figure 9-2). Neurons wrapped with myelin sheath are called **myelinated** (**MY**-eh-lih-**nayt**-ed). They are also called white matter. Neurons that are not covered with myelin are called **unmyelinated** (**UN-my**-eh-lih-**nayt**-ed). They are also called gray matter.

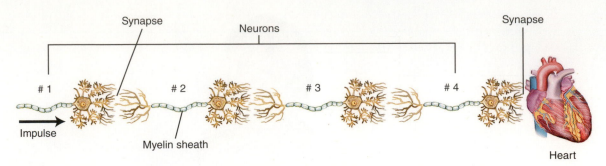

**Figure 9-2** Neurons placed end-to-end. An electrical impulse travels form one neuron to the next until it reaches its destination, which in this case is the heart.

**Neuroglia** (noo-**ROG**-glee-ah) are found between the neurons, connecting them and providing support and protection. Neuroglia do not carry electrical impulses. Astrocytes and microglia are two examples of neuroglia.

---

**In Brief**

Neurons and neuroglia are nerve cells.

Some neurons are myelinated; some neurons are unmyelinated.

Neurons transport electrical impulses.

Neuroglia support and protect neurons.

---

**Helping You Remember**

Neurons are like electrical wires. The myelin sheath is like the wrapping on an electric wire. Electric impulses move through an electrical wire, and nerve impulses travel from neuron to neuron. If the electric wire is broken, the impulses won't travel. Similarly, if the neuron is torn, the nerve impulses will not be transmitted.

## Nerves

Nerves are made up of neurons bunched together. They can be seen with the naked eye. There are two kinds of nerves. One kind carries impulses **to** the brain and spinal cord. For example, when the skin of your back is itchy, a message travels from the skin through a nerve to the spinal cord and then to the brain. When the message about the itch reaches the brain, the information is analyzed. An appropriate message is sent back from the brain through a second kind of nerve, which carries messages **from** the brain and spinal cord. These messages travel down the spinal cord and stimulate the muscles of the arms and hands. The muscles then respond to the message by scratching the skin. When a group of nerves is bundled together within the brain or spinal cord, the bundle is called a **tract**.

## Synapse

A **synapse** (**SIN**-apps) is the space between two neurons or between a neuron and an organ (Figure 9-2). When an electrical impulse reaches the end of a neuron, a neurotransmitter is released. The neurotransmitter carries the impulse across the space (the synapse) and onto the next neuron, or onto the organ the impulse is meant to stimulate. Some examples of neurotransmitters are **acetylcholine** (ah-**see**-tul-**KOL**-een), **dopamine** (**DOH**-pah-meen), **endorphins** (**EN**-dor-fins), **serotonin** (**ser**-oh-**TOH**-nin), and **norepinephrine** (**nor**-ep-ih-**NEF**-rin). These neurotransmitters have a variety of functions, including muscle movement, mood, and stress release.

### PRACTICE FOR LEARNING: Nerve Cells and Nerves

Circle true if the statement is correct. Circle false if the statement is not correct.

| | | |
|---|---|---|
| **1.** The myelin sheath acts as an insulator, keeping the nerve impulse on track. | True | False |
| **2.** Neurons carry electrical impulses. | True | False |
| **3.** Neurons wrapped with myelin sheath are said to be myelinated. | True | False |
| **4.** Myelinated neurons are also called white matter. | True | False |
| **5.** Electrical impulses travel to and away from the brain and spinal cord. | True | False |
| **6.** Neurons are organs made up of nerves. | True | False |
| **7.** Dopamine is a neurotransmitter. | True | False |
| **8.** The synapse carries serotonin to another neuron. | True | False |
| **9.** A synapse is the gap between two neurons. | True | False |

Answers: 1. True. 2. True. 3. True. 4. True. 5. True. 6. False. 7. True. 8. False. 9. True.

## 9.4 Central Nervous System

### The Brain

### PRACTICE FOR LEARNING: Parts of the Brain

Write the different parts of the brain in the correct space in Figure 9-3. To help you, the number beside the word tells you where it goes on the figure. Be sure to pronounce each word as you write it. Repeat the pronunciation several times if you find the word hard to say.

1. cerebrum (seh-**REE**-brum)
2. thalamus (**THAL**-ah-mus)
3. hypothalamus (**high**-poh-**THAL**-ah-mus)
4. midbrain (**MID**-brayn)
5. pons (**PONZ**)
6. medulla oblongata (meh-**DULL**-ah **ob**-long-**GAH**-tah)
7. cerebellum (**ser**-eh-**BELL**-um)

The brain is protected by the skull, which is also called the cranium. The brain is made up of billions of neurons and is divided into several parts. Each part has its own function.

## Parts of the Brain

The cerebrum is the largest part of the brain. It is divided into right and left hemispheres. The hemispheres are connected in the middle of the cerebrum by the **corpus callosum** (**KOR**-pus kah-**LOH**-sum). The left hemisphere controls the right side of the body and the right hemisphere controls the left side of the body. Each hemisphere is divided into lobes. The lobes are named after the cranial bones covering them: **frontal** lobe, **parietal** lobe, **temporal** lobe, **occipital** lobe.

The cerebrum is covered by gray matter called the **cerebral cortex** (seh-**REE**-bral **KOR**-tecks). The cerebrum is involved in movement, sensation, as well as thought, reasoning, and judgment.

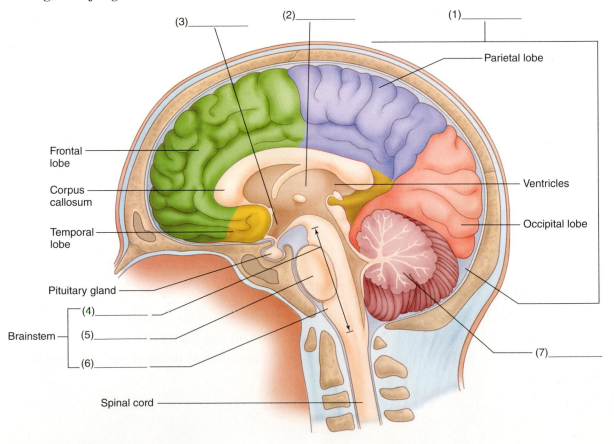

**Figure 9-3** Structures of the brain.

The thalamus and hypothalamus are two other important structures of the brain.

The thalamus, deep inside the brain, receives stimuli such as pain, touch, and temperature. It sends this information to the cerebral cortex for analysis and interpretation. It is the thalamus that first makes the body aware of a stimulus such as hot temperature. However, the sensation must be sent to the cerebral cortex before a proper response to the abnormal temperature can be made.

The hypothalamus is located below the thalamus. It regulates appetite, thirst, and temperature. It is also associated with emotions and behavior.

The midbrain, pons, and medulla oblongata are together called the **brainstem**. The brainstem regulates basic life functions such as waking, respiration, heart rate, and blood pressure. It also serves as a pathway for impulses traveling to and from the brain and spinal cord.

The cerebellum lies under the cerebrum. It is important in maintaining balance and muscle coordination. Cerebellar dysfunction may cause abnormal gait (the manner or style of walking).

---

**In Brief**   **Parts of the Brain**

cerebrum, cerebral cortex, thalamus, hypothalamus, cerebellum, brainstem (midbrain, pons, medulla oblongata)

---

**PRACTICE FOR LEARNING: Brain**

Name the part of the brain described below.

**1.** outer gray matter covering the cerebrum

_____

**2.** sends information to the cerebral cortex for analysis and interpretation

_____

**3.** maintains balance and muscle coordination

_____

**4.** includes pons, midbrain, and medulla _____

**5.** regulates appetite and thirst _____

> **Answers: 1. cerebral cortex. 2. thalamus. 3. cerebellum. 4. brainstem.**
> **5. hypothalamus.**

## Protective Coverings

**PRACTICE FOR LEARNING: Protective Coverings**

Write the structures listed below in the correct spaces in Figure 9-4. To help you, the number beside the word tells you where it goes on the figure. Be sure to pronounce each word as you write it. Repeat the pronunciation several times if you find the word hard to say.

1. dura mater (**DOO**-rah **MAY**-ter)

2. arachnoid membrane (ah-**RACK**-noid **MEM**-brayn)

3. pia mater (**PEE**-yah **MAY**-ter)

4. cerebrospinal (**ser**-eh-broh-**SPYE**-nal) fluid

5. ventricles (**VEN**-trih-kulz)

The most obvious protection for the brain and spinal cord are the skull bones and vertebrae. However, three membranes called **meninges** (meh-**NIN**-jeez) also serve as protective coverings (Figure 9-4).

The outermost covering is the **dura mater** (**DOO**-rah **MAY**-ter). It is tough and thick. The middle layer is the **arachnoid membrane** (ah-**RACK**-noid **MEM**-brayn). The inner

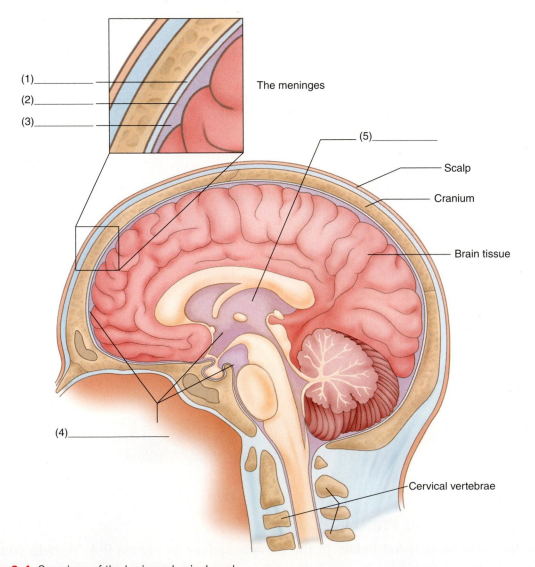

**Figure 9-4** Coverings of the brain and spinal cord.

covering is the **pia matter** (**PEE**-yah- **MAY**-ter). Below the dura is the subdural space, and below the arachnoid membrane is the subarachnoid space.

Another form of protection is the **cerebrospinal fluid** (CSF), a colorless liquid that continuously circulates within the subarachnoid space around the brain and spinal cord, inside the spinal cord, and in hollow cavities inside the brain called **ventricles**. CSF protects by acting as a shock absorber.

## Spinal Cord

The **spinal cord** is shown in Figure 9-1. It is a half-inch-thick cable made up of nerves bunched together. The nerves are soft tissue. They are protected by the bones of the vertebral column. Spinal nerves branch out from both sides of the spinal cord, extending to most parts of the body.

| | |
|---|---|
| **In Brief** | **Spinal cord** is made up of nerves. |
| | **Nerves** branch from the spinal cord to the rest of the body. |
| | **Vertebral column** is bone protecting the spinal cord. |

| | |
|---|---|
| **Helping You Remember** | The spinal cord and spinal column are not the same structure. The spinal cord is made up of nerves; the spinal column is made up of bone. The spinal column is also known as the vertebral column, spine, or backbone. |

## 9.5  Peripheral Nervous System (PNS)

Nerves leave the brain and spinal cord and extend to almost all body structures. This includes structures that are away from the center, which are called peripheral structures. In this case, peripheral means away from the brain and spinal cord. Figure 9-5 illustrates some spinal nerves as they extend from the spinal cord to peripheral sites. The names given to these nerves relate to the organ or structure the nerve serves. For example, the ulnar nerve stimulates the muscles attaching to the ulnar bone of the arm. The tibial nerve stimulates the muscles over the tibia or shin bone. The sciatic nerve stimulates the lower back, buttocks, thigh, and lower leg.

| | |
|---|---|
| **In Brief** | **PNS** includes nerves extending from the brain and spinal cord to body organs. |

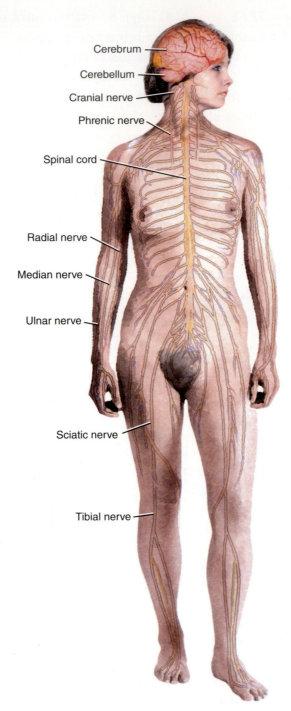

Cerebrum
Cerebellum
Cranial nerve
Phrenic nerve
Spinal cord
Radial nerve
Median nerve
Ulnar nerve
Sciatic nerve
Tibial nerve

**Figure 9-5**  Peripheral nerves branch from the brain and spinal cord.

## 9.6 New Roots, Suffixes, and Prefixes

Use these additional roots, suffixes, and prefixes when studying the terms in this chapter.

| ROOT | MEANING |
|------|---------|
| ech/o | sound |
| ment/o | mind |
| myelin/o | myelin sheath |
| narc/o | stupor |
| poli/o | gray matter |
| spin/o | spinal cord |
| | (when referring to the skeletal system, **spin/o** means spine; backbone; spinal column; vertebral column) |

| SUFFIX | MEANING |
|--------|---------|
| -us | thing |

## 9.7 Learning the Terms

Following these steps will make it easier for you to learn medical terms:

1. Pronounce the term repeatedly until it is easy for you.
2. Write it down. Ensure the spelling is correct.
3. Also write the definition. If possible, relate the word to a word, thought, or picture that will help you remember it.
4. Analyze the term with the method taught in this text.

### Roots

| ROOT caus/o | | MEANING burning |
|-------------|--------------|-----------------|
| Term | Term Analysis | Definition |
| causalgia (kaw-**ZAL**-jah) | -algia = pain | burning pain |

| ROOT cerebr/o (see also encephal/o) | | MEANING brain |
|---|---|---|
| Term | Term Analysis | Definition |
| cerebral angiography (seh-**REE**-bral **an**-jee-**OG**-rah-fee) | -al = pertaining to<br>-graphy = process of recording; process of producing images<br>angi/o = vessel | process of producing an image of the blood vessels of the brain |
| cerebrovascular (**ser**-eh-broh-**VAS**-kyoo-lar) | -ar = pertaining to<br>vascul/o = vessel | pertaining to the brain and blood vessels |
| cerebrospinal fluid (CSF) (**ser**-eh-broh- **SPYE**-nal) | -al = pertaining to<br>spin/o = spinal cord | fluid in and around the brain and spinal cord |

| ROOT encephal/o | | MEANING brain |
|---|---|---|
| Term | Term Analysis | Definition |
| echoencephalography (EEG) (**eck**-oh-en-**sef**-ah-**LOG**-rah-fee) | -graphy = process of recording; process of producing images<br>echo- = sound | use of ultrasound to create an image of the brain for diagnostic purposes |
| encephalitis (en-**sef**-ah-**LYE**-tis) | -itis = inflammation | inflammation of the brain |
| electroencephalography (ee-**leck**-troh-en-**sef**-ah-**LOG**-rah-fee) | -graphy = process of recording; process of producing images<br>electr/o = electric | process of recording the electrical activity of the brain |
| encephalopathy (en-**sef**-ah-**LOP**-ah-thee) | -pathy = disease | any disease of the brain |

| ROOT hydr/o | | MEANING water |
|---|---|---|
| Term | Term Analysis | Definition |
| hydrocephalus (**high**-droh-**SEF**-ah-lus) | -us = condition; thing<br>cephal/o = head | accumulation of cerebrospinal fluid in the brain (Figure 9-6) |

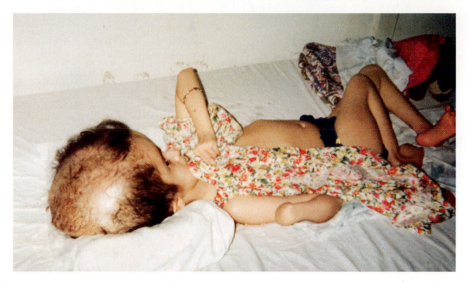

**Figure 9-6** Hydrocephalus. (Courtesy of Dr. Russell Cox)

| ROOT<br>**magnet/o** | | MEANING<br>**magnet** |
|---|---|---|
| *Term* | *Term Analysis* | *Definition* |
| **magnetic resonance imaging (MRI)** (mag-**NET**-ik **RES**-oh-nance **IM**-ah-jing) | -ic = pertaining to<br>resonance = magnification<br>imaging = picture | a picture of the brain produced by using magnetic waves (Figure 9-7) |

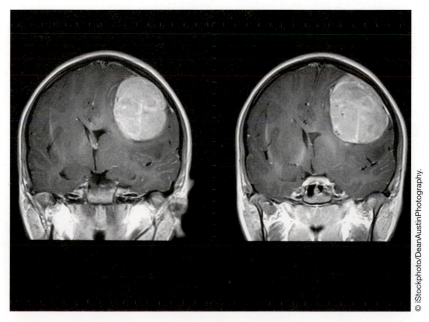

© iStockphoto/DeanAustinPhotography.

**Figure 9-7** MRI of the brain with a visible tumor in the upper right side.

| ROOT mening/o | | MEANING membrane; meninges (membranes around the brain and spinal cord) |
|---|---|---|
| Term | Term Analysis | Definition |
| meningitis (men-in-JIGH-tis) | -itis = inflammation | inflammation of the membranes surrounding the brain and spinal cord |

| ROOT myel/o | | MEANING spinal cord |
|---|---|---|
| Term | Term Analysis | Definition |
| poliomyelitis (poh-lee-oh-my-eh-LYE-tis) | -itis = inflammation poli/o = gray matter | inflammation of the gray matter of the spinal cord. Also known as polio. |

**Helping You Remember**   In the skeletal system, myel/o means bone marrow. In the nervous system, myel/o means spinal cord.

| ROOT neur/o | | MEANING nerve |
|---|---|---|
| Term | Term Analysis | Definition |
| neuromuscular (noo-row-MUS-kyoo-lar) | -ar = pertaining to muscul/o = muscle | pertaining to the nerve and muscle; myoneural |
| neurology (noo-ROL-oh-jee) | -logy = study of | the study of the nervous system including diseases and treatment |
| neurologist (noo-ROL-oh-jist) | -logist = specialist; one who studies | a specialist in the study of the diagnosis and treatment of nervous system disorders |

| SUFFIX -cele | | MEANING hernia (protrusion or displacement of an organ through a structure that normally contains it) |
|---|---|---|
| *Term* | *Term Analysis* | *Definition* |
| meningocele (meh-**NIN**-goh-**seel**) | mening/o = meninges; membrane | displacement of the meninges from its normal position through an abnormal opening in the skull or vertebra. (See spina bifida in Section 9.8.) |

| ROOT radicul/o | | MEANING nerve roots (attaches spinal nerve to spinal cord) |
|---|---|---|
| *Term* | *Term Analysis* | *Definition* |
| cervical radiculopathy (**SER**-vih-kal reh-**dick**-you-**LOP**-eh-thee) | -al = pertaining to<br>cervic/o = neck<br>-pathy = disease | disease of the nerve roots of the neck |

## Suffixes

| SUFFIX -esthesia | | MEANING sensation |
|---|---|---|
| *Term* | *Term Analysis* | *Definition* |
| anesthesia (**an**-es-**THEE**-zee-ah) | an- = no; not | loss of sensation |
| anesthesiologist (**an**-es-**thee**-zee-**OL**-oh-jist) | -logist = specialist; one who studies | a medical doctor who specializes in the administration of anesthetic |
| anesthetist (an-**EES**-the-tist) | -ist = specialist | a specialist in the administration of anesthetic agents |
| dysesthesia (**dis**-es-**THEE**-zee-ah) | dys- = bad; painful; difficult; poor; abnormal | painful sensation in response to normal stimulation |
| paresthesia (**par**-es-**THEE**-zee-ah) | para- = abnormal | abnormal sensation such as numbness and tingling |

| SUFFIX -lepsy | | MEANING seizure |
| --- | --- | --- |
| *Term* | *Term Analysis* | *Definition* |
| narcolepsy (**NAR**-koh-lep-see) | narc/o = stupor | sleep disorder involving sudden and uncontrollable brief episodes of falling asleep during the day |

| SUFFIX -phasia | | MEANING speech |
| --- | --- | --- |
| *Term* | *Term Analysis* | *Definition* |
| aphasia (ah-**FAY**-zee-ah) | a- = no; not; lack of | no speech |
| dysphasia (dis-**FAY**-zee-ah) | dys- = bad; poor; difficult; painful; abnormal | poor speech |

| SUFFIX -plegia | | MEANING paralysis |
| --- | --- | --- |
| *Term* | *Term Analysis* | *Definition* |
| hemiplegia (**hem**-ee-**PLEE**-jee-ah) | hemi- = half | paralysis affecting either the right or left side of the body |
| paraplegia (**par**-ah-**PLEE**-jee-ah) | para- = beside; near; abnormal | paralysis of the lower part of the body and legs |
| tetraplegia (**TET**-rah-**PLEE**-jee-ah) | tetra- = four | paralysis of all four limbs; quadriplegia |

## Prefixes

| PREFIX de- | | MEANING lack of; removal |
| --- | --- | --- |
| *Term* | *Term Analysis* | *Definition* |
| dementia (deh-**MEN**-she-ah) | -ia = condition ment/o = mind | mental deterioration; lack of brain function including memory, judgment, reasoning, and personality changes |

## 9.8 | Pathology

### Alzheimer (**ALZ**-high-mer) Disease

Alzheimer disease (AD) is a type of dementia. It is caused by the degeneration of brain cells. The disease results in the loss of memory, judgment, and reasoning. The disease gets worse over time, which means it is progressive. There are personality and behavior disorders.

### Amyotrophic (ah-**mye**-oh-**TROH**-fick) Lateral Sclerosis

Amyotrophic lateral sclerosis (**ALS**) is also known as Lou Gehrig disease. This is a progressive disease affecting the nerves in the brain and spinal cord responsible for movement. Muscular degeneration results. It often starts with weakness and twitching in the extremities. Eventually, the disease affects the ability to control the muscles needed to breathe, eat, and speak.

### Brain Tumors; Intracranial Tumors

There are two types of intracranial (within the skull) tumors: **gliomas** (gligh-**OH**-mahz) and **meningiomas** (meh-**nin**-jee-**OH**-mahz).

- Gliomas are malignant tumors of brain tissue (Figure 9-8). They can be fast or slow growing.
- Meningiomas are benign tumors. They are located outside the brain tissue but still within the cranium. They are slow growing.

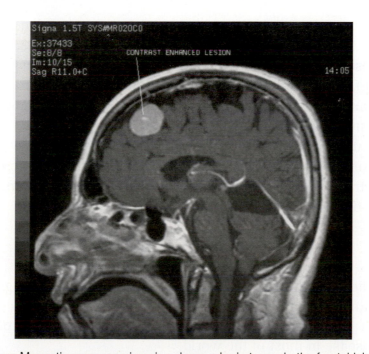

**Figure 9-8** Brain tumor. Magnetic resonance imaging shows a brain tumor in the frontal lobe.

## Levels of Consciousness (LOC)

Consciousness is the state of awareness of self and the environment. Disease, injury, or ingestion of drugs, alcohol, or medication can alter levels of consciousness (ALOC). The various levels of consciousness are listed below:

- **Conscious**: the person is attentive, awake, and aware of their surroundings.
- **Drowsy**: the person is tired, dozy, but can easily be aroused.
- **Lethargy** (**LETH**-ar-jee): state of being sluggish, drowsy, listless, and the person has to try hard to focus on his or her surroundings. The word "lethargic" is used to describe the conscious state of the patient.
- **Stupor** (**STOO**-por): a lower level of consciousness characterized by the person responding only to powerful stimuli.
- **Syncope** (**SING**-koh-pee): also known as fainting, is the brief loss of consciousness caused by the decreased flow of blood to the brain.
- **Coma** (**KOH**-mah): unconscious and unable to be aroused.

## Multiple Sclerosis (**MUL**-tih-pul Skler-**OH**-sis)

Multiple sclerosis (MS) is a condition in which the myelin sheath covering the neurons of the brain and spinal cord are destroyed. This is called demyelination ("lack of myelin sheath"). The lack of myelin sheath prevents impulses from being transmitted through the axon. This results in muscle weakness, paralysis, and other physical disabilities.

## Parkinson (**PAR**-kin-son) Disease (PD)

A disease that results in bradykinesia (slow movement), muscular rigidity, and resting tremors (shaking), also called pill-rolling tremors. Resting tremors involve the thumb and fingers and are present at rest, but disappear when the part moves. Parkinson is a chronic, progressive condition.

The cause is unknown. However, the abnormal movements are due to a decrease in levels of dopamine, in the brain. Treatment is with drugs to increase the levels of dopamine. This treatment is palliative, which means that it does not cure but eases symptoms of the disease.

## Poliomyelitis

Poliomyelitis (polio) is an infection caused by a virus. It is highly contagious. It attacks the nervous system and may cause paralysis. There is no cure. Polio can only be prevented by immunization with a weakened polio vaccine. Widespread use of the vaccine has eliminated the disease in most of the world.

**Postpoliomyelitis** has been identified in people who have had polio. The condition is characterized by muscle fatigue and weakness 15 years or more after they have recovered from polio.

## Sciatica (sigh-**AT**-ih-kah)

Inflammation of the sciatic nerve resulting in pain extending from the back into the buttocks and down the leg. It is often caused by a slipped disc in the lumbar area.

## Seizure Disorder; Epilepsy (**EP**-ih-lep-see)

A condition that causes the electrical impulses in the brain to become disorganized, uncoordinated, and excessive. The result is cerebral dysfunction, which causes abnormal movement, sensations, and changes in consciousness. The term "seizure" is used to describe these abnormalities.

An **electroencephalography** can detect the electrical impulses in the brain and register them as brain waves. It is commonly known as an **EEG**. Figure 9-9 illustrates normal and abnormal brain waves. Normal brain waves are the same in height and width. Abnormal brain waves, as seen in seizure disorder, are not the same in height and width.

### Types of Seizures

**Absence** (**AB**-senz) seizures, also known as **petit mal** (pe-**TEE MAHL**) seizures, are brief attacks lasting 1 to 30 seconds. The seizure takes the form of blank stares, eye abnormalities, and changes in the level of consciousness.

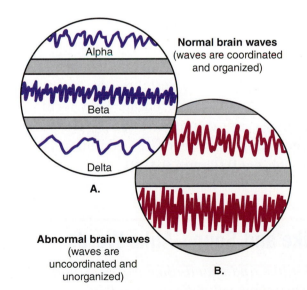

**Figure 9-9** Brain waves. A. Normal brain waves are usually consistent in height and width. Alpha waves are typical of a normal person who is awake and in a resting state. Beta waves are typical of a brain experiencing intense activity. Delta waves are typical of a normal person in deep sleep. B. Abnormal brain waves. Note the inconsistent height and width of the brain waves as seen in patients with seizure disorders.

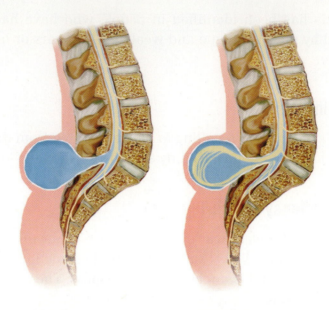

**A. Meningocele**          **B. Meningomyelocele**

**Figure 9-10** Meningocele and meningomyelocele due to spina bifida.

**Tonic-clonic** seizure, also known as **grand mal** seizure, alternates between the tonic phase, where the muscles become rigid, and the clonic phase, where the muscles uncontrollably jerk.

## Spina Bifida (SPYE-nah BIF-ih-da)

A defect in fetal development. The vertebrae do not form a complete circle around the spinal cord. It is a **congenital** (kon-**JEN**-ih-tal) condition, which means that it is present at birth.

In cases where the opening in the vertebrae is severe, the meninges and/or the spinal cord may protrude outside the vertebrae. They form a sac-like structure. If the sac contains only meninges, the condition is called **meningocele** (Figure 9-10A). If the sac contains meninges and spinal cord, the condition is called **meningomyelocele** (meh-**ning**-goh-**MY**-eh-loh-**seel**) (Figure 9-10B).

## 9.9   Look-Alike and Sound-Alike Words

*Below is a list of look-alike and sound-alike words. Study the spelling and definitions of each set of words. Questions will follow in the Review Exercises.*

### TABLE 9-1  Look-Alike and Sound-Alike Words

| | |
|---|---|
| aphasia | no speech |
| aphagia | no eating |
| aphakia | no lens (anatomical structure of the eye) |
| ataxia | no coordination |
| attacks | to become sick |
| clonus | twitching of a muscle |
| conus | resembling a cone shape |
| CNS | central nervous system |
| C&S | culture and sensitivity (a laboratory test) |
| elicit | to bring on; to elicit a response |
| illicit | illegal |
| gait | style of walking or running |
| gate | entrance or opening |

## 9.10  Review Exercises

### EXERCISE 9-1  Look-Alike and Sound-Alike Words

*Read the sentences carefully and circle the word in parentheses that correctly completes the meaning. Use Table 9-1 if it helps you.*

1. Jacob was admitted to the hospital with loss of blood to the speech centers in the brain due to a motor vehicle accident. On physical examination, at the time of admission, there was noted (**aphakia/aphagia/aphasia**).

2. Expect (**attacks/ataxia**) of delirium tremens following alcohol withdrawal. If there is cerebellar dysfunction, expect (**attacks/ataxia**).

3. The (**clonus/conus**) medullaris is the end portion of the spinal cord.

4. Continual (**clonus/conus**) indicates disruption of nerve impulses to the muscle.

5. To confirm inflammation of the (**CNS/C&S**), Dr. Lorenco withdrew CSF for (**CNS/C&S**).

6. To (**elicit/illicit**) a Babinski reflex on a newborn, stimulate the sole of the foot. The big toe should fan out.

7. Maria was caught with (**elicit/illicit**) drugs in the hospital.

8. Observe the patient carefully. Abnormal (**gate/gait**) may be the result of cerebellar damage.

9. A (**gait/gate**) was required to prevent the Alzheimer patient from wandering.

### EXERCISE 9-2  Matching Word Parts with Meaning

*Match the word part in Column A with its meaning in Column B.*

| | Column A | Column B |
|---|---|---|
| _____ | **1.** poli/o | A. brain |
| _____ | **2.** para- | B. hernia |
| _____ | **3.** tetra- | C. painful |
| _____ | **4.** cerebr/o | D. mind |
| _____ | **5.** ment/o | E. gray matter |
| _____ | **6.** -cele | F. vessel |
| _____ | **7.** -ar | G. four |
| _____ | **8.** dys- | H. membrane |
| _____ | **9.** -esthesia | I. abnormal |
| _____ | **10.** mening/o | J. pertaining to |
| _____ | **11.** hemi- | K. speech |
| _____ | **12.** -phasia | L. half |
| _____ | **13.** vascul/o | M. sensation |
| _____ | **14.** de- | N. condition |
| _____ | **15.** -ia | O. lack of |

### EXERCISE 9-3  Short Answer—Anatomy

*Answer the following questions in the space provided.*

1. (A) Name the organs that make up the central nervous system. (B) The peripheral nervous system.

   _____

   _____

2. Write one function for the following structures:

   **a.** cerebrum _____

   **b.** thalamus _____

   **c.** hypothalamus _____

   **d.** brainstem _____

**3.** What type of tissue makes up the spinal cord?

_____

**4.** What type of tissue protects the spinal cord?

_____

**5.** Name three portions of the brainstem.

_____

## EXERCISE 9-4   Labeling—Structures of the Brain

_Using the body structures listed below, label Figure 9-11. Write your answer in the numbered space provided below, or if you prefer, on the diagram._

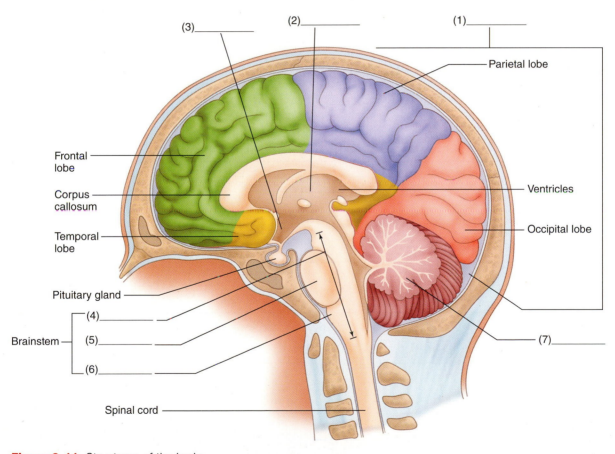

**Figure 9-11** Structures of the brain.

cerebellum _____

cerebrum _____

hypothalamus _____

medulla oblongata _____

midbrain _____

pons _____

thalamus _____

1. _____

2. _____

3. _____

4. _____

5. _____

6. _____

7. _____

## EXERCISE 9-5   Definitions—Anatomy

*Define the following terms. Use your dictionary if necessary.*

**1. neurons**

_____

**2. nerves**

_____

**3. myelin sheath**

_____

**4. gray matter**

_____

**5. pons**

_____

**6. cerebral cortex**

_____

**7. cerebellum**

_____

**8. spinal cord**

_____

**9. vertebral column**

_____

**10. peripheral nerves**

_____

## EXERCISE 9-6 Pathology

*Match the disease in Column A with its meaning in Column B.*

| | Column A | Column B |
|---|---|---|
| _____ | **1.** Alzheimer disease | A. may result in displaced meninges and/or spinal cord |
| _____ | **2.** multiple sclerosis | |
| _____ | **3.** Parkinson disease | B. characterized by resting tremors and muscle rigidity |
| _____ | **4.** spina bifida | |
| _____ | **5.** seizure disorder | C. disorganized, uncoordinated, and excessive electrical impulses in the brain |
| _____ | **6.** meningomyelocele | |
| _____ | **7.** hydrocephalus | D. type of dementia |
| _____ | **8.** lethargy | E. a complication of spina bifida |
| _____ | **9.** sciatica | F. characterized by demyelination of brain and spinal cord |
| _____ | **10.** tonic-clonic seizure | |
| _____ | **11.** absence seizure | G. accumulation of cerebrospinal fluid in the brain |
| _____ | **12.** poliomyelitis | |
| _____ | **13.** syncope | H. contagious disease caused by a virus |

I. uncoordinated movement alternating between muscular rigidity and jerky movement

J. uncoordinated electrical impulses in the brain of a short duration, 1–30 seconds

K. fainting

L. sluggish, drowsy, listless

M. usually caused by a slip disc in the lumbar vertebrae

## EXERCISE 9-7 Definitions—Learning the Terms

*Define the following terms:*

**1. cerebrovascular**

_____

**2. poliomyelitis**

_____

3. **neurology**

_____

4. **anesthesia**

_____

5. **dysesthesia**

_____

6. **paresthesia**

_____

7. **dysphasia**

_____

8. **tetraplegia**

_____

9. **paraplegia**

_____

10. **cerebrospinal fluid**

_____

## EXERCISE 9-8  Building Medical Words

_I. Use encephal/o to build medical words for the following definitions._

    **a.** inflammation of the brain _____

    **b.** any disease of the brain _____

_II. Use neur/o to build medical words for the following definitions._

    **a.** pertaining to the nerve and muscle _____

    **b.** study of the nervous system _____

_III. Use -esthesia to build medical words for the following definitions._

    **a.** loss of sensation _____

    **b.** painful sensations in response to normal stimulation

    _____

    **c.** abnormal sensations such as numbness and tingling

    _____

_IV. Use -plegia to build medical words for the following definitions._

    **a.** paralysis affecting either the right or left side of the body

    _____

**b.** paralysis of the lower part of the body and legs _____

**c.** paralysis of all four limbs _____

## EXERCISE 9-9 Definitions in Context

*Define the bold terms in context. Use your dictionary if necessary.*

Alita Lopez is a 62-year-old woman who was diagnosed with a brain tumor two months prior to admission. She suffered from **dysphasia**, abnormal **gait**, and **migraines** prior to admission. **MRI** showed increased **cerebrospinal fluid** in the left ventricle. Ms. Lopez underwent **neurosurgery** to relieve the **intracranial** pressure caused by the tumor. She was then treated with **chemotherapy** and **radiotherapy**.

**a.** dysphasia _____

**b.** gait _____

**c.** migraines _____

**d.** MRI _____

**e.** cerebrospinal fluid _____

**f.** neurosurgery _____

**g.** intracranial _____

**h.** chemotherapy _____

**i.** radiotherapy _____

## EXERCISE 9-10 Spelling

*Circle any words that are spelled incorrectly in the list below. Then correct the spelling in the space provided.*

**1.** disesthesia _____

**2.** myelin sheath _____

**3.** siezure _____

**4.** Parkinsin diease _____

**5.** resonence _____

**6.** thalmus _____

**7.** cerebellum _____

8. conjenital _____

9. medulla oblongata _____

10. Alzheimer disease _____

## Animations

Visit the companion website to view the video on **protective coverings** of the brain and spinal cord.

Also watch the following videos: **Spinal Cord Injuries**; **Parkinson Disease**.

## 9.11  Pronunciation and Spelling

*Listen, read, and study, so you can speak and write.*

1. Listen to each word on the audio file provided on the Student Companion Website.

2. Pronounce each word carefully.

3. Spell each word in the space provided.

| Word | Pronunciation | Spelling |
|------|--------------|----------|
| anesthesia | **an**-es-**THEE**-zee-ah | |
| aphasia | ah-**FAY**-zee-ah | |
| cerebellum | **ser**-eh-**BELL**-um | |
| cerebrospinal | **ser**-eh-broh-**SPYE**-nal | |
| cerebrovascular | **ser**-eh-broh-**VAS**-kyoo-lar | |
| cerebrum | seh-**REE**-brum | |
| dementia | deh-**MEN**-she-ah | |
| demyelination | dee-**my**-eh-lih-**NAY**-shun | |
| dysesthesia | **dis**-es-**THEE**-zee-ah | |
| dysphasia | dis-**FAY**-zee-ah | |
| electroencephalography | ee-**leck**-troh-en-**sef**-ah-**LOG**-rah-fee | |
| encephalitis | en-**sef**-ah-**LYE**-tis | |
| encephalopathy | en-**sef**-ah-**LOP**-ah-thee | |
| hemiplegia | **hem**-ee-**PLEE**-jee-ah | |

| Word | Pronunciation | Spelling |
|------|---------------|----------|
| hypothalamus | **high-**poh-**THAL-**ah-mus | |
| medulla oblongata | meh-**DULL-**ah **ob-**long-**GAH-**tah | |
| meninges | meh-**NIN-**jeez | |
| meningocele | meh-**NIN-**goh-seel | |
| meningoencephalitis | meh-**NIN-**goh-en-**sef-**ah-**LYE-**tis | |
| myelin sheath | **MY-**eh-lin **SHEETH** | |
| neurology | noo-**ROL-**oh-jee | |
| neurons | **NOO-**ronz | |
| paraplegia | **par-**ah-**PLEE-**jee-ah | |
| paresthesia | **par-**es-**THEE-**zee-ah | |
| poliomyelitis | **poh-**lee-oh-**my-**eh-**LYE-**tis | |
| pons | **PONZ** | |
| thalamus | **THAL-**ah-mus | |

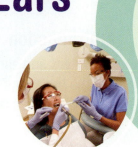

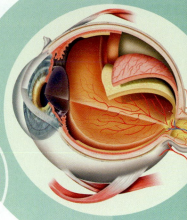

# CHAPTER 10

# The Eyes and Ears

## Chapter Outline

## Learning Objectives

*After studying this chapter and completing the review exercises, you should be able to:*

1. Name and describe the structures and functions of the eye and its accessory structures.
2. Describe the pathway of vision to the brain.
3. Pronounce, spell, define, and write the medical terms related to the eyes.
4. Describe common diseases related to the eyes.
5. Name and describe the structures and functions of the ear.
6. Describe the pathway of hearing to the brain.

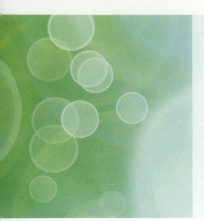

7. Pronounce, spell, define, and write the medical terms related to the ears.
8. Describe common diseases related to the ear.
9. Listen, read, and study so you can speak and write.

## Introduction

Our eyes and ears connect us with the world. The eyes send signals to one part of the brain, and we see. The ears send signals to another part of the brain, and we hear. This chapter explains these amazing organs.

## 10.1 Major Structures of the Eyeball

**PRACTICE FOR LEARNING: Eyeball**

Write the words below in the correct spaces in Figure 10-1. To help you, the number beside the word tells you where it goes on the figure. Be sure to pronounce each word as you write it. Repeat the pronunciation several times if you find the word hard to say.

1. Ciliary (**SIL**-ee-ahr-ee) body and muscle
2. Conjunctiva (kon-**JUNK**-tih-vah)
3. Iris (**EYE**-ris)
4. Pupil (**PYOO**-pil)
5. Cornea (**KOR**-nee-ah)
6. Lens (**LENZ**)
7. Sclera (**SKLEHR**-ah)
8. Choroid (**KOH**-roid)
9. Optic nerve (**OP**-tick **NERV**)
10. Macula lutea (**MACK**-yoo-lah **LOO**-tee-ah)
11. Retina (**RET**-ih-nah)

## 10.2 Layers of the Eyeball, Lens, and Cavities

The eyeball has three layers: outer, middle, and inner. They are described below.

### Outer Layer

The outer layer of the eye is made up of the cornea and the sclera. The cornea is transparent. This means that it is clear and lets light into the eye. The sclera is the white of the eye. It is fibrous and not transparent, and therefore light does not pass through it.

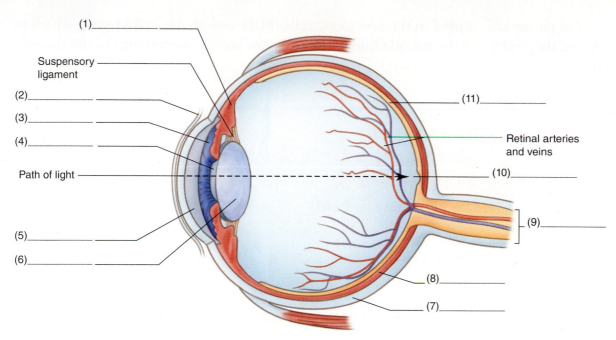

**Figure 10-1** Major structures of the eye.

Find the sclera on Figure 10-1. Using your finger, make a circle by following the sclera. Notice how the sclera joins the cornea at the front of the eye and then becomes the sclera again as the circle is completed.

## Middle Layer

Figure 10-1 also illustrates the middle layer of the eyeball. It is called the **uvea** (**YOO-vee-ah**). The uvea has three parts: the choroid, ciliary body, and the iris.

Find the choroid on Figure 10-1. Again, using your finger, follow the outline of the middle layer. The choroid is vascular and provides blood to the entire eye.

The ciliary body produces aqueous humor. The ciliary muscles move the lens to focus on near and far objects.

The iris is the colored portion of the eye. There is an opening in the middle of the iris called the pupil. It regulates the amount of light that enters the eye. In bright light, the pupil constricts (narrows) to protect the eye from bright light. In dimmer light, the pupil dilates (widens).

## Inner Layer

The inner layer of the eye is called the retina (Figure 10-1). Once again use your finger and trace the outline of the retina on the diagram. The retina contains cells called **rods** (**RODZ**) and **cones** (**KOHNZ**). These structures are named for their shape. They receive light rays and transform them into electrical impulses that travel to the brain along the optic nerve. This allows vision to occur.

The cones are located in the fovea centralis (**FOH**-vee-ah sen-**TRAL**-iss), which is a pit in the middle of the macula lutea. The rods are located peripheral to the macula lutea.

---

**In Brief**

**Outer layer**
Sclera, cornea

**Middle layer, or uvea**
Choroid, ciliary body, iris

**Inner layer**
Retina (rods and cones)

---

**PRACTICE FOR LEARNING: Outer Layer, Middle Layer, Inner Layer**

Write your answer in the space provided.

1. Write the structures that make up the following layers of the eye:

   **a.** outer layer _____

   **b.** middle layer _____

   **c.** inner layer _____

2. The middle layer is also known as the _____.

3. Name the location of the cones and rods. _____

4. State a function of rods and cones. _____

> Answers: 1. a. cornea, sclera. b. choroid, ciliary body, iris. c. retina containing rods and cones. 2. uvea. 3. cones are located in the fovea centralis. Rods are located peripheral to the macula lutea. 4. changes light rays into electrical impulses.

## Lens, Anterior Cavity, Posterior Cavity

Some structures of the eyeball are not considered to be part of any one layer of the eye. They are the lens, anterior cavity, and posterior cavity. You can see these in Figure 10-2. The lens is located behind the iris. It bends light rays.

There is a cavity in front of the lens and one behind it. The one in front is the **anterior cavity** (**KAV**-ih-tee). It is filled with a watery fluid called **aqueous humor** (**AY**-kwee-us **HYOO**-mer). The aqueous humor maintains the proper pressure within the eye. This is called intraocular pressure (IOP). As new aqueous humor is produced by the ciliary body, the old is drained into the bloodstream through a meshwork called the **trabeculae** (trah-**BECK**-yoo lee) and a canal called the canal of **Schlemm** (**SHLEM**). (Figure 10-3)

The **posterior cavity** is behind the lens. It is filled with gel called **vitreous** (**VIT**-ree-us) humor. It maintains the round shape of the eyeball and holds the retina in place, firmly against the choroid.

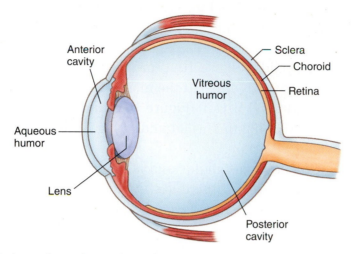

**Figure 10-2**  Lens, anterior cavity, and posterior cavity.

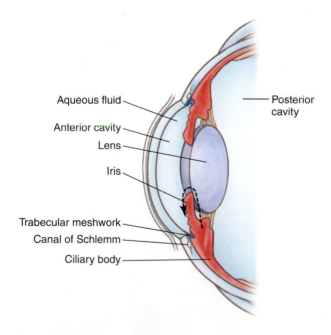

**Figure 10-3**  Flow of aqueous humor in the anterior cavity. As aqueous humor is produced, the old is drained into the blood stream through the trabeculae and Canal of Schlemm.

**In Brief**

The **lens** is behind the iris.

The **anterior cavity** is in front of the lens and contains aqueous humor.

The **posterior cavity** is behind the lens and contains vitreous humor.

## 10.3 | Accessory Structures

The accessory structures are located outside the eyeball. These include the **orbital cavity**, **eyelids**, **conjunctiva**, **lacrimal apparatus**, and **extraocular muscles**.

The orbital cavity is the eye socket. It is a depression in the skull bone into which the eyeball fits.

The upper and lower eyelids (Figure 10-4) protect the eye from foreign matter. The eyelids meet at the **canthus** (**KAN**-thus) at the medial and lateral corners of the eye.

The conjunctiva (**kon**-junk-**TYE**-vah) (Figure 10-1 and Figure 10-4) is a transparent layer of mucous membrane lining the eyelid and covering the front of the eye exposed to the air. It also provides protection.

The lacrimal apparatus includes glands and a system of ducts. The glands continually produce tears (Figure 10-4) and the ducts transport tears across the eye to clean and lubricate the eye. Excess tears flow through ducts into the nose. This is why your nose runs when you cry.

The **extraocular** (**ecks**-trah-**OCK**-yoo-lar) muscles (Figure 10-5) are located outside the eyeball. These muscles move the eye upward, downward, medially, and laterally. They are named according to their location and orientation. An example is the **superior rectus** (**RECK**-tuss) muscle. Its location is superior to the eyeball. Its orientation is rectus, which means straight. The other locations are **inferior**, **lateral**, and **medial**. The other orientation is **oblique** (oh-**BLEEK**), which means slanted (Figure 10-5). The extraocular muscles include:

- Superior and inferior rectus muscle
- Superior and inferior oblique muscles
- Lateral and medial rectus muscles

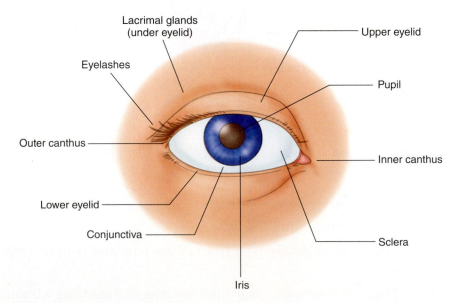

**Figure 10-4** Accessory structures of the eye.

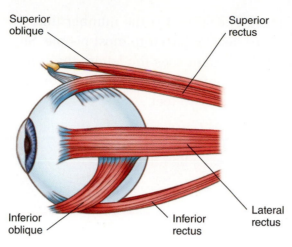

**Figure 10-5** Extraocular muscles.

## PRACTICE FOR LEARNING: Lens, Anterior and Posterior Cavities

Write one function for the following:

**1.** lens _____

**2.** vitreous humor _____

**3.** aqueous humor _____

> Answers: 1. refraction. 2. maintains round shape of the eyeball; holds the retina against the choroid; refraction. (any one answer is correct). 3. maintains intraocular pressure; refraction (either answer is correct).

## 10.4  Refraction

The eye bends light rays so that they come together at the retina at the same time. This is illustrated in Figure 10-6. This bending of light is called **refraction** (ree-**FRACK**-shun). Without the proper amount of refraction, vision will be blurred.

**Visual acuity** (ah-**KYOO**-ih-tee) is the eye's ability to see. A visual acuity test measures the patient's ability to see the smallest letters on a chart (a Snellen chart) from 20 feet away. The results are stated as two numbers. The first is 20, as it is the distance

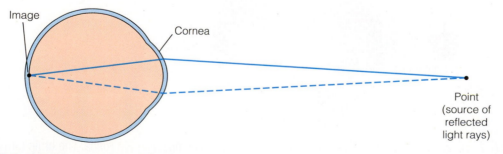

**Figure 10-6** Refraction: bending of light rays.

the patient is from the chart. The second is the number that shows the patient's ability to see the letters on the chart, as compared to most people. So, for example, a measure of 20/20 would mean that the patient sees the letters that someone with normal vision would see at 20 feet. A measure of 20/40 would mean that the patient sees at 20 feet what a normal patient would see at 40 feet.

| **In Brief** | **Refraction** means bending |
| --- | --- |

## 10.5  Visual Pathway

Sight is possible because various structures work together. Light rays must travel unobstructed through the cornea, aqueous humor, pupil, lens, and vitreous humor. The light rays are bent by each structure or fluid, and then focus on the retina. The light rays must focus precisely on the same point on the retina to produce a clear, sharp image. The rods and cones then change the image into electrical impulses. These impulses travel along the optic nerve to the brain. The brain then makes us aware of the object we are looking at. Figure 10-7 illustrates light traveling through this visual pathway.

| **In Brief** | **Path that light travels** $\longrightarrow$ cornea $\longrightarrow$ aqueous humor $\longrightarrow$ pupil $\longrightarrow$ lens $\longrightarrow$ vitreous humor $\longrightarrow$ retina (light rays change to electrical impulses) $\longrightarrow$ optic nerve $\longrightarrow$ brain |
| --- | --- |

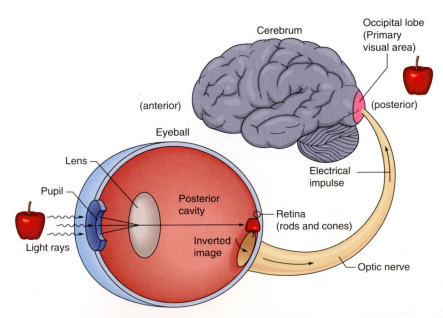

**Figure 10-7** Visual pathway. Notice the image of the apple is upside down on the retina. The brain turns the image right side up and clear vision is obtained.

## 10.6  New Roots, Suffixes, and Prefixes of the Eye

Use these additional roots, suffixes, and prefixes when studying the terms in this chapter.

| ROOT | MEANING |
| --- | --- |
| ambly/o | dull; dim |
| ametr/o | out of proportion |
| anis/o | unequal |
| dipl/o | double |
| nyct/o | night |

| SUFFIX | MEANING |
| --- | --- |
| -ician | specialist; one who specializes; expert |
| -metrist | specialist in the measure of |
| -pexy | surgical fixation |
| -phobia | fear |

| PREFIX | MEANING |
| --- | --- |
| eso- | inward |
| exo- | outside |
| extra- | outside |
| presby- | old age |

## 10.7  Learning the Terms of the Eye

Following these steps will make it easier for you to learn medical terms:

1. Pronounce the term repeatedly until it is easy for you.
2. Write it down. Ensure the spelling is correct.
3. Also write the definition. If possible, relate the word to a word, thought, or picture that will help you remember it.
4. Analyze the term with the method taught in this text.

## Roots

| ROOT<br>blephar/o (see also palpebr/o) | | MEANING<br>eyelid |
|---|---|---|
| *Term* | *Term Analysis* | *Definition* |
| **blepharoptosis**<br>(**blef**-ah-rop-**TOH**-sis) | -ptosis = drooping; sagging | drooping eyelid. Also known simply as "ptosis." |

| ROOT<br>conjunctiv/o | | MEANING<br>conjunctiva (membrane lining the eyelids and anterior part of eye) |
|---|---|---|
| *Term* | *Term Analysis* | *Definition* |
| **conjunctivitis**<br>(**kon**-junk-tih-**VYE**-tiss) | -itis = inflammation | inflammation of the conjunctiva |

| ROOT<br>core/o | | MEANING<br>pupil |
|---|---|---|
| *Term* | *Term Analysis* | *Definition* |
| **anisocoria**<br>(an-**iss**-oh-**KOR**-ee-ah) | -ia = condition<br>anis/o = unequal | condition in which the pupils are of unequal size |

| ROOT<br>corne/o (see also kerat/o) | | MEANING<br>cornea |
|---|---|---|
| *Term* | *Term Analysis* | *Definition* |
| **corneal abrasion**<br>(**KOR**-nee-al ab-**RAY**-zhun) | -eal = pertaining to<br>-ion = process<br>ab- = away from<br>ras/o = scrape | scraping of the superficial layers of the cornea |

| ROOT<br>irid/o; ir/o | | MEANING<br>iris |
|---|---|---|
| *Term* | *Term Analysis* | *Definition* |
| **iridectomy**<br>(**ir**-ih-**DECK**-toh-mee) | -ectomy = excision; surgical removal | excision of the iris |
| **iritis**<br>(eye-**RYE**-tiss) | -itis = inflammation | inflammation of the iris |

| ROOT kerat/o | | MEANING cornea |
|---|---|---|
| *Term* | *Term Analysis* | *Definition* |
| **keratoplasty** (ker-**AT**-oh-**plas**-tee) | -plasty = surgical reconstruction; surgical repair | surgical reconstruction of the cornea; corneal transplant |

| ROOT ocul/o (see also ophthalm/o) | | MEANING eye |
|---|---|---|
| *Term* | *Term Analysis* | *Definition* |
| **extraocular muscles** (**ecks**-trah-**OCK**-yoo-lar) | -ar = pertaining to extra- = outside | muscles located outside the eyeball |

| ROOT ophthalm/o | | MEANING eye |
|---|---|---|
| *Term* | *Term Analysis* | *Definition* |
| **exophthalmia** (**eck**-sof-**THAL**-mee-ah) | -ia = condition ex- = outward | outward protrusion of the eyeball |
| **ophthalmologist** (**ahf**-thal-**MOL**-eh-jist) | -logist = specialist | a medical doctor who specializes in the study of the diagnosis and medical and surgical treatment of eye disorders |
| **ophthalmoscopy** (**ahf**-thal-**MOS**-koh-pee) | -scopy = process of visually examining | process of visually examining the eye. Also known as funduscopy (fun-**DUSS**-keh-pee) |

**Note:** The fundus is the back portion of the eye. It includes the retina and macula lutea.

| | | |
|---|---|---|
| **ophthalmology** (**ahf**-thal-**MOL**-eh-jee) | -logy = study of | medical speciality dealing with the study of the eye including disease and treatment |
| **xerophthalmia** (**zer**-off-**THAL**-me-ah) | -ia = condition ophthalm/o = eye | drying of the surfaces of the eye including the conjunctiva |

| ROOT opt/o | | MEANING vision; sight |
| --- | --- | --- |
| Term | Term Analysis | Definition |
| **optician**<br>(op-**TISH**-an) | -ician = specialist; one who specializes; expert | expert who fills prescriptions for eyeglasses and contact lenses |

**Note:** Opticians are not medical doctors and do not carry out medical and surgical treatments of eye conditions.

| | | |
| --- | --- | --- |
| **optometrist**<br>(op-**TOM**-eh-trist) | -metrist = specialist in the measurement of | specialist in the testing of visual function and in the diagnosis and nonsurgical treatment of eye conditions |

**Note:** Optometrists prescribe eyeglasses and contact lenses and are licensed in some areas to prescribe medication. They do not have a degree in medicine.

| ROOT palpebr/o | | MEANING eyelid |
| --- | --- | --- |
| Term | Term Analysis | Definition |
| **palpebral**<br>(**PAL**-peh-bral) | -al = pertaining to | pertaining to the eyelid |

| ROOT phac/o; phak/o | | MEANING lens |
| --- | --- | --- |
| Term | Term Analysis | Definition |
| **aphakia**<br>(ah-**FAY**-kee-ah) | a- = absence; no; not; lack of; | absence of a lens |

| ROOT phot/o | | MEANING light |
| --- | --- | --- |
| Term | Term Analysis | Definition |
| **photophobia**<br>(foh-toh-**FOH**-bee-ah) | -phobia = fear | intolerance or sensitivity to light |

| ROOT retin/o | | MEANING retina |
| --- | --- | --- |
| Term | Term Analysis | Definition |
| retinopathy (ret-ih-**NOP**-eh-thee) | -pathy = disease | any disease of the retina |
| retinopexy (**RET**-ih-noh-**peck**-see) | -pexy = surgical fixation | surgical fixation of the retina |

## Suffixes

| SUFFIX -opia | | MEANING visual condition; vision |
| --- | --- | --- |
| Term | Term Analysis | Definition |
| amblyopia (**am**-blee-**OH**-pee-ah) | ambly/o = dull; dim | dimness of vision |
| ametropia (**am**-eh-**TROH**-pee-ah) | ametr/o = out of proportion | error of refraction in which images do not focus properly on the retina |
| hemianopia (**hem**-ee-an-**OH**-pee-ah) | hemi- = half an- = no; not | lack of vision in one-half of the visual field. Also known as hemianopsia (**hem**-ee-an-**OP**-see-ah). |
| nyctalopia (**nick**-tah-**LOH**-pee-ah) | nyct/o = night | night blindness; a person with normal day vision has difficulty seeing at night |
| diplopia (dih-**PLOH**-pee-ah) | dipl/o = double | double vision |
| presbyopia (**pres**-bee-**OH**-pee-ah) | presby- = old age | impaired vision due to advanced age |

| SUFFIX -tropia; tropion | | MEANING turning |
| --- | --- | --- |
| Term | Term Analysis | Definition |
| entropion (en-**TROH**-pee-on) | en- = in | inward turning of the **eyelid**; inversion of the eyelid |

| Term | Term Analysis | Definition |
|------|---------------|------------|
| esotropia (es-oh-**TROH**-pee-ah) | eso- = inward | inward turning of the **eyeball** (Figure 10-8B); cross-eyes |
| exotropia (eck-soh-**TROH**-pee-ah) | exo- = outward | outward turning of the **eyeball** (Figure 10-8C) |

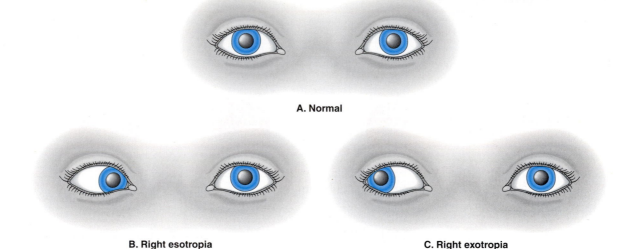

A. Normal

B. Right esotropia          C. Right exotropia

**Figure 10-8** Normal vision compared with types of strabismus. A. Normal vision. B. Right esotropia. C. Right exotropia.

**Note:** Esotropia and exotropia are also known as strabismus.

## 10.8 Pathology of the Eye

### Cataracts (**KAT**-ah-rakts)

Fogging of the lens (Figure 10-9). Normally, the lens is clear. When the lens is foggy, the light rays cannot focus on the retina. As a result, vision becomes blurred. Cataracts can be treated by destroying the diseased lens. This can be done by using ultrasound (high frequency sound waves). The removed lens is replaced with an artificial (prosthetic) intraocular lens (IOL).

### Errors of Refraction

Errors in the bending of light rays in the eye, resulting in blurred vision. Types are myopia, hyperopia, and astigmatism.

### Myopia (my-**OH**-pee-ah)

Nearsightedness. Only near objects can be seen clearly. Light rays focus in front of the retina because they are bent too quickly or because the eyeball is too long. Illustrated in Figure 10-10A.

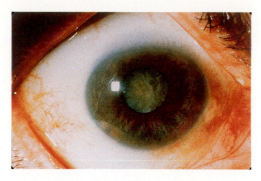

**Figure 10-9** Cataract. Courtesy of the National Eye Institute. NIH

### Hyperopia (**high**-per-**OH**-pee-ah)

Farsightedness. Only far-away objects can be seen clearly. Light rays focus behind the retina because they are bent too slowly or because the eyeball is too short. Illustrated in Figure 10-10B.

### Astigmatism (ah-**STIG**-mah-tiz-um)

Blurred vision, both near and far. The curve of the cornea is uneven. Thus, light rays do not reach a point of focus. Illustrated in Figure 10-10C.

All errors of refraction can be treated in a nonsurgical or surgical manner. Nonsurgical treatment is the prescription of eyeglasses with the appropriate lens to correct the visual distortion (Figures 10-10A and B). Surgical treatment involves using a laser to reshape the curvature of the cornea so that the light rays will focus on the retina. Some types of laser surgery are LASIK and LASEK.

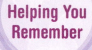

**Helping You Remember**   LASIK and LASEK are acronyms. These are words formed from the initial letter of the major parts of a compound term. LASIK means Laser-Assisted In-Situ Keratomileusis. LASEK means Laser-Assisted Subepithelial Keratectomy.

## Glaucoma (glaw-**KOH**-mah)

Damage to the retina and optic nerve due to increased intraocular pressure. The intraocular pressure increases because the aqueous humor produced is greater than the amount that flows out of the eye. Thus, aqueous humor builds up inside the anterior cavity. This distorts the shape of the eye and impairs vision (Figure 10-11c). The first level of treatment is eyedrops. If this is unsuccessful, surgery is done to increase the outflow of aqueous humor. Glaucoma can lead to blindness.

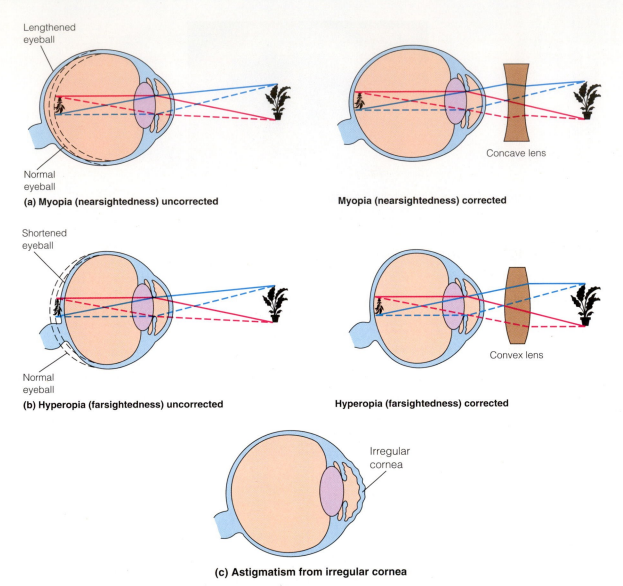

**Figure 10-10** Errors of refraction. A. Myopia (nearsightedness). B. Hyperopia (farsightedness). C. Astigmatism.

## Macular Degeneration (**MAK**-yoo-ler)

Deterioration of the macula lutea. Also known as age-related macular degeneration (AMD) because in some people, deterioration of the macula comes with the aging process. There is loss of central vision. It progresses to blindness (Figure 10-11D).

## Retinal Tears (**TAYRZ**) (do Not confuse with **TEERZ**)

Holes that develop on the retina. With age, the vitreous humor shrinks. As it shrinks, the humor pulls tightly on the retina and results in the creation of holes along the retinal wall. If not treated, they will result in the detachment (separation) of the retina from the layers underneath (Figure 10-12). If not treated, this will lead to blindness.

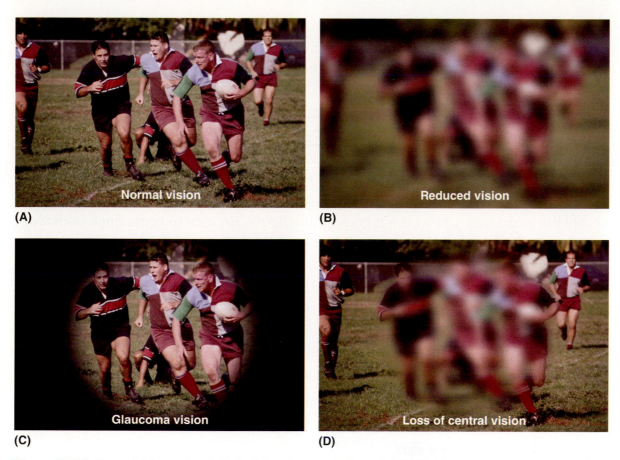

**Figure 10-11**  Normal vision and pathologic vision changes. A. Normal vision. B. Vision reduced by cataracts. C. The loss of peripheral vision due to untreated glaucoma. D. The loss of central vision due to macular degeneration.

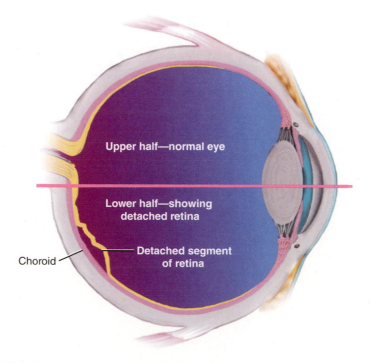

**Figure 10-12**  Retinal detachment.

Tears (**TEERZ**) refer to the droplets of fluid that fall from the eye.
Tears (**TAYRZ**) are holes that develop due to a pulling force.

## 10.9   Major Structures of the Ear

**PRACTICE FOR LEARNING: Ear**

Write the words below in the correct spaces in Figure 10-13. To help you, the number beside the word tells you where it goes on the figure. Be sure to pronounce each word as you write it. Repeat the pronunciation several times if you find the word hard to say.

1. external ear
2. middle ear
3. inner ear
4. auricle (**AW**-rih-kul) or pinna (**PIN**-ah)
5. external auditory meatus (**AW**-dih-tor-ee mee-**AY**-tus)
6. tympanic (tim-**PAN**-ick) membrane or eardrum
7. ossicles (**OSS**-ih-kulz)
8. cochlea (**KOCK**-lee-ah)

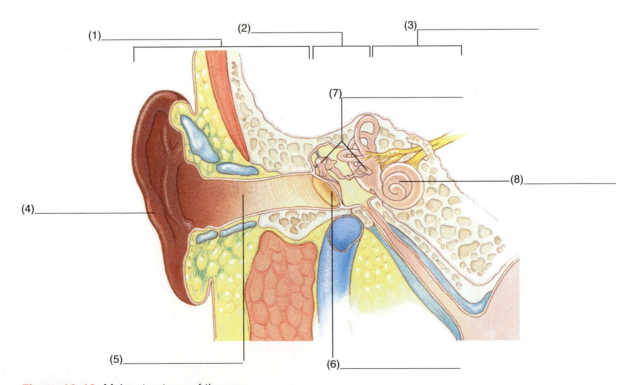

**Figure 10-13** Major structures of the ear.

## External Ear

The external ear can be seen in Figure 10-13. It includes the auricle (also called the pinna or earflap), the external auditory meatus, and the tympanic membrane (TM) or eardrum.

The auricle gathers the sounds. Sound travels down the external auditory meatus to the eardrum. The sound makes the eardrum vibrate. The sound waves from this vibration travel to the middle ear.

Glands in the external auditory meatus secrete a wax called **cerumen** (seh-**ROO**-men). It protects the ear from infection by trapping microorganisms.

**In Brief**

**External Ear**

Includes: auricle, external auditory meatus, tympanic membrane
Function: gathers and transmits sound to middle ear

## Middle and Inner Ears

PRACTICE FOR LEARNING: **Middle Ear and Inner Ears**

Write the words below in the correct spaces in Figure 10-14. To help you, the number beside the word tells you where it goes on the figure. Be sure to pronounce each word as you write it. Repeat the pronunciation several times if you find the word hard to say.

1. **malleus** (**MAL**-ee-uss)
2. **incus** (**ING**-kuss)
3. **stapes** (**STAY**-peez)
4. **oval window**
5. **eustachian tube** (yoo-**STAY**-shun)
6. **cochlea** (**KOCK**-lee-ah)
7. **vestibule** (**VES**-tih-byool)

The middle ear consists of three tiny bones called **ossicles** (**OSS**-ih-kulz). They are the malleus, the incus, and the stapes. The stapes is connected to the oval window. The eustachian tube connects the middle ear to the throat.

The inner ear consists of the cochlea and vestibule. These structures look like winding passageways that resemble a maze, so the inner ear is also called the **labyrinth** (**LAB**-ih-rinth). The inner ear is responsible for balance and hearing. Balance is maintained through the action of fluid in the inner ear. When we are off balance, the fluid is disturbed, and messages are sent to the brain telling it that the body is not in the right position. The brain then corrects the body's position to get back into balance.

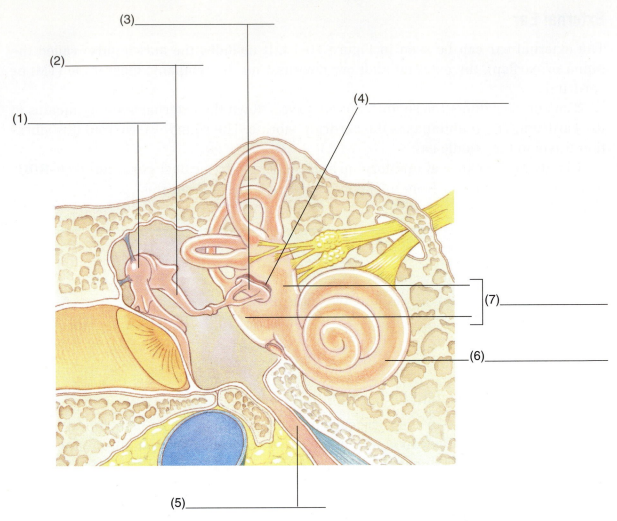

**Figure 10-14**  Middle and inner ear.

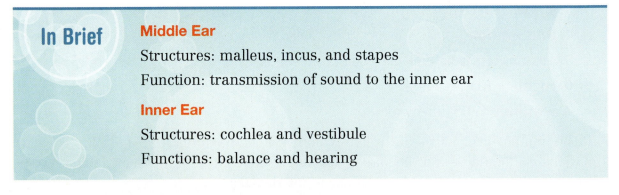

**In Brief**

**Middle Ear**

Structures: malleus, incus, and stapes

Function: transmission of sound to the inner ear

**Inner Ear**

Structures: cochlea and vestibule

Functions: balance and hearing

**PRACTICE FOR LEARNING: Structures of the Ear**

**1.** Circle the structure that does not fit into a given category.

    **a.** external ear: pinna, malleus, tympanic membrane

    **b.** middle ear: ossicles, malleus, external auditory meatus, stapes

    **c.** inner ear: vestibule, cochlea, auricle

**2.** Name the three ossicles found in the middle ear.

_____

**3.** Name the structure that connects the middle ear to the throat.

_____

**4.** What is the other name for the inner ear?

_____

Answers: 1. a. malleus; b. external auditory meatus; c. auricle. 2. malleus, incus, stapes. 3. eustachian tube. 4. labyrinth.

## 10.10  Auditory Pathway

Hearing is possible because sound waves travel through the external auditory meatus and hits the tympanic membrane. The sound is transmitted through the middle ear to the inner ear, where it reaches the cochlea. Fluid inside the cochlea is set in motion, which disturbs tiny hair cells inside the cochlea. These hair cells react to the vibration by moving, like tall grass swaying in the wind. The movement of the hair cells stimulates the underlying nerve cells, which create nerve impulses that travel along the auditory nerve to the brain for interpretation (Figure 10-15).

**In Brief**    **Path that sound travels** ⟶ pinna or auricle ⟶ external auditory meatus ⟶ tympanic membrane ⟶ ossicles (malleus, incus, stapes) ⟶ cochlea ⟶ auditory nerve ⟶ brain

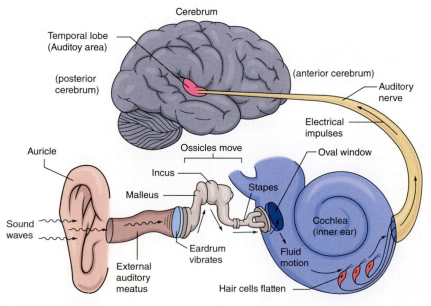

**Figure 10-15** Auditory pathway.

## 10.11  New Roots, Suffixes, and Prefixes of the Ear

Use these additional suffixes when studying the terms in this chapter.

| SUFFIX | MEANING |
|---|---|
| -metry | process of measuring |
| -ory | pertaining to |

## 10.12  Learning the Terms of the Ear

### Roots

| ROOT<br>audi/o (see also audit/o) | | MEANING<br>hearing |
|---|---|---|
| Term | Term Analysis | Definition |
| audiometry<br>(aw-dee-**OM**-eh-tree) | -metry = process<br>of measuring | process of measuring a patient's<br>hearing ability |

| ROOT<br>audit/o | | MEANING<br>hearing |
|---|---|---|
| Term | Term Analysis | Definition |
| auditory<br>(**AW**-dih-tor-ee) | -ory = pertaining to | pertaining to hearing |

| ROOT<br>aur/o | | MEANING<br>ear |
|---|---|---|
| Term | Term Analysis | Definition |
| aural<br>(**AW**-ral) | -al = pertaining to | pertaining to the ear |

**Helping You Remember**   Do not confuse oral with aural. Oral means "pertaining to the mouth." Aural means "pertaining to the ear."

| ROOT labyrinth/o | | MEANING inner ear; labyrinth |
| --- | --- | --- |
| Term | Term Analysis | Definition |
| labyrinthitis (**lab**-ih-rin-**THIGH**-tiss) | -itis = inflammation | inflammation of the inner ear |

| ROOT myring/o (see also tympan/o) | | MEANING tympanic membrane; eardrum |
| --- | --- | --- |
| Term | Term Analysis | Definition |
| myringotomy (**mir**-ing-**GOT**-oh-me) | -tomy = process of cutting; to cut | process of cutting into the eardrum to remove fluid from the middle ear |
| myringoplasty (mih-**RING**-goh-**plas**-tee) | -plasty = surgical reconstruction, surgical repair | surgical reconstruction of the tympanic membrane only. There is no repair of the ossicles.Compare with tympanoplasty below. |

| ROOT ot/o | | MEANING ear |
| --- | --- | --- |
| Term | Term Analysis | Definition |
| otalgia (oh-**TAL**-jee-ah) | -algia = pain | earache |
| otitis media (oh-**TYE**-tis **ME**- dee-ah) | -itis = inflammation media = middle | inflammation of the middle ear |
| otorrhea (**oh**-toh-**REE**-ah) | -rrhea = discharge; flow | discharge from the ear |

| ROOT staped/o | | MEANING stapes |
| --- | --- | --- |
| Term | Term Analysis | Definition |
| stapedioplasty (stah-**PEE**-dee-oh-**plas**-tee) | -plasty = surgical reconstruction; surgical repair | a surgical reconstruction of the stapes. It includes a stapedectomy (**stah**-peh-**DECK**-teh-mee) followed by replacement of the stapes with a prosthetic (pros-**THET**-ick) (artificial) stapes. |

| ROOT tympan/o | | MEANING tympanic membrane |
|---|---|---|
| *Term* | *Term Analysis* | *Definition* |
| **tympanometry** (**tim**-peh-**NOM**-eh-tree) | -metry = process of measuring | use of air pressure in the ear canal to test for disorders of the middle ear |
| **tympanoplasty** (**TIM**-peh-noh-**plas**-tee) | -plasty = surgical repair; surgical reconstruction | surgical reconstruction of a torn eardrum and/or the ossicles of the middle ear. If necessary, drainage tubes are inserted to manage middle ear disease. |

## Suffixes

| SUFFIX -cusis | | MEANING hearing |
|---|---|---|
| *Term* | *Term Analysis* | *Definition* |
| **presbycusis** (**pres**-bih-**KYOO**-sis) | presby- = old age | diminished hearing due to old age |

## 10.13 Pathology of the Ear

### Hearing Impairment

Hearing impairment is diminished or total loss of hearing with impaired ability to distinguish between speech sounds. There are two types of deafness. **Conductive deafness** is caused by the obstruction of the path traveled by sound waves from the external ear to the inner ear. Examples of obstruction are a buildup of earwax or a foreign body such as a raisin lodged in the ear canal. Treatment is by removing the obstruction.

The second type of deafness is **sensorineural** (**sen**-seh-ree-**NOOR**-al) **deafness**. This is caused by damage to the auditory nerve. This occurs with age. It can also be caused by loud noises from machinery or music, tumors, or infections. Hearing aids may be helpful for treating sensorineural deafness. If not, then a cochlear implant may be needed.

### Meniere Disease (meh-**NYAR**)

A condition of the inner ear. It includes hearing loss, a feeling of pressure in the ear, dizziness or **vertigo** (**VER**-tih-goh), and ringing in the ears or **tinnitus** (**TIN**-ih-tuss). **Nystagmus** (niss-**TAG**-muss), an involuntary, rapid, rhythmic movement of the eyeball may also be present.

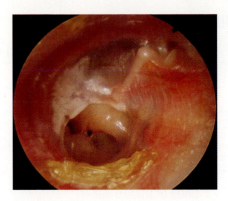

**Figure 10-16** Perforated tympanic membrane. Courtesy of Dr. andrew B. Silva, Pediatric Otolaryngology.

## Otitis Media

Inflammation is the most common disorder of the middle ear. When the infection is of sudden onset and short duration, the diagnosis is **acute**. When the infection is of gradual onset and long duration, the diagnosis is **chronic**. If there is a buildup of a watery fluid in the middle ear, it is known as **serous** (**SEER**-uss) otitis media. If there is a buildup of pus in the middle ear, it is known as **purulent** (**PYOO**-roo-lent) otitis media. Tympanometry is a diagnostic procedure used to determine whether the middle ear is filled with fluid. Antibiotics are the usual treatment. Should they not clear the infection, then a myringotomy is performed to drain the fluid and a tiny tube called a tympanostomy (**tim**-peh-**NOSS**-teh-mee) tube is placed in the eardrum to prevent the fluid from building up.

## Otosclerosis (**oh**-toh-skleh-**ROH**-sis)

A bony formation around the oval window resulting in the inability of the stapes to transmit sound through the oval window and into the inner ear. This results in deafness. Treatment is stapedioplasty.

## Perforated Tympanic Membrane

Rupture of the tympanic membrane (Figure 10-16). It often results in hearing loss. If surgery is necessary to restore hearing loss, the procedure is called tympanoplasty.

## 10.14 Look-Alike and Sound-Alike Words

Below is a list of look-alike and sound-alike words. Study the spelling and definitions of each set of words. Questions will follow in the Review Exercises.

**TABLE 10-1  Look-Alike and Sound-Alike Words**

| | |
|---|---|
| aura | warning signs to the patient that a seizure is starting |
| aural | pertaining to the ear |
| oral | pertaining to the mouth |
| here | the place you are in |
| hear | to hear sound |
| malleus | bone of middle ear |
| malleolus | bony bumps on the lower leg, commonly called the ankle |
| palpable | to feel |
| palpebral | pertaining to the eyelid |
| serious | not joking; causing great harm |
| serous | watery fluid |
| tears | (TEERZ) droplets of fluid that fall from the eye |
| tears | (TAYRZ) holes that develop due to a pulling force |
| tendinitis | inflammation of the tendon |
| tinnitus | ringing in the ears |

## 10.15  Review Exercises

### EXERCISE 10-1  Look-Alike and Sound-Alike Words

*Read the sentences carefully and circle the word in parentheses that correctly completes the meaning. Use Table 10-1 if it helps you.*

1. On (**aural/oral**) examination, the tympanic membrane was red and inflamed.

2. When the tuning fork is placed (**hear/here**), the patient cannot (**hear/here**) the sound.

3. The swelling over the (**malleus/malleolus**) was caused by a sprained ankle.

4. The (**malleus/malleolus**), incus, and stapes are bones in the middle ear.

5. No (**palpable/palpebral**) neck masses; no (**serious/serous**) abnormalities. However, he did have a discharge from his right ear and was admitted with a diagnosis of (**serious/serous**) otitis media.

6. The patient thinks his (**tendonitis/tinnitus**) is caused by loud noises.

## EXERCISE 10-2 Matching Word Parts with Meaning

*Match the word part in Column A with its meaning in Column B.*

| | Column A | Column B |
|---|---|---|
| _____ | **1.** aur/o | A. cornea |
| _____ | **2.** nyct/o | B. lens |
| _____ | **3.** anis/o | C. light |
| _____ | **4.** -ptosis | D. tympanic membrane |
| _____ | **5.** eso- | E. double |
| _____ | **6.** opt/o | F. hearing |
| _____ | **7.** myring/o | G. fear |
| _____ | **8.** dipl/o | H. night |
| _____ | **9.** -phobia | I. vision |
| _____ | **10.** presby- | J. ear |
| _____ | **11.** phot/o | K. eye |
| _____ | **12.** audi/o | L. unequal |
| _____ | **13.** kerat/o | M. drooping |
| _____ | **14.** phac/o | N. inward |
| _____ | **15.** ophthalm/o | O. old age |

## EXERCISE 10-3 Matching—Structure and Function

*Match the structures listed below with its function. Write your answer in the space provided.*

aqueous humor   pupil
cochlea     tympanic membrane
cornea     vestibule
macula lutea   vitreous humor

**1.** maintains intraocular pressure _____

**2.** location of cones in the retina _____

**3.** regulates amount of light entering the eye _____

**4.** maintains shape of eyeball _____

**5.** entry point of light into the eye _____

**6.** transmits sound to the middle ear _____

**7.** function is balance _____

**8.** function is hearing _____

## EXERCISE 10-4   Short Answer—Anatomy and Physiology

*I. Arrange the following structures of the ear so that they indicate the correct sequence in the transmission of sound waves to the brain from the external ear.*

auditory nerve          external auditory meatus          pinna or auricle
brain                         ossicles                              tympanic membrane
cochlea

1. _____

2. _____

3. _____

4. _____

5. _____

6. _____

7. _____

*II. Arrange the following structures of the eye so that they indicate the correct sequence in the transmission of light rays to the brain from the external eye.*

aqueous humor          lens                retina
brain                         optic nerve      vitreous humor
cornea                      pupil

1. _____

2. _____

3. _____

4. _____

5. _____

6. _____

7. _____

8. _____

## EXERCISE 10-5   Labeling—Eye

*Using the body structures listed below, label Figure 10-17. Write your answer in the numbered spaces provided below, or if you prefer, on the diagram.*

choroid _____

ciliary body _____

conjunctiva _____

cornea  _____

iris  _____

lens  _____

macula lutea  _____

optic nerve  _____

pupil  _____

retina  _____

sclera  _____

1. _____

2. _____

3. _____

4. _____

5. _____

6. _____

7. _____

8. _____

9. _____

10. _____

11. _____

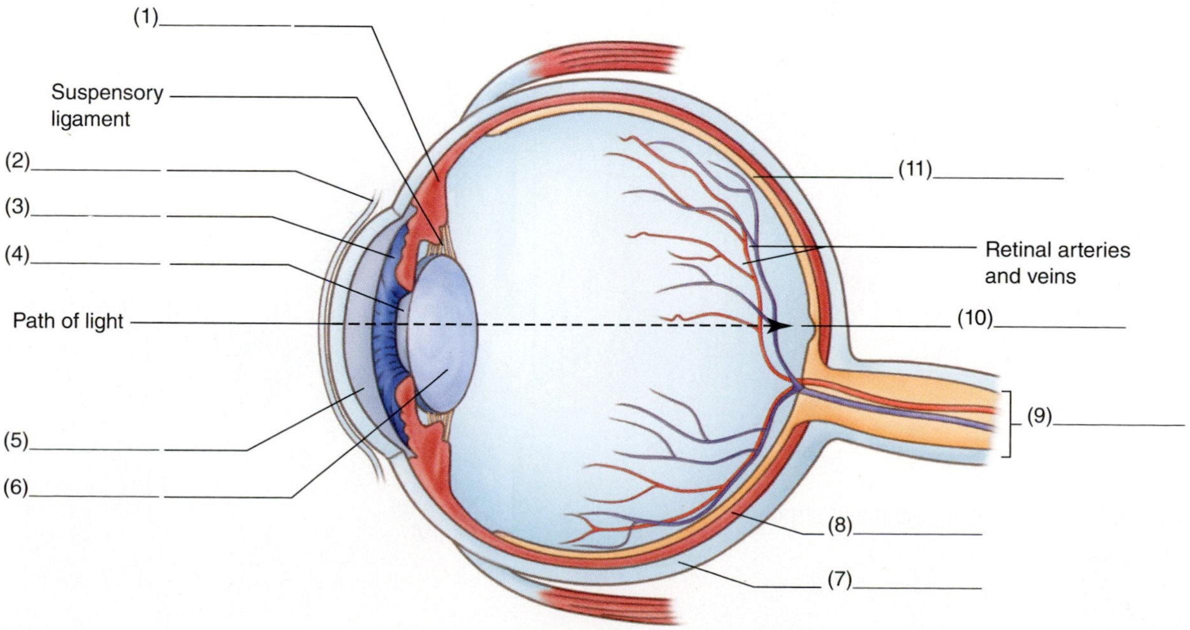

**Figure 10-17**  Labeling the major structures of the eye.

## EXERCISE 10-6   Labeling—Ear

*Using the body structures listed below, label (Figure 10-18). Write your answers in the numbered spaces provided below.*

auricle

cochlea

eustachian tube

external auditory meatus

ossicles

tympanic membrane

1. _____

2. _____

3. _____

4. _____

5. _____

6. _____

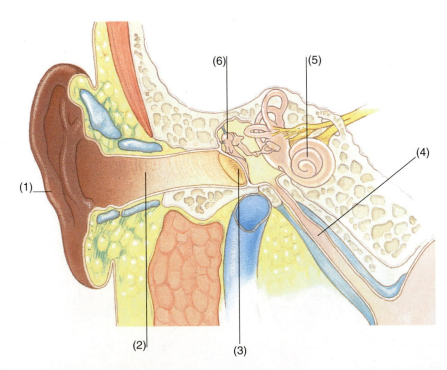

**Figure 10-18** Labeling the major structures of the ear.

**EXERCISE 10-7  Definitions—Pathology**

*Define the following.*

**1. retinal detachment**

_____

_____

_____

**2. serous otitis media**

_____

_____

_____

**3. perforated tympanic membrane**

_____

_____

_____

**4. Meniere disease**

_____

_____

_____

**5. myopia**

_____

_____

_____

**6. astigmatism**

_____

_____

_____

**7. cataracts**

_____

_____

_____

**8. glaucoma**

_____

_____

_____

## EXERCISE 10-8 Definitions—learning the Terms

_Define the following terms._

1. **blepharoptosis** _____

2. **ophthalmoscopy** _____

3. **ophthalmologist** _____

4. **optician** _____

5. **optometrist** _____

6. **aphakia** _____

7. **photophobia** _____

8. **retinopathy** _____

9. **diplopia** _____

10. **presbyopia** _____

11. **esotropia** _____

12. **auditory** _____

13. **aural** _____

14. **audiometry** _____

15. **myringotomy** _____

16. **otorrhea** _____

17. **presbycusis** _____

18. **otalgia** _____

### EXERCISE 10-9  Building Medical Words

*I. Using the suffix -opia, build the medical word meaning:*

    **a.** double vision _____

    **b.** nearsightedness _____

    **c.** dimness of vision _____

    **d.** impaired vision due to old age _____

*II. Using the suffix -tropia, build the medical word meaning:*

    **a.** turning inward of the eyeball _____

    **b.** outward turning of the eyeball _____

*III. Using the root ot/o, build the medical word meaning:*

    **a.** pain in the ear _____

    **b.** discharge from the ear _____

### EXERCISE 10-10  Definitions in Context

*Define the bolded terms in context. Use your medical dictionary if necessary.*

#### Report #1 Discharge Summary

ADMISSION DIAGNOSIS: LEFT **CATARACT** FOR EXTRACTION.

HISTORY: Mrs. Serowan had noted progressive **deteriorating** vision in the right eye over a number of years. Remainder of medical history is unremarkable.

PHYSICAL EXAMINATION: Best corrected **visual acuity** was 20/70 in the right eye.

COURSE IN HOSPITAL: On June 21, **ultrasound** was used to destroy the cataract. A **prosthetic intraocular lens** was inserted. On the first postoperative day, she was discharged home.

    a. **cataract** _____

    b. **deteriorating** _____

    c. **visual acuity** _____

    d. **ultrasound** _____

    e. **prosthetic intraocular lens** _____

Report #2 Operative Report

PREOPERATIVE DIAGNOSIS: **OTITIS MEDIA**.

OPERATION PROPOSED: BILATERAL **MYRINGOTOMY** AND TUBE INSERTION.

POSTOPERATIVE DIAGNOSIS: **RECURRENT** OTITIS MEDIA.

OPERATION PERFORMED: **BILATERAL** MYRINGOTOMY WITH TUBE INSERTION.

OPERATIVE NOTE: The patient was brought to the operating room, placed in the **supine** position, and given a general anesthetic. Using the operative **microscope**, the right **external auditory meatus** was cleaned of a small amount of **cerumen** revealing an abnormal **tympanic membrane** with a buildup of pus-filled material. A myringotomy was performed and the infectious material was suctioned out. A tube was inserted to drain any further fluid buildup. The procedure was then performed on the left side with a similar technique. A buildup of watery fluid was noted. The patient was then taken to the recovery room in good condition.

a. **otitis media** _____

b. **myringotomy** _____

c. **recurrent** _____

d. **bilateral** _____

e. **supine** _____

f. **microscope** _____

g. **external auditory meatus** _____

h. **cerumen** _____

i. **tympanic membrane** _____

### EXERCISE 10-11 Spelling

*Circle any words that are spelled incorrectly in the list below. Then correct the spelling in the space provided*

**1.** tinnitis _____

**2.** maleus _____

**3.** aqueus _____

**4.** glaucoma _____

**5.** vitreus _____

**6.** otorhea _____

**7.** conjunctiva _____

**8.** palpebra _____

**9.** kornea _____

**10.** serumen _____

## Animations

Visit the companion website to view the video on **How We Hear**.
Also watch the following videos: **Cataracts**; **Serous Otitis Media**.

## 10.16  Pronunciation and Spelling

*Listen, read, and study, so you can speak and write.*

1. Listen to each word on the audio file provided on the Student Companion Website.

2. Pronounce each word carefully.

3. Spell each word in the space provided.

| Word | Pronunciation | Spelling |
|------|---------------|----------|
| amblyopia | am-blee-OH-pee-ah | |
| aphakia | ah-FAY-kee-ah | |
| aqueous humor | AY-kwee-us HYOO-mer | |
| audiometry | aw-dee-OM-eh-tree | |
| ametropia | am-eh-TROH-pee-ah | |
| anisocoria | an-iss-oh-KOR-ee-ah | |
| auditory | AW-dih-tor-ee | |
| aural | AW-ral | |
| auricle | AW-rih-kul | |
| blepharoptosis | blef-ah-rop-TOH-sis | |
| cataracts | KAT-ah-rackts | |
| cochlea | KOCK-lee-ah | |
| conjunctivitis | kon-junk-tih-VYE-tiss | |
| corneal abrasion | COR-nee-al ab-RAY-zhun | |
| diplopia | dih-PLOH-pee-ah | |

| Word | Pronunciation | Spelling |
|------|---------------|----------|
| esotropia | **es**-oh-**TROH**-pee-ah | |
| eustachian tube | yoo-**STAY**-shun | |
| exotropia | **eck**-soh-**TROH**-pee-ah | |
| glaucoma | glaw-**KOH**-mah | |
| incus | **INK**-uss | |
| iridectomy | **ir**-ih-**DECK**-toh-mee | |
| iritis | eye-**RYE**-tiss | |
| labyrinthitis | **lab**-ih-rin-**THIGH**-tiss | |
| malleus | **MAL**-ee-uss | |
| Meniere disease | meh-**NYAR** | |
| myopia | my-**OH**-pee-ah | |
| ophthalmologist | **ahf**-thal-**MOL**-eh-jist | |
| ophthalmoscopy | **ahf**-thal-**MOS**-koh-pee | |
| optician | op-**TISH**-an | |
| optometrist | op-**TOM**-eh-trist | |
| otalgia | oh-**TAL**-jee-ah | |
| otitis media | oh-**TYE**-tis **ME**-dee-ah | |
| otorrhea | **oh**-toh-**REE**-ah | |
| palpebral | **PAL**-peh-bral | |
| photophobia | **foh**-toh-**FOH**-bee-ah | |
| presbycusis | **pres**-bih-**KYOO**-sis | |
| presbyopia | **pres**-bee-**OH**-pee-ah | |
| purulent | **PYOO**-roo-lent | |
| retinopathy | **ret**-ih-**NOP**-ah-thee | |
| retinopexy | **RET**-ih-noh-**peck**-see | |
| stapes | **STAY**-peez | |
| tinnitus | **TIN**-ih-tuss | |
| tympanic | tim-**PAN**-ick | |
| tympanoplasty | **tim**-pah-no-**PLAS**-tee | |
| vertigo | **VER**-tih-goh | |
| vestibule | **VESS**-tih-byool | |

## CHAPTER 11

# Digestive System

## Chapter Outline

## Learning Objectives

*After studying this chapter and completing the review exercises, you should be able to:*

1. Name and locate the organs of the digestive system.
2. Describe the structures and functions of the organs of the digestive system.
3. Describe the peritoneum.
4. Pronounce, spell, define, and write the medical terms related to the digestive system.
5. Describe common diseases related to the digestive system.
6. Listen, read, and study so you can speak and write.

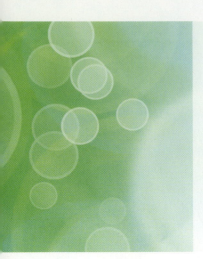

## Introduction

Figure 11-1 shows you the digestive system. The main part is a long tube called the **digestive tract**. It is also known as the **gastrointestinal tract**. It is about 16 feet (5 m) long. It starts at the mouth and ends at the anus. The inside wall is lined with **mucous membrane**, also known as **mucosa** (myoo-**KOSA**).

The digestive tract takes in food. It then breaks it down so that the body can use it. This is called **digestion**. The food molecules then go into the blood and lymph systems. This is called the process of **absorption**. The waste materials that are left continue to the end of the digestive tract and are eliminated.

## 11.1 | Major Organs of the Digestive System

**PRACTICE FOR LEARNING: Major Organs of the Digestive System**

Write the words below in the correct spaces in Figure 11-1. To help you, the number beside the word tells you where it goes on the figure. Be sure to pronounce each word as you write it. Repeat the pronunciation several times if you find the word hard to say.

1. oral cavity (**OR**-al)
2. pharynx (**FAR**-inks)
3. esophagus (eh-**SOF**-ah-gus)
4. stomach (**STUM**-ick)
5. small intestine (in-**TESS**-tine)
6. large intestine (in-**TESS**-tine)
7. rectum (**RECK**-tum)
8. appendix (ah-**PEN**-dicks)
9. pancreas (**PAN**-kree-ass)
10. gallbladder (**GALL**-blad-er)
11. liver (**LIV**-er)
12. salivary gland (**SAL**-ih-vehr-ee)

Figure 11-1 shows you the six regions of the digestive tract. They are the oral cavity (mouth), the pharynx, the esophagus, the stomach, the small intestine, and the large intestine.

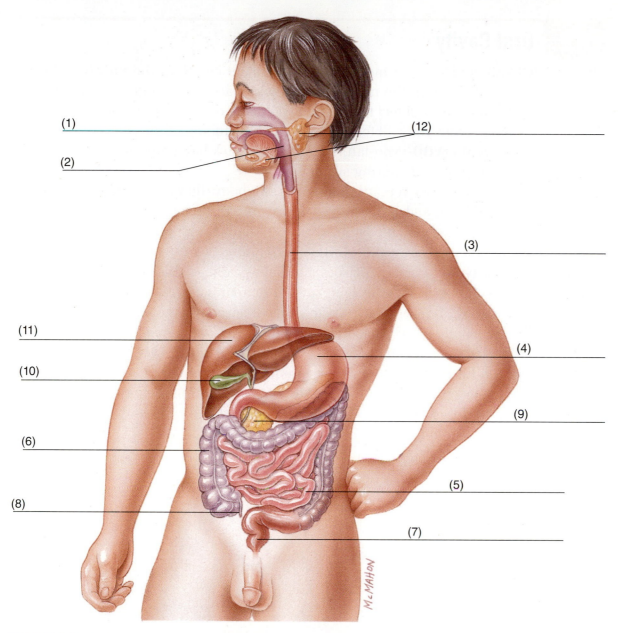

(1)

(2)

(12)

(3)

(11)

(10)

(4)

(9)

(6)

(8)

(5)

(7)

McMAHON

**Figure 11-1**  Major organs of the digestive system.

Four organs connected to the digestive system help out in the process of digestion. They are the salivary glands, the pancreas, the liver, and the gallbladder. Identify them in Figure 11-1.

## 11.2  Oral Cavity

The **oral** (**OR**-al) **cavity** is the mouth. The roof of the mouth is the **palate** (**PAL**-at). It separates the mouth from the nasal cavity. If you place your tongue on the anterior portion of the palate, you will feel the hard palate made of bone. Drag your tongue over the posterior palate, and you will feel the soft palate made up of muscle. At the back of the palate is the **uvula** (**YOO**-vyoo-lah). It looks like a sack hanging from the soft palate. It closes off the nasal passage during swallowing.

The **tongue** is the most versatile muscle in the body. Its primary functions are to provide a sense of taste and to assist in swallowing. It is also very important in the production of speech. The tongue is attached to the bottom of the mouth by a mucous membrane cord called the **frenulum** (**FREN**-yoo-lum).

There are four types of **teeth**: incisors, bicuspids, canines, and molars. Between the ages of 6 months and 2 years, children grow 20 temporary teeth. They are also called deciduous teeth. They are eventually replaced by 32 permanent teeth. At the core of the tooth is **pulp**. It is made up of blood vessels and nerves, which extend into the root of the tooth through the root canal. Covering the pulp is the **dentin** (**DEN**-tin). Around the dentin and above the gums is hard, white **enamel**. The root of the tooth is anchored to bone and held in place by **cementum** (seh-**MEN**-tum). The front teeth tear the food, and the back teeth **masticate** (**MAS**-tih-kayt) or chew food (Figure 11-2).

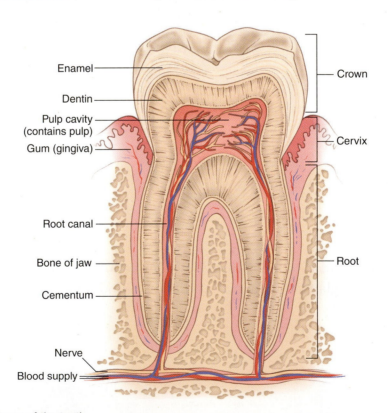

**Figure 11-2**  Structures of the tooth.

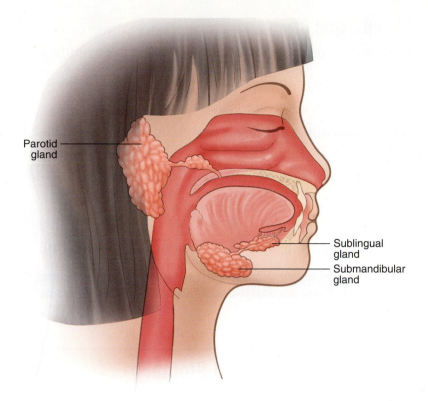

**Figure 11-3**  Salivary glands.

Salivary glands produce saliva. Saliva drains into the oral cavity via salivary ducts. Saliva contains an antibacterial substance that protects the mouth against germs. Saliva also starts the digestion (breakdown) of carbohydrates. There are three pairs of salivary glands: the **parotid** (pah-**ROT**-id), the **submandibular** (**sub**-man-**DIB**-yoo-lar), and **sublingual** (sub-**LING**-gwal) (Figure 11-3).

| **In Brief** | **Oral cavity is the mouth.** |
| --- | --- |
| | **Palate** separates the nasal cavity from the oral cavity. |
| | **Uvula** closes off the nasal passage during swallowing. |
| | **Tongue** is for speech, taste, and swallowing. |
| | **Teeth** are made up of pulp, dentin, and enamel. |
| | Function: mastication. |
| | **Salivary glands:** parotid, submandibular, sublingual. |
| | Function: produce saliva |
| | **Saliva** starts digestion |

**PRACTICE FOR LEARNING: Oral Cavity**

Choose the correct answer or answers from the choices in parentheses.

1. The sac-like structure at the back of the mouth is the (uvea/uvula).
2. The roof of the mouth is the (gingiva/labia/palate).
3. Which of the following is **not** a salivary gland? (submandibular/carotid/parotid).
4. The blood vessels and nerves of the tooth are located in the (dentin/pulp/gums).
5. Deciduous teeth are also known as (permanent/temporary) teeth.
6. The root canal contains (blood vessels/enamel/nerves/dentin).

> Answers: 1. uvula. 2. palate. 3. carotid. 4. pulp. 5. temporary. 6. blood vessels; nerves.

## 11.3  Pharynx, Esophagus, and Stomach

During chewing, the food is mixed with saliva, producing a softened ball of food called a **bolus** (**BO**-lus). The bolus is pushed by the tongue into the throat, or pharynx, which is a 5-inch (12.5-cm) tube. This pushing commences the process of swallowing, which moves the bolus into the esophagus.

The esophagus is a 10-inch (25-cm) tube. It begins at the pharynx, extends to the diaphragm, and passes through an opening in the diaphragm called the **esophageal hiatus** (eh-**sof**-ah-**JEE**-ul high-**AYE**-tus). The esophagus continues through the diaphragm to the stomach. The muscles of the esophagus cause wave-like contractions called **peristaltic** (**per**-ih-**STAL**-tick) **waves**. These waves push the bolus down the esophagus and into the stomach.

As the bolus nears the stomach, it encounters a closed area caused by a tight circular muscle called a **sphincter** (**SFINK**-ter). The sphincter opens to allow the bolus into the stomach and then closes again to prevent stomach contents from reentering the esophagus. The sphincter is called the **lower esophageal sphincter** (**LES**). It is also known as the **cardiac** sphincter or the **gastroesophageal** sphincter. Once the bolus passes through the sphincter into the stomach, the food is broken down by enzymes. It becomes a semiliquid called **chyme** (**KYM**).

The stomach is J-shaped, with four regions: the **cardia** (**KAR**-dee-ah), **fundus** (**FUN**-dus), **body**, and **antrum** (**AN**-trum). The inner lining of mucous membrane consists of a series of folds called **rugae** (**ROO**-jee), which stretch to accommodate food (Figure 11-4).

Food (called chyme at this point) leaves the stomach for the small intestine through another sphincter called the **pyloric** (pie-**LOR**-ick) **sphincter**.

The function of the stomach is to break down food.

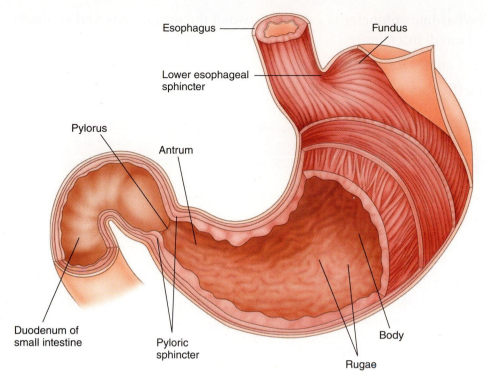

**Figure 11-4** Structures of the stomach.

**In Brief**

**Pharynx** is also known as the throat.

**Peristalsis** pushes the bolus through the esophagus.

**Esophagus** is located between the pharynx and stomach.

**Esophageal hiatus** is a normal opening in the diaphragm.

**Sphincters** are circular muscles that keep food moving in one direction.

**Stomach** regions are the cardia, antrum, body, and fundus.

**Bolus** is a wet ball of food.

**Chyme** is partially digested food.

**Rugae** are folds in stomach.

Function of stomach: breaks down food

## PRACTICE FOR LEARNING: Pharynx, Esophagus, Stomach

Choose the correct answer from the choices in parentheses.

1. Hiatus refers to a(n) (peristaltic wave/muscle/opening).

2. Which of the following is **not** a part of the stomach? (body/ frenulum/rugae/cardia)

3. The esophageal hiatus is located in the (stomach/esophagus/diaphragm).

**4.** The cardiac sphincter is located between the (esophagus and stomach/stomach and small intestine).

**5.** Food enters the small intestine as a semiliquid substance called (bolus/chyme).

**6.** The (fundus/hiatus/sphincter/antrum) is defined as a tight circular muscle.

Answers: 1. opening. 2. frenulum. 3. diaphragm. 4.esophagus and stomach. 5. chyme. 6. sphincter.

## 11.4  Small Intestine

**PRACTICE FOR LEARNING: Small Intestine**

Write the words below in the correct spaces in Figure 11-5. To help you, the number beside the word tells you where it goes on the figure. Be sure to pronounce each word as you write it. Repeat the pronunciation several times if you find the word hard to say.

**1.** duodenum (**doo**-oh-**DEE**-num)

**2.** jejunum (jeh-**JOO**-num)

**3.** ileum (**ILL**-ee-um)

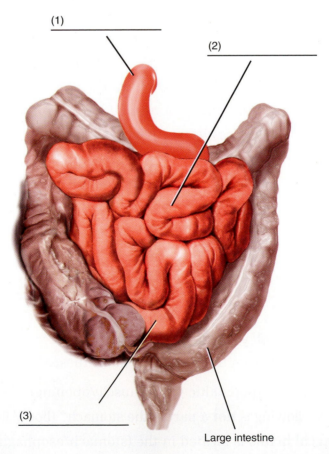

(1) _____

(2) _____

(3) _____

Large intestine

**Figure 11-5** Small intestine.

Figure 11-5 illustrates the small intestine coiled within the abdominopelvic cavity. It is also called the small **bowel**. It is 11 feet (3.35 m) long and has three regions: The duodenum is the proximal (first) section, the jejunum is the middle section, and the ileum is the distal (last) section. The small intestine leads to the large intestine. Although the diameter of the small intestine is only about 1 inch (2.54 cm), it expands to accommodate food as it passes through.

The function of the small intestine is to absorb nutrients from digested food and pass them into the bloodstream. The remaining waste products enter the large intestine.

**In Brief**

**Small intestine**

Includes: duodenum, jejunum, ileum

Function: break down, absorb, and transport foodstuffs

## 11.5   Large Intestine

### PRACTICE FOR LEARNING: Large Intestine

Write the words below in the correct spaces in Figure 11-6. To help you, the number beside the word tells you where it goes on the figure. Be sure to pronounce each word as you write it. Repeat the pronunciation several times if you find the word hard to say.

**1.** appendix (ah-**PEN**-dicks)

**2.** cecum (**SEE**-kum)

**3.** ascending colon (ah-**SEN**-ding **KOH**-lon)

**4.** transverse colon (tranz-**VERS KOH**-lon)

**5.** descending colon (dee-**SEN**-ding **KOH**-lon)

**6.** sigmoid colon (**SIG**-moid **KOH**-lon)

**7.** rectum (**RECK**-tum)

**8.** anal canal (**AY**-nul)

**9.** anus (**AY**-nus)

The large intestine is about 5 feet (1.8 m) long. It is also called the large bowel. As illustrated in Figure 11-6, the large intestine has three regions. First is a pouch called the cecum. The appendix, which has no known function, hangs down from the cecum. The next region is the colon. It forms a long, square arch consisting of four areas: The ascending colon, transverse colon, descending colon, and sigmoid colon. The last region of the large intestine is the rectum. It is about 8 inches long and is lined with mucous folds.

The final segment of the rectum is the anal canal.

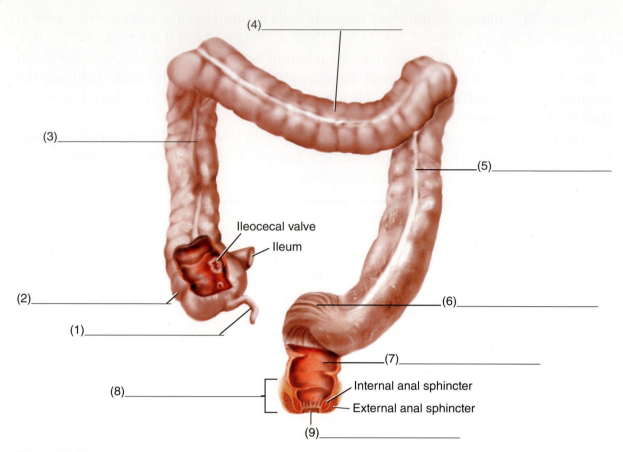

Ileocecal valve

Ileum

Internal anal sphincter

External anal sphincter

**Figure 11-6** Large intestine.

The functions of the large intestine are to absorb water, vitamin K, some B vitamins and **defecation** (**def**-eh-**KAY-**shun), the elimination of wastes.

**In Brief**

**Large intestine**

Includes: cecum, colon, rectum

**Colon**

Includes: ascending colon, transverse colon, descending colon, sigmoid colon

**Bowel** refers to the large and small intestines.

Functions: Defecation

Absorption of water, Vitamin K and B

**PRACTICE FOR LEARNING: Small and Large Intestines**

Choose the correct answer from the choices in parentheses:

1. Food leaves the stomach and enters the (jejunum/duodenum/ileum).

2. The small **and** large intestines are also known as (bowel/colon/peritoneum).

3. A function of the large intestine is (mastication/defecation).

4. The transverse colon is part of the (small/large) intestine.

5. The duodenum is part of the (small/large) intestine.

6. A function of the small intestine is (mastication/defecation/absorption) of nutrients.

7. The appendix is located on the _____ side of the abdomen.

> Answers: 1. duodenum. 2. bowel. 3. defecation. 4. large intestine. 5. small intestine. 6. absorption. 7. right.

## 11.6  Liver, Gallbladder, Biliary Ducts, and Pancreas

The liver weighs about 4 pounds (1.75 kg). It is located below the diaphragm in the right upper quadrant (RUQ) of the abdomen (Figure 11-7). The liver has many functions, including the production of bile; elimination of toxic substances; and breakdown of proteins, fats, and carbohydrates (CHO).

The biliary tract includes the liver, the gallbladder (GB), and the biliary ducts. The biliary ducts include the hepatic ducts, the common hepatic duct, the cystic duct, and the common bile duct (CBD) (Figure 11-7).

Bile is a greenish-yellow fluid produced in the liver. Look at the bile ducts in Figure 11-7. Bile goes from the liver through the right and left hepatic ducts, through the common hepatic duct, and into the cystic duct, which leads to the gallbladder. Bile is stored in the gallbladder. The function of bile is to break down fats in the duodenum. When bile is required, it travels through the cystic duct and into the common bile duct (CBD) where the common hepatic and cystic ducts meet. The CBD drains into the duodenum.

The liver is essential to life. However, the gallbladder may be surgically removed without too much disruption to body function. After removal of the gallbladder, the bile may be stored in the biliary ducts, and biliary processes proceed normally.

The pancreas is illustrated in Figure 11-7. It is a long, fish-shaped organ lying behind the stomach. It secretes pancreatic juice, which contains enzymes to break down food in the duodenum.

The pancreas also secretes the hormones **insulin** (**IN**-suh-lin) and **glucagon** (**GLOO**-kah-gon). These hormones work together to regulate the amount of sugar in the bloodstream. See Chapter 19, under Pancreas, for details of sugar regulation.

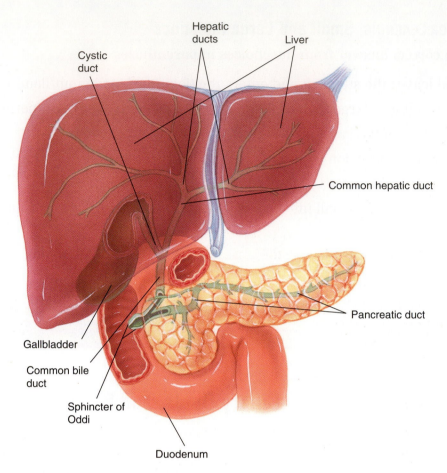

**Figure 11-7**  Liver, gallbladder, pancreas, and biliary tract.

**In Brief**

**Liver**

Location: RUQ

Functions: produces bile; breaks down proteins, carbohydrates, and fats; eliminates toxic waste

**Gallbladder**

Location: Under the liver

Function: Stores bile

**Pancreas**

Location: Lies behind the stomach

Function: Secretes enzymes and hormones

## 11.7   Peritoneum

Figure 11-8 illustrates the **peritoneum** (**per**-ih-toh-**NEE**-um). It is a membrane lining the abdominopelvic cavity and covering the abdominopelvic organs. It has two layers. The space between the two layers is called the **peritoneal** (**per**-ih-toh-**NEE**-al) **cavity**. It is filled with peritoneal fluid, a watery substance that prevents friction between the two layers.

**In Brief**

**Peritoneum**

Membrane lining the abdominal and pelvic cavities and covering its organs

Peritoneal fluid fills the peritoneal cavity.

PRACTICE FOR LEARNING: **Biliary Tract and the Peritoneum**

Choose the correct answer from the choices in parentheses:

1. The hepatic ducts carry bile from the (gallbladder/liver).
2. A greenish-yellow fluid stored in the gallbladder is (glucagon/bile).
3. The (pancreas/liver) regulates blood sugar.

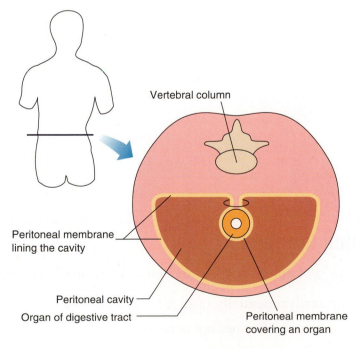

**Figure 11-8**  Peritoneal membrane.

**4.** The peritoneum lines the (thoracic/abdominal) cavity.

**5.** Fats are broken down by (bile/insulin) in the (duodenum/liver).

Answers: 1. liver. 2. bile. 3. pancreas. 4. abdominal. 5. bile; duodenum.

## 11.8   New Roots, Suffixes, and Prefixes

Use these additional roots, suffixes, and prefixes when studying the medical terms in this chapter.

| ROOT | MEANING |
|---|---|
| aer/o | air |
| cec/o | cecum (first portion of the large intestine) |
| intestin/o | intestine |

| SUFFIX | MEANING |
|---|---|
| -aise | ease |
| -flux | flow |
| -hexia | habit |
| -tripsy | crushing |
| -y | process; condition |

| PREFIX | MEANING |
|---|---|
| meso- | middle |
| re- | back |

## 11.9   Learning the Terms

Following these steps will make it easier for you to learn medical terms:

**1.** Pronounce the term repeatedly until it is easy for you.

**2.** Write it down. Ensure the spelling is correct.

**3.** Also write the definition. If possible, relate the word to a word, thought, or picture that will help you remember it.

**4.** Analyze the term with the method taught in this text.

## Roots

| ROOT append/o; appendic/o | | MEANING appendix |
|---|---|---|
| Term | Term Analysis | Definition |
| appendicitis (ah-**pen**-dih-**SIGH**-tis) | -itis = inflammation | inflammation of the appendix |

| ROOT bucc/o | | MEANING cheek |
|---|---|---|
| Term | Term Analysis | Definition |
| buccal mucosa (**BUCK**-ahl myoo-**KOH**-sa) | -al = pertaining to  mucosa = mucous membrane | pertaining to the mucous membrane of the cheek |

| ROOT cac/o (see mal-) | | MEANING bad |
|---|---|---|
| Term | Term Analysis | Definition |
| cachexia (kah-**KECK**-see-ah) | -hexia = habit | state of ill health and malnutrition; wasting away of muscle; emaciation (ee-**may**-she-**AY**-shun)  Cachexia is associated with severe cancers. |

| ROOT cholangi/o | | MEANING bile duct; bile vessel |
|---|---|---|
| Term | Term Analysis | Definition |
| cholangiogram (koh-**LAN**-jee-**oh**-gram) | -gram = record | record (image) of the bile ducts produced by x-rays |

| ROOT cholecyst/o | | MEANING gallbladder |
|---|---|---|
| Term | Term Analysis | Definition |
| cholecystectomy (**koh**-lee-sis-**TECK**-toh-mee) | -ectomy = excision; surgical removal | excision of the gallbladder |
| cholecystitis (**koh**-lee-sis-**TYE**-tis) | -itis = inflammation | inflammation of the gallbladder |

| ROOT choledoch/o | | MEANING common bile duct |
| --- | --- | --- |
| Term | Term Analysis | Definition |
| choledochotomy (**koh**-led-oh-**KOT**-oh-mee) | -tomy = to cut into; incision; process of cutting | incision into the common bile duct |

| ROOT col/o | | MEANING colon |
| --- | --- | --- |
| Term | Term Analysis | Definition |
| colitis (koh-**LYE**-tis) | -itis = inflammation | inflammation of the colon |
| colic (**KOLL**-ick) | -ic = pertaining to | severe abdominal pain; pertaining to the colon |

**Helping You Remember**

The roots *chol/e* and *col/o* are often confused. They are pronounced the same but have entirely different meanings: *chol/e* means gall and *col/o* means colon. Therefore, the term for inflammation of the gallbladder is spelled <u>chol</u>ecystitis, not <u>col</u>ecystitis.

| ROOT enter/o | | MEANING small intestine; intestine |
| --- | --- | --- |
| Term | Term Analysis | Definition |
| gastroenteritis (**gas**-troh-**en**-ter-**EYE**-tis) | -itis = inflammation<br>gastr/o = stomach | inflammation of the stomach and intestines often accompanied by nausea (a sick feeling) and vomiting |
| mesentery (**MEZ**-en-**ter**-ee) | meso- = middle | membrane attaching the intestines to the posterior abdominal wall. The mesentery is situated in the middle of the intestines. It holds the intestines in place. |

| ROOT gastr/o | | MEANING stomach |
|---|---|---|
| *Term* | *Term Analysis* | *Definition* |
| gastroenterologist (**gas**-troh-**en**-ter-**OL**-oh-jist) | -ist = specialist<br>enter/o = intestine | specialist in the study and treatment of diseases of the digestive tract |
| gastroesophageal reflux disease (GERD) (**gas**-troh-eh-**sof**-ah-**JEE**-ul **REE**-flucks) | -eal = pertaining to<br>esophag/o = esophagus<br>-flux = flow<br>re- = back | backward flow of stomach contents into the esophagus<br>When this happens, the esophageal mucosa (mucous membrane) is damaged by the acid from the stomach. |
| nasogastric intubation (**nay**-zo-**GAS**-trick **in**-too-**BAY**-shun) | -ic = pertaining to<br>nas/o = nose<br>intubation = insertion of a tube into a body cavity or canal | placement of a tube through the nose and into the stomach for feeding purposes |

| ROOT gingiv/o | | MEANING gums; gingival |
|---|---|---|
| *Term* | *Term Analysis* | *Definition* |
| gingivitis (**jin**-jih-**VYE**-tis) | -itis = inflammation | inflamed gums |

**Helping You Remember**   Inflammation is spelled with two "m's." Inflamed is spelled with one "m."

| ROOT gloss/o (see also lingu/o) | | MEANING tongue |
|---|---|---|
| *Term* | *Term Analysis* | *Definition* |
| glossitis (glos-**EYE**-tis) | -itis = inflammation | inflammation of the tongue |

| ROOT hepat/o | | MEANING liver |
|---|---|---|
| Term | Term Analysis | Definition |
| hepatitis (hep-ah-TYE-tis) | -itis = inflammation | inflammation of the liver |

**Helping You Remember**

Do not confuse *ile/o*, which means "intestine," with *ili/o*, which means "hip." To remember, think of the "e" in ile/o corresponding to the "e" in intestine and the "i" in ili/o corresponding to the "i" in hip.

| ROOT ile/o | | MEANING ileum(distal portion of the small intestine) |
|---|---|---|
| Term | Term Analysis | Definition |
| ileectomy (ill-ee-ECK-toh-mee) | -ectomy = excision; surgical removal | excision of the ileum |
| ileocecal junction (il-ee-oh-SEE-kal) | -al = pertaining to cec/o = cecum | pertaining to the area where the ileum joins the cecum |

| ROOT labi/o | | MEANING lips |
|---|---|---|
| Term | Term Analysis | Definition |
| labial (LAY-bee-al) | -al = pertaining to | pertaining to the lips |

| ROOT lapar/o | | MEANING abdomen |
|---|---|---|
| Term | Term Analysis | Definition |
| laparoscope (LAP-ah-roh-skohp) | -scope = instrument used to visually examine | instrument used to visually examine the inside of the abdomen |

| ROOT | | MEANING |
| --- | --- | --- |
| **lingu/o** | | **tongue** |
| *Term* | *Term Analysis* | *Definition* |
| **sublingual** (sub-**LING**-gwal) | -al = pertaining to<br>sub- = under | pertaining to under the tongue |

| ROOT | | MEANING |
| --- | --- | --- |
| **lith/o** | | **stone; calculus** |
| *Term* | *Term Analysis* | *Definition* |
| **lithotripsy** (**LITH**-oh-**trip**-see) | -tripsy = crushing | crushing of gallstones into pebbles tiny enough to be eliminated without surgical removal |

| ROOT | | MEANING |
| --- | --- | --- |
| **orex/o** | | **appetite** |
| *Term* | *Term Analysis* | *Definition* |
| **anorexia** (**an**-oh-**RECK**-see-ah) | -ia = condition<br>an- = no; not; lack of | loss of appetite |

**Helping You Remember**

Do not confuse anorexia with anorexia nervosa.

Anorexia is a loss of appetite due to an underlying condition.

Anorexia nervosa is a psychological eating disorder of self-starvation.

| ROOT | | MEANING |
| --- | --- | --- |
| **or/o (see also stomat/o)** | | **mouth** |
| *Term* | *Term Analysis* | *Definition* |
| **oral** (**OR**-al) | -al = pertaining to | pertaining to the mouth |

| ROOT stomat/o; stom/o | | MEANING mouth |
|---|---|---|
| Term | Term Analysis | Definition |
| stomatitis (sto-mah-TYE-tis) | -itis = inflammation | inflammation of the mouth |
| xerostomia (zeer-oh-STOH-me-ah) | -ia = condition xer/o = dry | dryness of the mouth due to a dysfunction of the salivary glands, as they fail to produce sufficient saliva. Often seen as a side effect to medication. |

## Suffixes

| SUFFIX -emesis | | MEANING vomiting |
|---|---|---|
| Term | Term Analysis | Definition |
| hyperemesis (high-per-EM-eh-sis) | hyper- = excessive; above normal | excessive vomiting |
| hematemesis (hee-mah-TEM-eh-sis) | hemat/o = blood | vomiting of blood |
| melanemesis (mel-ah-NEM-eh-sis) | melan/o = black | black vomit. The vomit looks like coffee grounds because food mixes with the blood. |

| SUFFIX -pepsia | | MEANING digestion |
|---|---|---|
| Term | Term Analysis | Definition |
| dyspepsia (dis-PEP-see-ah) | dys- = difficult; painful; bad | indigestion |

| SUFFIX -phagia | | MEANING eating; swallowing |
|---|---|---|
| Term | Term Analysis | Definition |
| aerophagia (ayr-oh-FAY-jee-ah) | aer/o = air | excessive swallowing of air while drinking or eating. This causes abdominal distention and eructation (eh-ruck-TAY-shun). Commonly known as burping.<br><br>In some cases, flatulence (FLAT-yoo-lence) may be present. This is the passage of gas through the digestive tract. |
| aphagia (ah-FAY-jee-ah) | a- = no; not; lack of | inability to swallow |
| dysphagia (dis-FAY-jee-ah) | dys- = difficult; painful; bad | difficulty in swallowing |
| polyphagia (pol-ee-FAY-jee-ah) | poly- = many | excessive eating |

| SUFFIX -stomy | | MEANING surgical creation of a new opening |
|---|---|---|
| Term | Term Analysis | Definition |
| colostomy (koh-LOSS-toh-mee) | col/o = colon | surgical creation of a new opening between the colon and the abdominal wall. Wastes are then eliminated through this opening. Can be temporary or permanent (Figure 11-9). |

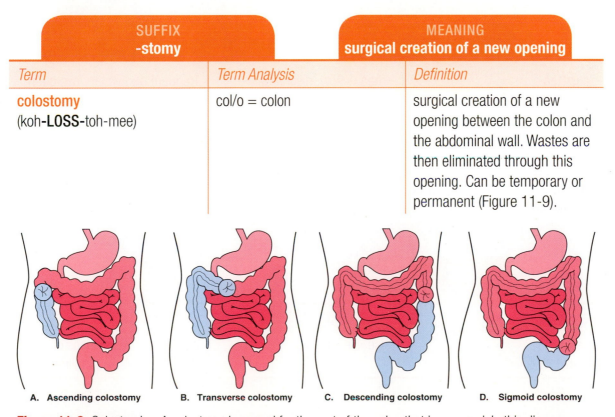

A. Ascending colostomy    B. Transverse colostomy    C. Descending colostomy    D. Sigmoid colostomy

**Figure 11-9** Colostomies: A colostomy is named for the part of the colon that is removed. In this diagram, the areas of intestine that are removed are shown in blue.

| Term | Term Analysis | Definition |
|------|---------------|------------|
| **ileostomy** (**ill**-ee-**OS**-toh-mee) | ile/o = ileum; distal portion of small intestine | surgical creation of a new opening between the ileum and abdominal wall. Wastes are eliminated through this new opening. |
| **duodenojejunostomy** (**doo**-oh-**dee**-no-jay-joon-**OSS**-teh-mee) | duoden/o = duodenum; proximal portion of small intestine jejun/o = jejunum; middle portion of small intestine | surgical creation of a new opening between the duodenum and jejunum |

**Note:** The joining of two structures inside the body that are normally separate is called **anastomosis** (ah-**nas**-teh-**MOH**-sis). Duodenojejunostomy is an anastomosis between the duodenum and jejunum. When a new opening is made between two or more organs, both word roots are used in the medical term. Compare this with ileostomy. In this procedure, the ileum is attached to the abdominal wall, not another organ, so only one combining form is used.

## Prefixes

| PREFIX **dia-** | | MEANING **through; complete** |
|------|---------------|------------|
| Term | Term Analysis | Definition |
| **diarrhea** (**dye**-ah-**REE**-ah) | -rrhea = flow; discharge | frequent and watery excretion of stool. Stool is the waste products eliminated from the body. Stool is also known as feces (**FEE-s**eez). |

**Note:** When a person has no control over when feces are discharged, they are said to be **incontinent** (in-**KON**-tih-nent).

| PREFIX **mal-** | | MEANING **bad** |
|------|---------------|------------|
| Term | Term Analysis | Definition |
| **malaise** (mah-**LAYZ**) | -aise = ease | a feeling of uneasiness or discomfort. A sign of illness. |

## 11.10 | Pathology

### Cholecystolithiasis (koh-leh-sis-toh-lih-THIGH-eh-sis) or cholelithiasis (koh-leh-lih-THIGH-eh-sis)

Calculi (stones) in the gallbladder are commonly called gallstones. If the calculi are located in the common bile duct, the condition is called **choledocholithiasis** (koh-**led**-eh-koh-lih-**THIGH**-eh-sis) (Figure 11-10). Treatment includes **laparoscopic** (**lap**-ah-roh-**skop**-ick) **cholecystectomy**, which removes the gallbladder through a small, minimally invasive incision or an **open cholecystectomy**, which removes the gallbladder through a larger, more invasive abdominal incision.

### Cirrhosis of the Liver

Cirrhosis (sih-**ROH**-sis) is a chronic degeneration of liver cells caused by alcoholism or hepatitis B or C. As the liver degenerates, normal hepatic cells become scarred and replaced with fat giving the liver a yellowish color (*cirrh/o* means "yellow").

Chronic liver damage results in abnormalities throughout the body such as high blood pressure, **jaundice** (yellow appearance of the skin), **ascites** (eh-**SIGH**-teez) (accumulation of fluid [edema] in the abdomen), and **edema** in the legs.

### Cleft Palate and Cleft Lip

**Cleft palate** is a birth defect in which the hard and/or soft palate fails to close during development. Because the nasal cavity is no longer separated from the oral cavity, eating

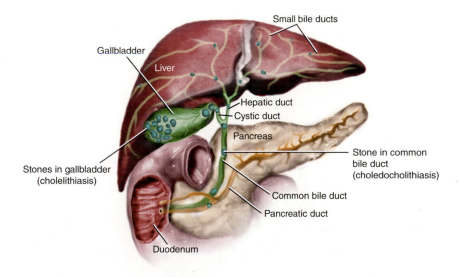

**Figure 11-10** Stones in the gallbladder and bile ducts.

and speaking are difficult. Treatment is surgical reconstruction of the palate. This is called **palatoplasty** (**pal**-ah-toh-**PLAS**-tee).

**Cleft lip** is a birth defect where both sides of the lip fail to join completely. It is also known as **harelip**. This results in an opening in the upper lip. This opening can be a small slit or can be a large opening extending toward the nose. The opening can be on one or both sides of the lip. Cleft lip and cleft palate can occur together or singly. They both can be corrected surgically.

## Crohn (KROHN) Disease

Crohn disease (CD) is a form of inflammatory bowel disease that can involve any part of the digestive tract. It is most often found in the ileum. The inflammation causes obstruction of intestinal contents.

In severe cases, the diseased bowel is removed and an artificial opening is created between the intestine and abdominal wall. (See colostomy in Section 11.9, Learning the Terms). If the artificial opening is between the colon and abdominal wall, the operation is called a **colostomy** (koh-**LOSS**-toh-mee). If the artificial opening is between the ileum and abdominal wall, the operation is called an **ileostomy** (**ill**-ee-**OSS**-toh-mee).

## Diverticulosis

Pocket(s) in the mucous membrane may occur at any point along the stomach and small and large intestines (Figure 11-11). One pocket is called a **diverticulum** (**dye**-ver-**TICK**-yoo-lum). The plural is **diverticula** (**dye**-ver-**TICK**-you-lah). **Diverticulosis** (**dye**-ver-**tick**-yoo-**LOH**-sis) describes a condition of many diverticula.

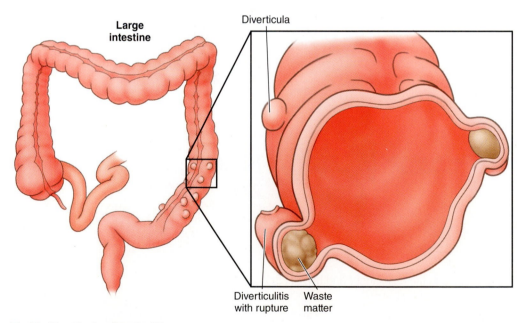

**Figure 11-11** Diverticula, diverticulitis.

Bacteria and bits of food are easily trapped in the diverticulum. This can cause inflammation, a condition called **diverticulitis** (**dye**-ver-**TICK**-yoo-**lye**-tiss).

Diverticulosis is often asymptomatic (no symptoms). However, sometimes it leads to diverticular bleeding, which can result in serious loss of blood. Also, if chronic diverticulitis does not respond to treatment, surgery may be necessary to remove the affected bowel.

## Hemorrhoids

Varicose veins in the anal canal. Varicose veins means the veins are dilated (widened) and filled with blood. Depending upon the location within the anus, they are called internal or external. Surgical treatment is **hemorrhoidectomy** (**hem**-ah-royd-**ECK**-teh-mee).

## Hernia

A protrusion or displacement of an organ through a structure that normally holds it in place. Herniae of the digestive tract occur when the abdominal muscles are unable to hold the intestines in place because of a weakness. The weakness can be congenital (present at birth) or acquired from lifting heavy objects or straining on defecation.

An **inguinal hernia** occurs when a small portion of bowel is displaced into the groin area (Figure 11-12A).

A **hiatal hernia** involves the displacement of the stomach through the hiatal opening in the diaphragm. (Figure 11-12B).

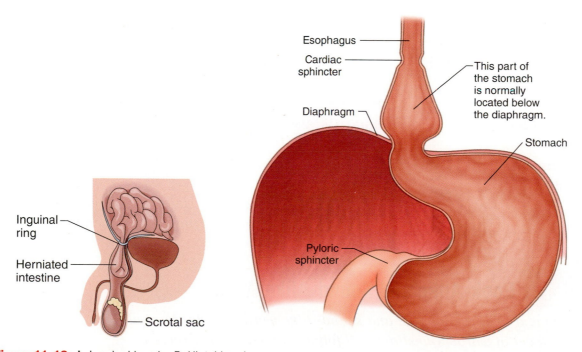

**Figure 11-12** A. Inguinal hernia. B. Hiatal hernia.

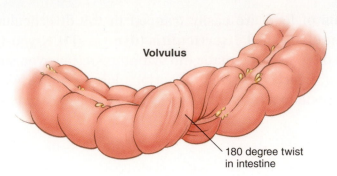

**Figure 11-13** Intestinal obstruction: Volvulus is a twisting of the bowel on itself.

## Intestinal Obstruction

Failure of the contents of the digestive tract to move toward the rectum because of a blockage. Several reasons for obstruction include:

- **Adhesions**, scar tissue that forms between organs and abdominal tissues causing them to stick together
- **Ileus** (**ILL**-ee-us), the temporary loss of peristalsis along the small intestine
- **Intussusception** (**in**-tuh-suh-**SEP**-shun), a telescoping of one segment of bowel into another
- **Volvulus** (**VOL**-vyoo-lus), a twisting of the intestine (Figure 11-13)

## Ulcers

Wearing away of the mucous membrane lining the digestive tract. This creates an open sore. The ulcer can literally eat a hole through the mucous membrane, causing bleeding to the digestive tract. This can result in complications such as hematemesis or **melanemesis**. It can also result in the passage of black or tarry stool, which is called **melena** (meh-**LEE**-nah). Ulcers are named after their location.

    **Aphthous** (**AFF**-thuss) **stomatitis** are ulcers in the mouth, also called **canker** sores.

    **Peptic** (**PEP**-tick) **ulcers** are of the stomach or duodenum. Also known as gastric or duodenal ulcers respectively.

    Antibiotics are used to treat ulcers caused by the bacteria *Helicobacter pylori*. Other drug treatment includes antacids and agents that protect the mucous membrane lining.

## 11.11   Look-Alike and Sound-Alike Words

*Below is a list of look-alike and sound-alike words. Study the spelling and definitions of each set of words. Questions will follow in the Review Exercises.*

## TABLE 11-1  Look-Alike and Sound-Alike Words

| | |
|---|---|
| **acidic** | pertaining to an acid |
| **acetic** | sour |
| **ascitic** | pertaining to ascites (accumulation of fluid in the abdomen) |
| **aphagia** | inability to swallow |
| **aphasia** | inability to speak or write |
| **aplasia** | lack of development |
| **cirrhosis** | a liver disease |
| **scirrhous** | pertaining to a hard cancerous tumor |
| **dysphagia** | difficulty swallowing |
| **dysphasia** | difficulty speaking |
| **hepatoma** | tumor of the liver |
| **hematoma** | bruise |
| **ingestion** | taking food or liquid into the body |
| **injection** | the placement of a substance into the body via a needle |
| **ileum** | the distal portion of the small intestine |
| **ilium** | the hip bone |
| **labial** | pertaining to the lip |
| **labile** | unstable |
| **liver** | large organ of the digestive system |
| **livor** | discoloration on different parts of the body after death |
| **palate** | roof of the mouth |
| **pallet** | a moveable platform for transporting objectives |
| **palette** | a thin board with a thumb holes, used by artists to mix their paint |
| **pellet** | a small round ball of food |
| **reflux** | to flow backward |
| **reflex** | involuntary response to a stimulus |

## 11.12 Review Exercises

### EXERCISE 11-1 Look-Alike and Sound-Alike Words

*Read the sentences carefully and circle the word in parentheses that correctly completes the meaning. Use Table 11-1 if it helps you.*

1. On examination of the gastrointestinal tract, there were no signs of (**dysphasia/ dysphagia**), nausea, vomiting, or hematemesis. However, on neurological exam some (**aphasia/aphagia**) was noted due to the stroke.

2. She complained of tiredness and malaise as well as symptoms of (**reflux/reflex**) and heartburn.

3. Chronic hepatitis and (**cirrhosis/scirrhous**) are possible (**liver/livor**) diseases. Suggest (**liver/livor**) biopsy.

4. The physician's impression was that a (**cirrhosis/scirrhous**) mass was in the distal (**ileum/ilium**).

5. This patient has been admitted with dyspeptic symptoms due to multiple drug (**ingestions/injections**).

6. She has no abdominal distention, vomiting, (**acidic/ascitic**) regurgitation, or dyspepsia.

7. The disease is characterized by enlarged lips and enlarged (**labial/labile**) glands.

8. The patient was admitted with a large (**hepatoma/hematoma**) due to multiple wounds to the neck and back.

### EXERCISE 11-2 Matching Word Parts With Meaning

*I. Match the word part in Column A with its meaning in Column B.*

| | Column A | Column B |
|---|---|---|
| _____ | **1.** -tripsy | A. gallbladder |
| _____ | **2.** cholecyst/o | B. common bile duct |
| _____ | **3.** stomat/o | C. gums |
| _____ | **4.** -flux | D. crushing |
| _____ | **5.** cholangi/o | E. lips |
| _____ | **6.** lapar/o | F. mouth |
| _____ | **7.** choledoch/o | G. liver |
| _____ | **8.** hepat/o | H. bile duct |
| _____ | **9.** gingiv/o | I. flow |
| _____ | **10.** labi/o | J. abdomen |

*II. Match the word part in Column A with its meaning in Column B.*

| Column A | Column B |
|----------|----------|
| _____ **1.** bucc/o | A. new opening |
| _____ **2.** cac/o | B. black |
| _____ **3.** –emesis | C. dry |
| _____ **4.** xer/o | D. cheek |
| _____ **5.** aer/o | E. flow; discharge |
| _____ **6.** -stomy | F. bad |
| _____ **7.** -hexia | G. mouth |
| _____ **8.** -rrhea | H. vomiting |
| _____ **9.** melan/o | I. air |
| _____ **10.** stom/o | J. habit |

## EXERCISE 11-3 Matching—Pathology

*I. Match the disease in Column A with its description in Column B.*

| Column A | Column B |
|----------|----------|
| _____ **1.** cholelithiasis | A. inflammatory bowel disease |
| _____ **2.** hernia | B. wearing away of the mucous membrane lining the digestive tract |
| _____ **3.** melanemesis | C. inflammation of the gums |
| _____ **4.** gingivitis | D. stones in the gallbladder |
| _____ **5.** Crohn disease | E. black vomit |
| _____ **6.** ulcer | F. displacement of an organ through a structure that normally contains it |

*II. Match the disease in Column A with its description in Column B.*

| Column A | Column B |
|----------|----------|
| _____ **1.** diverticula | A. abdominal edema |
| _____ **2.** hemorrhoids | B. displacement of intestine into the groin |
| _____ **3.** hiatal hernia | C. involves the salivary glands |
| _____ **4.** ascites | D. passage of bloody stools |
| _____ **5.** inguinal hernia | E. temporary loss of peristalsis |
| _____ **6.** ileus | F. displacement of stomach through an opening in the diaphragm |
| _____ **7.** xerostomia | G. varicose veins in anal canal |
| _____ **8.** melena | H. abnormal pockets in the mucous membrane of the stomach or bowel |

**EXERCISE 11-4  Labeling—Digestive Tract**

*Using the body structures listed below, label Figure 11-14. Write your answer in the numbered spaces provided below, or if you prefer, on the diagram.*

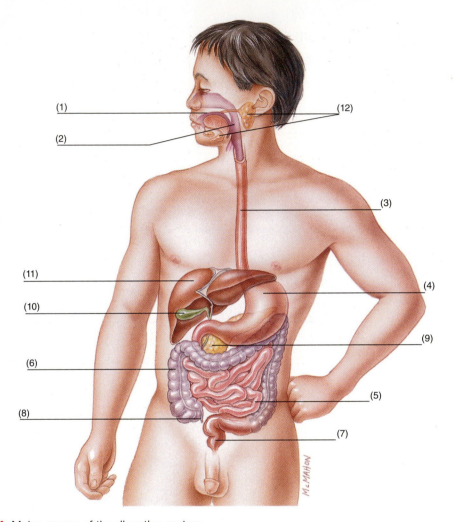

**Figure 11-14** Major organs of the digestive system.

appendix

esophagus

gallbladder

large intestine

liver

oral cavity

pancreas

pharynx _____

rectum _____

salivary gland _____

small intestine _____

stomach _____

1. _____

2. _____

3. _____

4. _____

5. _____

6. _____

7. _____

8. _____

9. _____

10. _____

11. _____

12. _____

## EXERCISE 11-5  Definitions—Anatomy and Physiology

*I. Define the following anatomical terms. Use your medical dictionary if necessary.*

1. **oral cavity** _____

2. **pharynx** _____

3. **duodenum** _____

4. **cecum** _____

5. **gallbladder** _____

  **6. bowel** _____

  **7. jejunum** _____

  **8. biliary tract** _____

  **9. cardiac sphincter** _____

**10. gingiva** _____

*II. Write the function of the following anatomical structures:*

  **1. small intestine** _____

  **2. bile** _____

  **3. large intestine** _____

  **4. esophagus** _____

  **5. saliva** _____

  **6. insulin** _____

  **7. cementum** _____

  **8. pharynx** _____

  **9. teeth** _____

**10. cardiac sphincter** _____

## EXERCISE 11-6   Definitions—Learning the Terms

*Define the following terms.*

  **1. glossitis** _____

  **2. anorexia** _____

  **3. colic** _____

  **4. colostomy** _____

  **5. malaise** _____

  **6. dyspepsia** _____

  **7. gastroesophageal reflux** _____

  **8. hyperemesis** _____

  **9. sublingual** _____

**10. lithotripsy** _____

## EXERCISE 11-7  Building Medical Words

*I. Use lith/o to build medical words for the following definitions.*

   **a.** condition of stones in the gallbladder _____

   **b.** condition of stones in the common bile ducts _____

   **c.** crushing of gallstones _____

*II. Use -emesis to build medical words for the following definitions.*

   **a.** excessive vomiting _____

   **b.** vomiting of blood _____

   **c.** black vomit _____

*III. Use -phagia to build medical words for the following definitions.*

   **a.** no eating _____

   **b.** difficulty in eating _____

   **c.** excessive eating _____

*IV. Use -itis to build medical words for the following definitions*

   **a.** inflammation of the appendix _____

   **b.** inflammation of the gallbladder _____

   **c.** inflammation of the colon _____

   **d.** inflammation of the stomach and intestines _____

   **e.** inflammation of the gums _____

   **f.** inflammation of the tongue _____

   **g.** inflammation of the liver _____

   **h.** inflammation of the mouth _____

*V. Use –stomy to build medical words for the following definitions*

   **a.** surgical creation of a new opening into the colon _____

   **b.** surgical creation of a new opening into the ileum _____

   **c.** surgical creation of a new opening between the first and second portion of the small intestine _____

## EXERCISE 11-8  Definitions in Context

*Define the bolded terms in context. Use your medical dictionary if necessary.*

1. The patient had an **x-ray** while in the emergency department that showed a normal **pharynx**, esophagus, stomach, and **duodenum**.

   **a.** x-ray _____

   **b.** pharynx _____

   **c.** duodenum _____

2. On his last admission, a **colonoscopy** showed worsening of his **Crohn disease**. He also had a **gastroscopy** showing mild **gastritis** but no **ulcer disease**.

   **d.** colonoscopy _____

   **e.** Crohn disease _____

   **f.** gastroscopy _____

   **g.** gastritis _____

   **h.** ulcer disease _____

3. The patient was admitted with **epigastric pain**, at which time she was diagnosed with **cholecystolithiasis**. We therefore decided to proceed with a **cholecystectomy**.

   **i.** epigastric pain _____

   **j.** cholecystolithiasis _____

   **k.** cholecystectomy _____

4. He has no visible **emesis** or **gastroesophageal reflux**.

   **l.** emesis _____

   **m.** gastroesophageal reflux _____

5. There was no **dysphagia**, **nausea**, **malaise**, or **hematemesis**.

   **n.** dysphagia _____

   **o.** nausea _____

   **p.** malaise _____

   **q.** hematemesis _____

**EXERCISE 11-9 Spelling**

*Circle any words that are spelled incorrectly in the list below. Then correct the spelling in the space provided.*

1. duodenum _____

2. malaise _____

3. Chron disease _____

4. melanemesis _____

5. cholitis _____

6. appendix _____

7. jegunum _____

8. peritoneum _____

9. coledocholithiasis _____

10. disphagia _____

## Animations

Visit the companion website to view the videos on **Digestion** and **Laparoscopic Examination**.

## 11.13 Pronunciation and Spelling

*Listen, read, and study, so you can speak and write.*

1. Listen to each word on the audio file provided on the Student Companion Website.

2. Pronounce each word carefully.

3. Spell each word in the space provided.

| Word | Pronunciation | Spelling |
|---|---|---|
| aerophagia | ayr-**oh**-FAY-**jee**-**ah** | |
| aphthous stomatitis | **AFF**-thuss **sto**-mah-**TYE**-tis | |
| anorexia | **an**-oh-**RECK**-see-ah | |
| appendicitis | ah-**pen**-dih-**SIGH**-tis | |
| biliary | **BILL**-ee-air-ee | |

| Word | Pronunciation | Spelling |
|------|---------------|----------|
| buccal mucosa | **BUCK**-ahl myoo-**KOH**-sa | |
| cachexia | kah-**KECK**-see-ah | |
| cholecystectomy | **koh**-lee-sis-**TECK**-toh-mee | |
| choledochotomy | **koh**-led-oh-**KOT**-oh-mee | |
| cirrhosis | sih-**ROH**-sis | |
| colitis | koh-**LYE**-tis | |
| colostomy | koh-**LOSS**-toh-mee | |
| Crohn disease | **KROHN** | |
| diverticulosis | **dye**-ver-**tick**-yoo-**LOH**-sis | |
| diarrhea | **dye**-ah-**REE**-ah | |
| duodenojejunostomy | **doo**-oh-**dee**-no-jay-joon-**OSS**-teh-mee | |
| dyspepsia | dis-**PEP**-see-ah | |
| dysphagia | dis-**FAY**-jee-ah | |
| esophagus | eh-**SOF**-ah-gus | |
| gastroenteritis | **gas**-troh-**en**-ter-**EYE**-tis | |
| gingivitis | **jin**-jih-**VYE**-tis | |
| hematemesis | **hee**-mah-**TEM**-eh-sis | |
| hyperemesis | **high**-per-**EM**-eh-sis | |
| ileectomy | **ill**-ee-**ECK**-toh-mee | |
| ileum | **ILL**-ee-um | |
| insulin | **IN**-suh-lin | |
| jejunum | jeh-**JOO**-num | |
| labial | **LAY**-bee-al | |
| malaise | mah-**LAYZ** | |
| melanemesis | **mel**-ah-**NEM**-eh-sis | |
| mesentery | **MEZ**-en-**ter**-ee | |
| oral | **OR**-al | |
| peritoneum | **per**-ih-toh-**NEE**-um | |
| stomatitis | **sto**-mah-**TYE**-tis | |
| sublingual | sub-**LING**-gwal | |

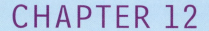

## CHAPTER 12

# Cardiovascular System

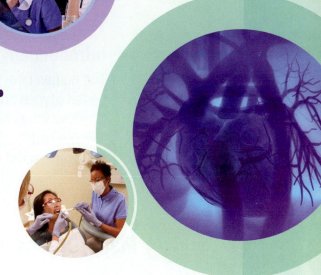

## Chapter Outline

## Learning Objectives

*After studying this chapter and completing the review exercises, you should be able to:*

1. Name and locate the major organs of the cardiovascular system.
2. Name, locate, and describe the structures of the heart and associated blood vessels.
3. Describe the function of the heart and blood vessels.
4. Name common blood vessels.
5. Trace blood flow through the heart and body.
6. Pronounce, spell, define, and write the medical terms related to the cardiovascular system.
7. Describe common diseases related to the cardiovascular system.
8. Listen, read, and study so you can speak and write.

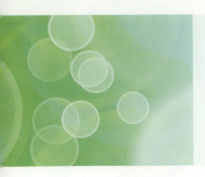

## Introduction

The human body is made up of 70 to 80 trillion cells. All of these cells need to be fed oxygen and nutrients. These are provided by the cardiovascular system (CVS), which is illustrated in Figure 12-1.

The body's cells must also get rid of waste materials. The CVS does this job too, at the same time it delivers oxygen and nutrients.

## 12.1   Major Organs of the Cardiovascular System

**PRACTICE FOR LEARNING: Major Organs of the CVS**

Write the words below in the correct spaces in Figure 12-1. To help you, the number beside the word tells you where it goes on the figure. Be sure to pronounce each word as you write it. Repeat the pronunciation several times if you find the word hard to say.

1. heart (**HART**)
2. arteries (**AR**-ter-eez)
3. arterioles (ar-**TEER**-ee-ohlz)
4. capillaries (ka-**PILL**-ah-reez)
5. venules (**VEN**-yoolz)
6. veins (**VAYNZ**)

The heart pumps blood. It beats 60 to 90 times every minute for your whole life. Each beat pumps blood throughout the body. The blood flows through blood vessels. Numbers 2 through 6 on Figure 12-1 are the different types of blood vessels.

## 12.2   Structures of the Heart

**PRACTICE FOR LEARNING: The Heart**

Write the structures listed below in the correct spaces in Figure 12-2. To help you, the number beside the word tells you where it goes on the figure. Be sure to pronounce each word as you write it. Repeat the word several times if you find the word hard to say.

1. superior vena cava (**VE**-nah **KAY**-vah)
2. pulmonary semilunar valve (**POOL**-mon-**ayr**-ee **seh**-me-**LOO**-nar **VALV**)
3. right atrium (**AY**-tree-um)
4. tricuspid valve (trigh-**KUS**-pid)
5. right ventricle (**VEN**-trih-kul)

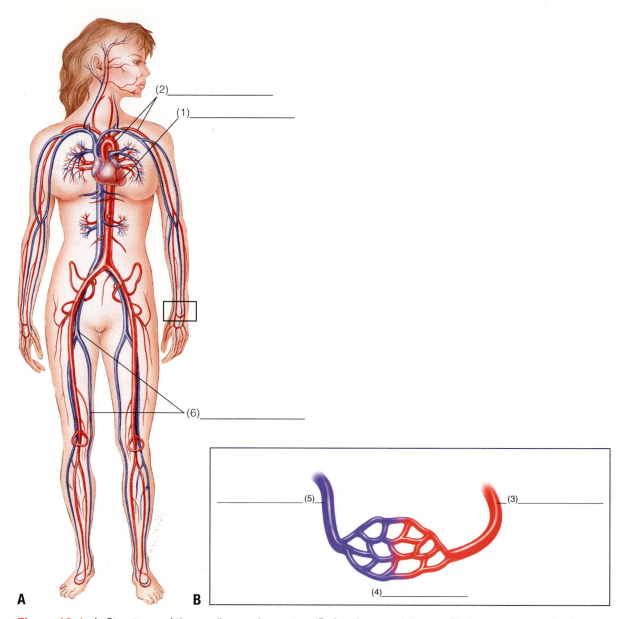

**Figure 12-1**  A. Structures of the cardiovascular system. B. Arteries, arterioles, capillaries, venules, and veins.

**6.** inferior vena cava (**VE**-nah **KAY**-vah)

**7.** septum (**SEP**-tum)

**8.** left ventricle (**VEN**-trih-kul)

**9.** bicuspid (bye-**KUS**-pid) or mitral (**MY**-tral) valve

**10.** aortic semilunar valve (ay-**OR**-tick **seh**-mee-**LOO**-nar **VALV**)

**11.** left atrium

**12.** aorta (ay-**OR**-tah)

Figure 12-2 shows you a big picture of the heart and the large blood vessels attached to it. The large blood vessels include the aorta, superior vena cava (SVC), inferior vena

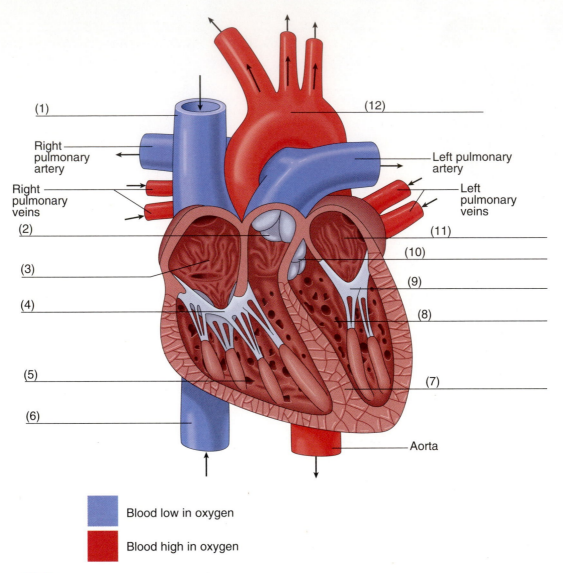

(1)

Right
pulmonary
artery

Right
pulmonary
veins

(2)

(3)

(4)

(5)

(6)

(12)

Left pulmonary
artery

Left
pulmonary
veins

(11)

(10)

(9)

(8)

(7)

Aorta

Blood low in oxygen

Blood high in oxygen

**Figure 12-2**  Heart and major blood vessels.

cava (IVC), and pulmonary artery. Review Figure 12-2 carefully before you move on to the rest of the chapter.

## Heart Chambers

Look at Figure 12-3. It shows that the heart contains four cavities. They are called chambers. The upper chambers are called **atria** (**AY**-tree-ah) (singular is atrium). The lower chambers are called ventricles (singular is ventricle).

Figure 12-3 also illustrates that the heart is separated into the right and left sections. The wall dividing them is called the septum.

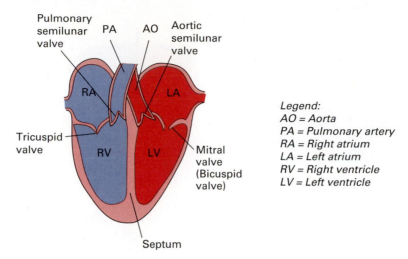

**Figure 12-3** Heart chambers.

## In Brief

**Atria** are the upper chambers.

**Ventricles** are the lower chambers.

**Septum** separates the right and left sides of the heart.

PRACTICE FOR LEARNING: **Heart Chambers**

Write the correct answer in the space provided.

1. Write the name for the upper chambers. _____

2. Write the name for the lower chambers. _____

3. Write the name for the partition that separates the right side of the heart from the left side. _____

> Answers: 1. atria. 2. ventricles. 3. septum.

## Heart Valves

There are four valves in the heart. They open to let blood in, and then they close tightly to ensure there is no backward flow of blood (Figure 12-4).

Two of the valves are called semilunar valves (Figure 12-4A). The semilunar valve at the entrance of the pulmonary artery is called the pulmonary semilunar valve. The one at the entrance of the aorta is called the aortic semilunar valve.

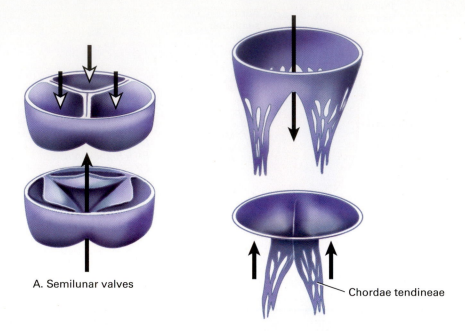

A. Semilunar valves

Chordae tendineae

B. Atrioventricular valves

**Figure 12-4**  Heart valves. A. Semilunar valves. B. Atrioventricular valves.

The other two valves are called **atrioventricular** (**ay**-tree-oh-ven-**TRICK**-yoo-lar) valves, or AV valves (Figure 12-4B). The AV valve between the right atrium and ventricle is called the tricuspid valve because it has three cusps, or flaps. The AV valve between the left atrium and ventricle has two cusps and is referred to as the bicuspid, or mitral valve.

Tough fibers called **chordae tendineae** (**KOR**-dee **TEN**-din-ee) attach the flaps of the AV valves to the heart wall. They ensure that the flaps close tightly.

**In Brief**

**Semilunar valves**
pulmonary valve
aortic valve

**Atrioventricular (AV) valves**
tricuspid valve
bicuspid valve

**PRACTICE FOR LEARNING: Valves and Chordae Tendineae**

Write the correct answer in the space provided.

1. Name the valve that separates the right atrium from the right ventricle.

   _____

2. How many flaps does the tricuspid valve have?

   _____

**3.** Write another name for the bicuspid valve.

_____

**4.** Write the name of the fibrous cords that attach the atrioventricular flaps to the heart wall. The term is difficult to spell. Make sure your spelling is correct.

_____

**5.** Write the name of the valve located at the entrance to the pulmonary artery.

_____

**6.** Write the name of the valve located at the entrance to the aortic artery.

_____

> **Answers: 1. tricuspid or atrioventricular (AV) valve. 2. three. 3. mitral valve. 4. chordae tendineae. 5. pulmonary semilunar valve. 6. aortic semilunar valve.**

## Walls of the Heart

The heart has three walls (Figure 12-5). The outer wall is the **epicardium** (**ep**-ih-**KAR**-dee-um). The middle wall is the **myocardium** (**my**-oh-**KAR**-dee-um). It is composed of the muscle that contracts the ventricles, pumping the blood out of the heart. The inner wall is the **endocardium** (**en**-do-**KAR**-dee-um).

## Pericardium

The heart is surrounded by a sac called the pericardium (**per**-ih-**KAR**-dee-um) (Figure 12-6). It has two layers. Pericardial fluid lies between the layers. This fluid prevents friction between the two layers when the heart beats.

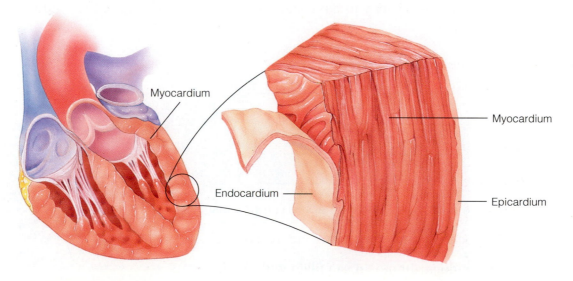

**Figure 12-5** Walls of the heart.

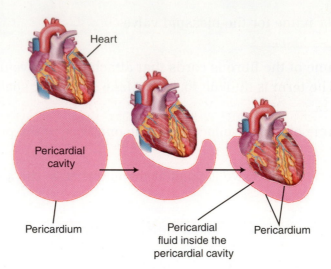

Heart

Pericardial
cavity

Pericardium

Pericardial
fluid inside the
pericardial cavity

Pericardium

**Figure 12-6** Pericardium.

**In Brief**

**Epicardium** outermost wall of the heart

**Myocardium** muscle wall of the heart

**Endocardium** innermost wall of the heart

**Pericardium** sac surrounding the heart

PRACTICE FOR LEARNING: **Heart Walls**

Write the correct answer in the space provided.

**1.** Name the three walls making up the heart.

_____, _____, _____.

**2.** Using the terminology you have learned, write the meaning of the following word parts.

**a.** my/o _____

**b.** cardi/o _____

**c.** -um _____

**d.** epi- _____

**e.** endo- _____

**3.** Mark the following statements as True or False.

**a.** The pericardium surrounds the heart. _____

**b.** The endocardium is a sac filled with fluid. _____

**c.** The pericardium is responsible for muscular contraction. _____

**d.** The pericardium has two layers. _____

## 12.3  How the Heart Beats

Electrical impulses stimulate the heart to beat. Unlike other nerve impulses, they do not come from the brain. They are created in special tissue in the atrium called the pacemaker. They then follow a trail through the heart to the **Purkinje** (per-**KIN**-jee) fibers, which extend throughout the ventricles. When the impulses reach the Purkinje fibers, the ventricles contract and push blood out of the heart into arteries.

The trail the impulses follow from the pacemaker to the ventricles is called the conduction pathway. It is illustrated in Figure 12-7. When the electrical impulses follow the conduction pathway properly, the heart will beat in a regular way, 60 to 90 beats per minute. This is called **normal sinus rhythm**.

The electrical activity of the heart can be recorded in a procedure called electrocardiography (Figure 12-8A). The record of such a test is called an **electrocardiogram**

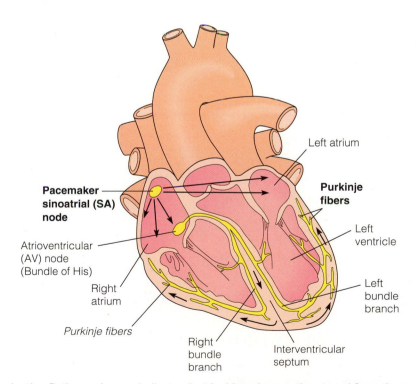

**Figure 12-7** Conduction Pathway. Arrows indicate electrical impulses as they travel from the pacemaker to the Purkinje fibers.

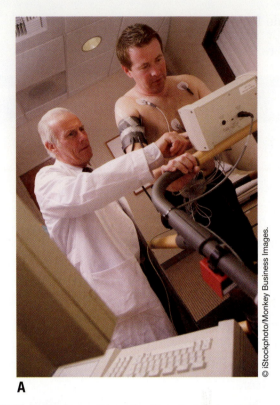

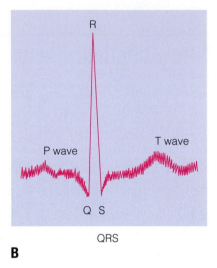

© iStockphoto/Monkey Business Images.

**A**            **B**

**Figure 12-8**   A. Electrocardiography. The electrical activities of the heart are recorded by electrodes placed on the skin. B. Normal electrocardiogram. P wave indicates strength of atrial contraction. QRS wave indicates strength of ventricular contraction. T wave indicates ventricular relaxation.

(ee-**leck**-troh-**KAR**-dee-oh-**gram**). It is usually referred to as an ECG or EKG. Figure 12-8B shows a record of a normal ECG. The spikes or waves on the record represent the strength of contraction of the atria and ventricles.

| **In Brief** | **Electrical impulses** travel through the heart from the pacemaker to the Purkinje fibers, causing the ventricles to contract and the heart to beat. An ECG monitors the electrical impulses as they travel through the heart. |
|---|---|

### PRACTICE FOR LEARNING: How the Heart Beats

**1.** What is the purpose of an electrocardiogram?

_____

**2.** When electrical impulses reach the Purkinje fibers, which heart structure contracts? _____

Answers: 1. to record the electrical activity through the heart. 2. ventricles.

## 12.4 Blood Pressure and Pulse

On each ventricular contraction, blood is pumped through an artery. It pushes on the artery wall. The pressure this creates is called blood pressure (BP).

Blood pressure is measured with an instrument called a **sphygmomanometer** (**sfig**-moh-man-**OM**-eh-ter). Figure 12-9 shows you what that instrument looks like. When the blood pressure (BP) is taken manually, as shown in Figure 12-9, a stethoscope (**STETH**-oh-skope) is used to listen to blood sounds. When using a digital sphygmomanometer, which is automated, no stethoscope is used.

A normal blood pressure reading is written like this: 115/75 mm Hg. The first number is the **systolic** (**SIS**-tohl-ick) pressure, the pressure against the arterial wall when the ventricles contract and pumps blood out of the heart. The second number is the **diastolic** (**dye**-as-**TOHL**-ick) pressure, the pressure against the arterial wall when the ventricles relax. High blood pressure is called **hypertension** (**high**-per-**TEN**-shun). Low blood pressure is called **hypotension** (**high**-poh-**TEN**-shun). If high blood pressure affects the heart, the condition is called **hypertensive heart disease**.

A BP reading between 120/80 to 139/89 is considered **prehypertension** (**pree**-high-per-**TEN**-shun). A reading over 140/90 is hypertension. BP of 90/60 is hypotension. Many experts now suggest that 115/75 is the optimum.

The arteries dilate and constrict in unison with the heartbeat. These movements, known as a pulse, can be readily detected at several sites. Figure 12-10 illustrates the following pulse sites: temporal, carotid, brachial, radial, femoral, popliteal, and dorsalis pedis.

---

**In Brief**    **Sphygmomanometer**

A device used to measure blood pressure. Optimum blood pressure reading is 115/75 mm Hg.

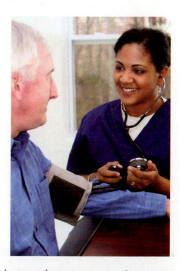

**Figure 12-9** Blood pressure reading using a sphygmomanometer.

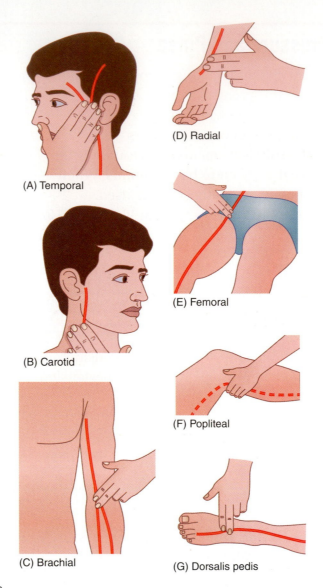

(A) Temporal

(B) Carotid

(C) Brachial

(D) Radial

(E) Femoral

(F) Popliteal

(G) Dorsalis pedis

**Figure 12-10** Pulse sites.

## PRACTICE FOR LEARNING: Blood Pressure and Pulse

**1.** Write the name of the device used to measure blood pressure.
_____.

**2.** Name the location of the following pulse sites:

(a) radial pulse _____.

(b) carotid pulse _____.

(c) dorsalis pedis pulse _____.

(d) popliteal pulse _____.

Answers: 1. sphygmomanometer. 2. (a) wrist/over the radius, (b) neck, (c) top of foot, (d) behind the knee.

## 12.5   Blood Vessels and Circulation

### Blood Vessels

Blood vessels carry blood throughout the body. **Arteries** (**AR**-ter-eez), **arterioles** (ar-**TEER**-ee-ohlz), **capillaries** (kah-**PILL**-ah-reez), **venules** (**VEN**-youlz), and **veins** (**VAYNZ**) are types of blood vessels (see Figure 12-1 at the beginning of the chapter).

#### Arteries

Arteries are thick, muscular, and elastic. They are capable of expanding to accommodate the surge of blood when the heart contracts. All arteries except the pulmonary artery carry oxygenated (**OCK**-see-jeh-**nay**-ted) blood.

Generally, arteries are named according to the organs they supply. For example, the artery carrying blood to the kidneys is called the renal artery (Figure 12-11).

#### Capillaries

Capillaries are located in the organs. They are extremely tiny and have thin walls. Capillaries are not named. The thin walls of the capillaries enable the transfer of oxygen to the organs and carbon dioxide from the organs.

#### Veins

Veins are similar to arteries, except the walls are less muscular and elastic. Therefore, they need help to push blood up toward the heart from the lower extremities. This assistance is provided by the contraction of the skeletal muscles and a system of tiny valves that prevent backflow of blood.

All veins except the pulmonary vein carry deoxygenated blood. Deoxygenated blood carries carbon dioxide and waste rather than oxygen.

Like arteries, many veins are named after the organs they are associated with. For example, the vein associated with the liver is the hepatic vein (Figure 12-12).

### Circulation

Figure 12-13 outlines the circulatory system. Using your finger, start on the right side of the heart and trace the flow of blood through the heart, lungs, and body.

Deoxygenated blood containing carbon dioxide and waste materials is pumped out of the right side of the heart through the pulmonary arteries to the lungs. There, the carbon dioxide and waste are absorbed by the lungs and breathed out. Oxygen is breathed in and absorbed by the blood. This **oxygenated** blood then flows back through the pulmonary veins to the left side of the heart, where it is pumped through the aorta and out into arteries. It flows from the arteries into smaller arteries called arterioles until it reaches an organ.

In each organ are the smallest blood vessels, called capillaries. The blood flows into the capillaries. Tissue cells in the organ absorb the oxygen from the blood in the capillaries, as well as nutrients that the blood has picked up from the digestive system

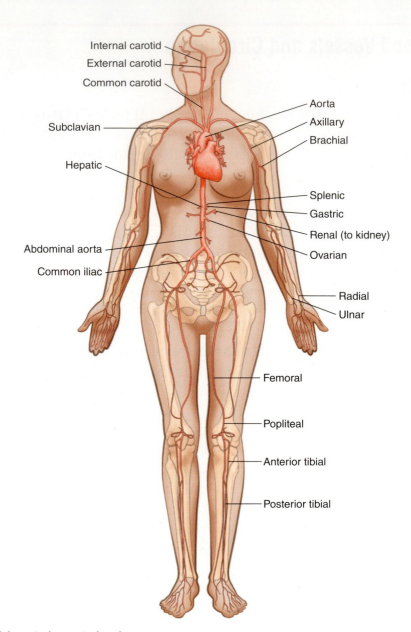

**Figure 12-11**  Major arteries, anterior view.

before it reaches the organ. At the same time, the organ's cells release carbon dioxide and waste into the capillaries. This deoxygenated blood then leaves the capillaries and flows through tiny vessels called venules (small veins) into bigger vessels called veins. The veins lead into the **inferior** and **superior venae cavae** (**VEE**-nee **KAY**-vee), which are much larger veins. They carry the blood back to the heart. The blood is then pumped to the lungs where the cycle is repeated.

The heart cannot feed itself from the blood that flows through it. Its walls are too thick and muscular. It has its own system of arteries and veins. These are the **coronary** arteries and veins. They supply the heart muscle with the oxygen and nutrients it needs to function properly. A heart attack or myocardial infarction (**my**-oh-**KAR**-dee-al in-**FARK**-shun) is a blockage in the coronary arteries. Because oxygen and nutrients can no longer reach the heart muscle, the muscle is damaged.

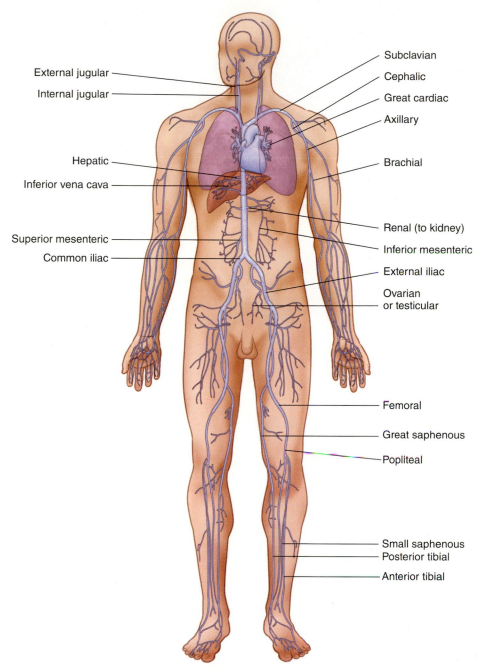

External jugular
Internal jugular

Subclavian
Cephalic
Great cardiac
Axillary

Hepatic
Inferior vena cava

Brachial

Superior mesenteric
Common iliac

Renal (to kidney)
Inferior mesenteric

External iliac
Ovarian
or testicular

Femoral

Great saphenous

Popliteal

Small saphenous
Posterior tibial

Anterior tibial

**Figure 12-12** Common Veins, anterior view.

| In Brief | Blood flow through the body: right side of heart ⟶ pulmonary arteries ⟶ lungs ⟶ pulmonary veins ⟶ left side of heart ⟶ aorta ⟶ arteries ⟶ arterioles ⟶ capillaries ⟶ venules ⟶ veins ⟶ inferior and superior venae cavae ⟶ right side of heart |

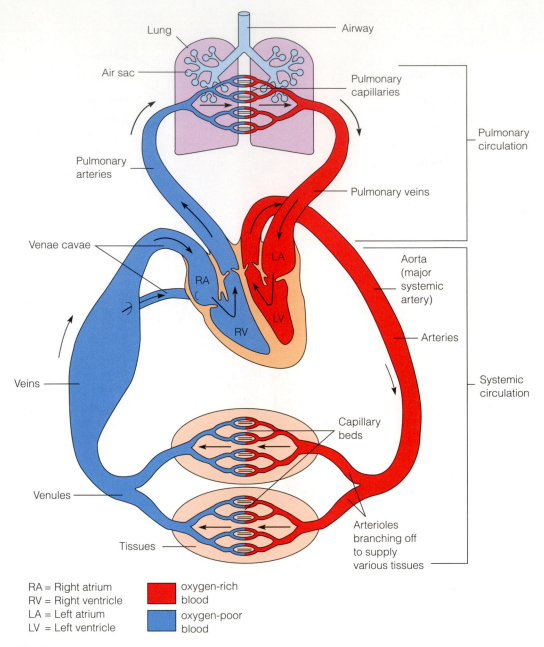

**Figure 12-13** Circulation of blood through the body.

RA = Right atrium
RV = Right ventricle
LA = Left atrium
LV = Left ventricle

oxygen-rich blood
oxygen-poor blood

## PRACTICE FOR LEARNING: Blood Vessels and Circulation

**1.** Name the three types of blood vessels. _____,
_____, and _____.

**2.** What are small arteries called? _____

**3.** What are small veins called? _____

4. Generally, all arteries carry (oxygenated/deoxygenated blood). Which artery is the exception?

5. Generally, all veins carry (oxygenated/deoxygenated blood). Which vein is the exception?

> **Answers: 1.** arteries, veins, capillaries. **2.** arterioles. **3.** venules. **4.** oxygenated; pulmonary artery. **5.** deoxygenated; pulmonary vein.

## 12.6  New Roots, Suffixes and Prefixes

Use these additional roots and suffix when studying the terms in this chapter.

| ROOT | MEANING |
|------|---------|
| constrict/o | to draw together; constrict |
| dilat/o | to expand; widen |

| SUFFIX | MEANING |
|--------|---------|
| -emia | blood condition |

## 12.7  Learning the Terms

Following these steps will make it easier for you to learn medical terms:

1. Pronounce the term repeatedly until it is easy for you.

2. Write it down. Ensure the spelling is correct.

3. Also write the definition. If possible, relate the word to a word, thought, or picture that will help you remember it.

4. Analyze the term with the method taught in this text.

### Roots

| ROOT<br>angi/o | | MEANING<br>blood vessel |
|----------------|---|-------------------------|
| *Term* | *Term Analysis* | *Definition* |
| angioplasty<br>(**AN**-jee-oh-**plas**-tee) | -plasty = surgical repair; surgical reconstruction | surgical repair of a blood vessel |

| ROOT arteri/o | | MEANING artery |
|---|---|---|
| Term | Term Analysis | Definition |
| arteriosclerosis (ar-**teer**-ee-oh-skleh-**ROH**-sis) | -sclerosis = hardening | hardening of the arteries due to the loss of elasticity in the arterial wall |
| arteriostenosis (ar-**teer**-ee-oh-steh-**NOH**-sis) | -stenosis = narrowing | narrowing of an artery |
| carotid endarterectomy (kah-**ROT**-id **end**-ar-ter-**ECK**-toh-mee) | carotid = artery in the neck -ectomy = excision; surgical removal endo- = within | excision of the inner lining of the carotid artery |

| ROOT ather/o | | MEANING fatty debris |
|---|---|---|
| Term | Term Analysis | Definition |
| atheroma (**ath**-er-**OH**-mah) | -oma = mass; tumor | name given to the fatty mass (plaque) that accumulates on the wall of an artery. The fatty mass contains cholesterol. |
| atherosclerosis (**ath**-er-oh-skleh-**ROH**-sis) | -sclerosis = hardening | hardening and narrowing of an artery due to an atheroma (Figure 12-16) |

| ROOT cardi/o | | MEANING heart |
|---|---|---|
| Term | Term Analysis | Definition |
| cardiac catheterization (**KAR**-dee-ack **kath**-eh-ter-eye-**ZAY**-shun) | -ac = pertaining to catheterization = a procedure to remove fluid from the body using a flexible tube called a catheter | diagnostic procedure in which a flexible tube called a catheter is inserted into a vein, sliding it upward into the heart to obtain diagnostic information about how well the heart is working. Figure 12-14 |

| Term | Term Analysis | Definition |
|------|---------------|------------|

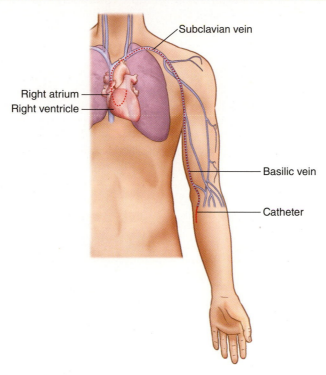

**Figure 12-14** Cardiac Catheterization.

| Term | Term Analysis | Definition |
|------|---------------|------------|
| **cardiologist** (**kar**-dee-**OL**-oh-jist) | -logist = specialist in the study of | specialist in the study of the heart including its diseases and treatment |
| **cardiomegaly** (**KAR**-dee-oh **MEG**-ah-lee) | -megaly = enlargement | enlarged heart |
| **cardiomyopathy** (**kar**-dee-oh-my-**OP**-ah-thee) | -pathy = disease my/o = muscle | disease of the heart muscle |
| **echocardiograph** (**eck**-oh-**KAR**-dee-oh-graf) | -graph = instrument used to record ech/o = sound | an instrument using ultrasound to record an image of the heart |
| **pancarditis** (**pan**-kar-**DYE**-tis) | -itis = inflammation pan- = all | inflammation of all the walls of the heart (this includes the epicardium, myocardium, and endocardium) |

| ROOT coron/o | | MEANING crown | |
|--------------|---|----------------|---|
| Term | Term Analysis | Definition | |
| **coronary arteries** (**KOR**-uh-**nehr**-ee) | -ary = pertaining to | the arteries that supply the heart with blood | |

**Helping You Remember**   The coronary arteries sit on top of the heart like a crown.

| ROOT cyan/o | | MEANING blue |
| --- | --- | --- |
| Term | Term Analysis | Definition |
| cyanosis (**sigh**-ah-**NOH**-sis) | -sis = state of; condition | condition of blueness of the skin |

| ROOT diaphor/e | | MEANING profuse sweating |
| --- | --- | --- |
| Term | Term Analysis | Definition |
| diaphoresis (**dye**-ah-foh-**REE**-sis) | -sis = state of; condition | state of profuse sweating |

**Helping You Remember**   Embolus comes from the Greek "embolos" meaning "plug." An embolos was used as a cork in a liquor bottle.

| ROOT embol/o | | MEANING plug |
| --- | --- | --- |
| Term | Term Analysis | Definition |
| embolus (**EM**-boh-lus) | -us = condition; thing | a blood clot or clump of foreign material moving through a blood vessel obstructing blood flow. Can be fatal. |

| ROOT isch/o | | MEANING hold back |
| --- | --- | --- |
| Term | Term Analysis | Definition |
| myocardial ischemia (**my**-oh-**KAR**-dee-al iss-**KEE**-me-ah) | -emia = blood condition<br>-al = pertaining to<br>my/o = muscle<br>cardi/o = heart | hold back or deficiency of blood to the heart muscle |

| ROOT phleb/o (see also ven/o) | | MEANING vein |
| --- | --- | --- |
| Term | Term Analysis | Definition |
| thrombophlebitis (throm-boh-fleh-BYE-tis) | -itis = inflammation<br>thromb/o = clot | inflammation of a vein with clot formation |

| ROOT rhythm/o | | MEANING rhythm |
| --- | --- | --- |
| Term | Term Analysis | Definition |
| arrhythmia (ah-RITH-mee-ah) | -ia = state of; condition<br>a- = no; not | deviation from normal sinus rhythm. For further detail, see arrhythmia in Section 12.8 below. |

**Helping You Remember**  The prefix *a-* changes to *ar-* in the word "arrhythmia" because the root begins with *r*.

| ROOT scler/o | | MEANING hardening |
| --- | --- | --- |
| Term | Term Analysis | Definition |
| sclerotherapy (skleh-roh-THER-ah-pee) | -therapy = treatment | injection of a solution into the vein for the purpose of destroying the vein's inner lining by hardening. Sclerotherapy is very effective in treating varicose veins and requires no hospitalization. |

| ROOT thromb/o | | MEANING clot |
| --- | --- | --- |
| Term | Term Analysis | Definition |
| thrombus (THROM-bus) | -us = condition; thing | a blood clot that obstructs a blood vessel |

| ROOT vas/o | | MEANING vessel |
| --- | --- | --- |
| Term | Term Analysis | Definition |
| vasoconstriction (vas-oh-kon-STRICK-shun) | -ion = process<br>constrict/o = to draw together; constrict | constriction or narrowing of the vessel walls |
| vasodilation (vas-oh-dye-LAY-shun) | -ion = process<br>dilat/o = expand; widen | widening of the vessel walls |

| ROOT ven/o | | MEANING vein |
| --- | --- | --- |
| Term | Term Analysis | Definition |
| venous (VEE-nus) | -ous = pertaining to | pertaining to a vein |

## Suffixes

| SUFFIX -centesis | | MEANING surgical puncture to remove fluid |
| --- | --- | --- |
| Term | Term Analysis | Definition |
| cardiocentesis (kar-dee-oh-sen-TEE-sis) | cardi/o = heart | surgical puncture of the heart to remove fluid |
| pericardial centesis (par-ee-KAR-dee-al sen-TEE-sis) | -al = pertaining to<br>peri- = around<br>cardi/o = heart | surgical puncture to remove fluid in the pericardium |

**Note:** "Centesis" can be used as a suffix or as a word standing alone. Both forms have the same meaning.

## Prefixes

| PREFIX brady- | | MEANING slow |
| --- | --- | --- |
| Term | Term Analysis | Definition |
| bradycardia (brad-ee-KAR-dee-uh) | -ia = condition; state of<br>cardi/o = heart | slow heartbeat; slower than 60 beats per minute |

| PREFIX de- | | MEANING lack of; removal |
| --- | --- | --- |
| Term | Term Analysis | Definition |
| **defibrillation** (dee-**fib**-rih-**LAY**-shun) | fibrillation = fast, uncoordinated heartbeat | stopping atrial or ventricular fibrillation using an electronic device called a defibrillator |

**Note:** A defibrillator applies an electric shock to a heart muscle. The defibrillator is placed on top of the chest muscle and activated. The electrical current momentarily stops the heart action so that the pacemaker can reestablish normal heart rhythm.

| PREFIX tachy- | | MEANING fast |
| --- | --- | --- |
| Term | Term Analysis | Definition |
| **tachycardia** (**tack**-ee-**KAR**-dee-ah) | -ia = condition; state of cardi/o = heart | fast heartbeat; faster than 100 beats per minute |

## 12.8  Pathology

### Aneurysm (**AN**-yoo-riz-um)

An abnormal bulge in the wall of an artery (Figure 12-15). It occurs most often in the aorta or in the brain.

A ruptured aneurysm occurs when the wall of the artery bursts. This causes internal hemorrhaging, which may result in death.

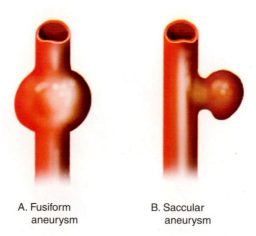

A. Fusiform aneurysm

B. Saccular aneurysm

**Figure 12-15** Aneruysms. A. Fusiform—bulging on both sides of the artery. B. Saccular—bulging on one side of the artery.

## Arrhythmia

An irregular heart rhythm that deviates from the normal sinus rhythm. Examples include:

- **Fibrillation** (**fib**-rih-**LAY**-shun), which is very fast uncoordinated heartbeats of the atria or ventricles. May reach 350 plus beats per minute.

- **Flutter**, which is very fast coordinated heartbeats. May reach up to 300 beats per minute.

- **Palpitation** (**pal**-pih-**TAY**-shun), which is an abnormal sensation in the chest. The patient feels like the heart is pounding. Heartbeats can be regular or irregular. Do not confuse with palpation (pal-**PAY**-shun), which means to feel.

- **Heart block**, which is the interruption of the electrical impulses which travel from the pacemaker through the conduction system to the Purkinje fibers. This results in failure of the ventricles to contract. Right bundle branch block (RBBB) and left bundle branch block (LBBB) are the most common heart blocks.

## Coronary Artery Disease

Coronary artery disease (CAD) is a complete or partial blockage within the coronary arteries resulting in decreased blood flow to the heart muscle (Figure 12-16). The blockage is caused by an accumulation of fatty plaques (atheroma) on the walls of the artery.

To improve the blood flow within the vessel, a balloon angioplasty may be performed. This pushes the plaque against the wall of the vessel (Figure 12-17). A stent, which is a wire-mesh tube, is inserted into the vessel to prevent the fat from accumulating again (Figure 12-18).

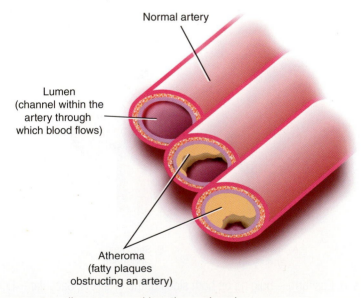

**Figure 12-16** Coronary artery disease caused by atherosclerosis.

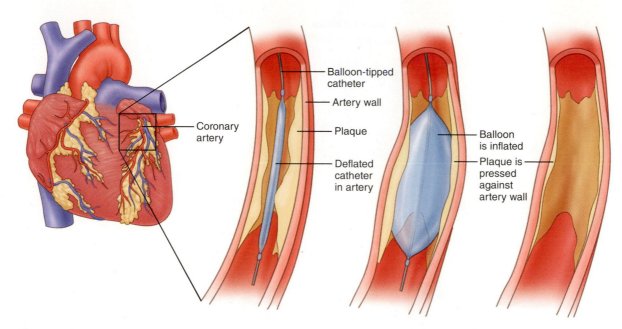

**Figure 12-17**  Balloon angioplasty flattens the fatty plaque against the vessel wall.

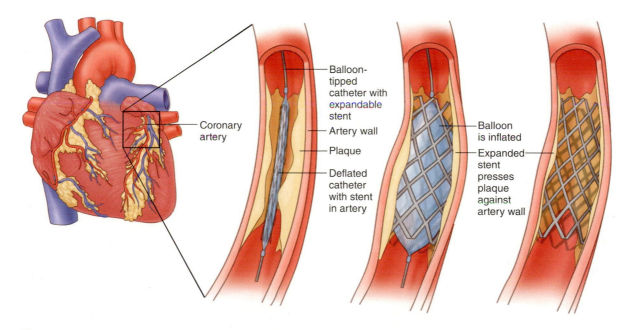

**Figure 12-18**  A stent is used to prevent the reattachment  of fatty plaque on the arterial wall.

## Cerebrovascular Accident; Stroke

Cerebrovascular accident (CVA) is a lack of blood to the brain, depriving it of oxygen and nutrients (Figure 12-19). Types of strokes include ischemic and hemorrhagic.

### Ischemic Stroke—there are three types:

**Thrombotic** (throm-**BOT**-ick): a thrombus (clot) blocks blood flow to the brain.

**Embolic** (em-**BOL**-ick): an embolus travels to a cerebral artery and blocks blood flow to the brain.

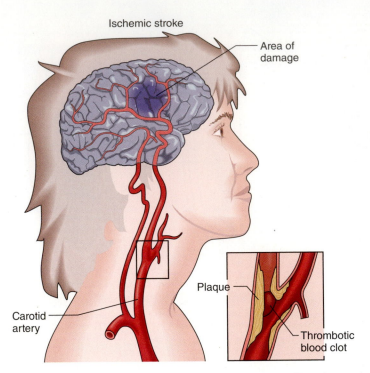

Ischemic stroke

Area of damage

Plaque

Carotid artery

Thrombotic blood clot

**Figure 12-19**  An ischemic stroke is caused by the lack of blood to the brain. The obstruction, as shown in this figure, is due to plaque (atheroma) or thrombus. An embolus, not shown here, can also cause an obstruction.

**Transient ischemic attack** (**TIA**): a temporary loss of blood flow to the brain resulting in neural abnormalities, which last from a few seconds to a number of hours.

### Hemorrhagic (**hem**-eh-**RADJ**-ick) stroke

An aneurysm bursts and results in a lack of blood to brain tissue. Often the aneurysm involves the cerebral artery.

## Cardiac Arrest

Cardiac arrest is when the heart unexpectedly stops pumping blood.

## Congestive Heart Failure

Congestive heart failure (CHF) is myocardial disease resulting in the failure of the heart to pump blood effectively through the blood vessels. This results in congestion (backing up) of blood in the blood vessels.

## Murmur (MER-mer)

An abnormal extra heart sound amongst normal heart sounds.

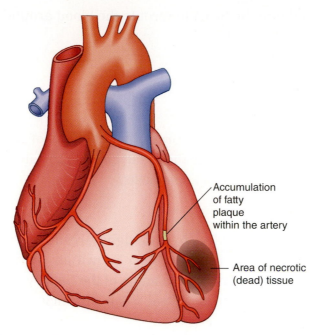

Accumulation
of fatty
plaque
within the artery

Area of necrotic
(dead) tissue

**Figure 12-20** Myocardial infarction (heart attack).

## Myocardial Infarction; Heart Attack

Myocardial infarction (MI) means death of the heart muscle. Look at Figure 12-20. When one or more of the coronary arteries are blocked because of coronary artery disease, blood flow to the heart muscle stops and the tissue dies. The heart is unable to function properly, and not enough blood is pumped to the body's tissues.

The primary symptom is **angina pectoris**, which means "pain over the chest area."

The treatment is a coronary artery bypass graft (CABG), also known as bypass surgery (Figure 12-21). In this procedure, the chest is opened and a piece of vein from the

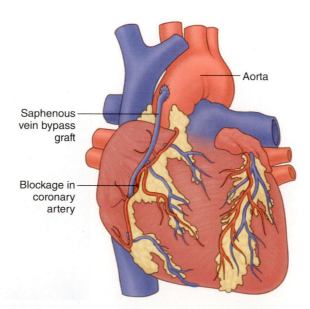

Aorta

Saphenous
vein bypass
graft

Blockage in
coronary
artery

**Figure 12-21** Coronary artery bypass graft uses a transplanted vein to reroute blood past the blocked artery.

leg or chest is implanted into the heart to reroute the blood around the obstruction. This restores blood to the heart muscle.

## Valvular Disorders

### Valvular Stenosis

A narrowing of one of the heart valves, preventing the flow of blood through the heart. The name of the heart valve affected is the name given to the stenosis. Examples: Aortic stenosis, mitral valve stenosis, tricuspid stenosis.

### Valvular Insufficiency

The inability of one of the heart valves to close tightly, resulting in a backflow or **regurgitation** (ree-**ger**-jih-**TAY**-shun) of blood. Also known as **valvular incompetence** or **valvular regurgitation**. Like stenosis, the name of the heart valve affected is the name given to the insufficiency. Examples: mitral valve insufficiency and pulmonary valve insufficiency.

## Varicose Veins

Dilated and twisted veins, usually involving the saphenous veins of the lower leg (Figure 12-22). The cause is damaged valves in the veins. They do not close, allowing the blood to flow backward. The blood forms pools, which dilate the veins. Sclerotherapy is a treatment for uncomplicated varicose veins.

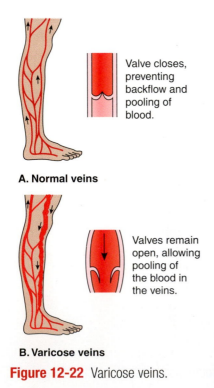

Valve closes, preventing backflow and pooling of blood.

**A. Normal veins**

Valves remain open, allowing pooling of the blood in the veins.

**B. Varicose veins**

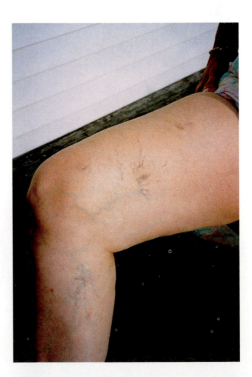

**C.**

**Figure 12-22** Varicose veins.

## 12.9 Look-Alike and Sound-Alike Words

*Below is a list of look-alike and sound-alike words. Study the spelling and definitions of each set of words. Questions will follow in the Review Exercises.*

### TABLE 12-1 Look-Alike and Sound-Alike Words

| | |
|---|---|
| arrhythmia | abnormal heart rhythm |
| erythremia | increase in the number of red blood cells |
| infarction | death of tissue |
| infection | to contaminate with a disease |
| venous | pertaining to a vein |
| Venus | one of the planets |
| palpation | to feel |
| palpitation | fast heartbeat |
| pericardium | structure around the heart |
| precordium | area in front of the heart |
| vain | concerned about one's own appearance; conceited; futile; unsuccessful result |
| vane | a device used to show the way the wind blows; weathervane |
| vein | a type of blood vessel |

## 12.10 Review Exercises

### EXERCISE 12-1 Look-Alike and Sound-Alike Words

*Read the sentences carefully and circle the word in parentheses that correctly completes the meaning. Use Table 12-1 if it helps you.*

**1.** Mr. Garcia, a 53-year-old-man, is admitted with an upper respiratory (**infection/infarction**) and pneumonia of two days' duration.

**2.** A diagnosis of renal (**infection/infarction**) due to narrowing of the renal arteries was made.

**3.** There are abnormal jugular (**venus/venous**) pulses; the carotid arterial pulses are normal.

4. On (**palpation/palpitation**) there was a mass noted over the breastbone.

5. Naleen was admitted with shortness of breath and (**palpations/palpitations**).

6. In open-heart surgery, a segment of the saphenous (**vain/vane/vein**) is removed and used as a graft.

7. In a (**vain/vane/vein**) attempt at hemostasis, the artery was clamped and ligated.

8. Previous pancarditis has resulted in inflammation of the (**precordium/ pericardium**), the structure surrounding the heart.

## EXERCISE 12-2 Matching Word Parts with Meaning

*Match word part in Column A with its meaning in Column B.*

| | Column A | Column B |
|---|---|---|
| _____ | 1. dilat/o | A. fatty debris |
| _____ | 2. -sclerosis | B. vessel |
| _____ | 3. -stenosis | C. crown |
| _____ | 4. pan- | D. narrowing |
| _____ | 5. endo- | E. hold back |
| _____ | 6. isch/o | F. widen |
| _____ | 7. vas/o | G. vein |
| _____ | 8. coron/o | H. hardening |
| _____ | 9. phleb/o | I. all |
| _____ | 10. ather/o | J. within |

## EXERCISE 12-3 Labeling

*Using the body structures listed below, label Figure 12-23. Write your answer in the numbered spaces provided below, or if you prefer, in the diagram.*

aorta _____

aortic semilunar valve _____

inferior vena cava _____

interventricular septum _____

left atrium _____

left ventricle _____

mitral valve _____

pulmonary semilunar valve

right atrium

right ventricle

superior vena cava

tricuspid valve

1. _____      7. _____

2. _____      8. _____

3. _____      9. _____

4. _____      10. _____

5. _____      11. _____

6. _____      12. _____

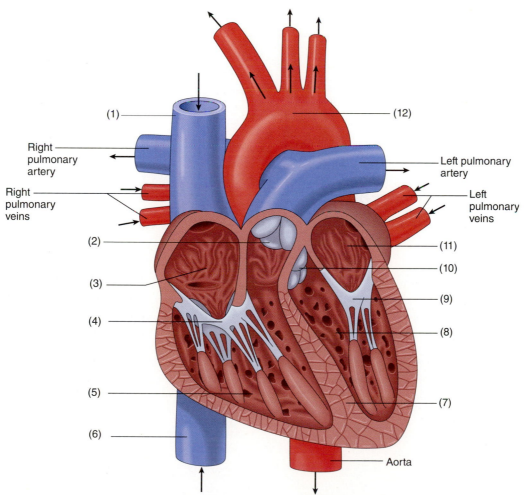

**Figure 12-23** Heart and major blood vessels.

## EXERCISE 12-4  Definitions—Learning the Terms

*Define the following terms.*

1. **arteriosclerosis** _____

2. **atheroma** _____

3. **arteriostenosis** _____

4. **embolus** _____

5. **thrombus** _____

6. **ischemia** _____

7. **vasoconstriction** _____

8. **bradycardia** _____

9. **angioplasty** _____

10. **coronary arteries** _____

11. **carotid endarterectomy** _____

12. **cardiomegaly** _____

13. **cyanosis** _____

14. **diaphoresis** _____

15. **cardiac catheterization** _____

## EXERCISE 12-5  Matching—Anatomy and Physiology

*Match the terms below with their descriptions that follow. Write your answer in the space provided.*

| | | |
|---|---|---|
| atria | electrocardiography | pulmonary vein |
| bicuspid | epicardium | sphygmomanometer |
| carotid arteries | pericardium | systolic pressure |
| chordae tendineae | pulmonary artery | tricuspid |
| coronary arteries | pulmonary valve | ventricles |
| diastolic pressure | | |

1. blood vessel carrying deoxygenated blood from the right side of the heart to the lungs _____

2. lower chamber of the heart _____

3. left atrioventricular valve _____

4. right atrioventricular valve _____

5. pressure against the arterial wall when the ventricles contract

   _____

6. anchors atrioventricular valves to the heart wall _____

7. instrument that measures blood pressure _____

8. upper chambers of the heart _____

9. process of recording the electrical activity of the heart

   _____

10. semilunar valve _____

11. pressure against the arterial wall when the ventricles relax

    _____

12. blood vessel in the neck carrying oxygenated blood toward the brain

    _____

13. sac surrounding the heart _____

14. blood vessel supplying the heart with oxygen _____

15. blood vessel carrying oxygenated blood from the lungs to the left atrium

    _____

16. outermost wall of the heart _____

## EXERCISE 12-6  Blood Flow Through Body

*Write the structures through which blood passes, in proper sequence, starting from the right side of the heart and finishing in the right side of the heart.*

_____

_____

_____

## EXERCISE 12-7 **Definitions—Pathology**

*Match the following conditions with their descriptions. Write your answer in the space provided.*

aneurysm
angina pectoris
bundle branch block
cardiac arrest
cerebrovascular accident
fibrillation

flutter
hemorrhagic stroke
hypertension
murmur
myocardial infarction

myocardial ischemia
thrombotic stroke
tricuspid stenosis
valvular insufficiency
varicose veins

**1.** chest pains _____

**2.** dilated, twisted veins of the leg _____

**3.** abnormal bulge in the wall of the artery _____

**4.** A stroke is also known as _____

**5.** condition where the heart muscle dies because of a lack of oxygen

_____

**6.** hold back of blood to heart muscle _____

**7.** sudden stoppage of the heart _____

**8.** high blood pressure _____

**9.** fast uncoordinated heart beat _____

**10.** fast coordinated heart beat _____

**11.** loss of blood to the brain due to clot formation _____

**12.** loss of blood to the brain due to a burst blood vessel _____

**13.** an abnormal extra heart sound amongst normal heart sounds

_____

**14.** electrical impulses leading to the Purkinje fibers are blocked

_____

**15.** regurgitation of blood through a heart valve _____

**16.** narrowing of the right AV valve preventing the flow of blood through the heart

_____

## EXERCISE 12-8 Definitions in Context

*Define the bolded terms in context. Use your medical dictionary if necessary.*

### Report #1 ECHOCARDIOGRAPHY REPORT

No **arrhythmia**. The right **atrium** is at the upper limits of normal. The **ventricle** is also normal. The **aortic valve** and **tricuspid** function normally. There was no evidence of a **thrombus** within the **coronary arteries**.

a. echocardiography _____

b. arrhythmia _____

c. atrium _____

d. ventricle _____

e. aortic valve _____

f. tricuspid _____

g. thrombus _____

h. coronary arteries _____

### Report #2 HISTORY AND PHYSICAL EXAMINATION

Lynnel says she had a severe attack of **angina pectoris** about two years ago and was hospitalized for **myocardial ischemia**.

About one day ago, she started having difficulty breathing plus **nausea** and vomiting. Because her breathing was very difficult, she went to the emergency department of the hospital and was found to have a **myocardial infarction**.

On physical examination, Lynnel does appear older than her stated age of 56. Her **blood pressure** is **182/80**. Her **pulse** is 130, and she has **tachycardia**.

Neck veins are **distended**. Abdomen is soft, not distended. No masses can be felt. There is **edema** in the lower extremities.

DIAGNOSES

1. MYOCARDIAL INFARCTION

2. **ATHEROSCLEROSIS**

3. **CARDIOVASCULAR DISEASE** DUE TO **HYPERTENSION**

a. angina pectoris _____

b. myocardial ischemia _____

c. nausea _____

d. myocardial infarction _____

e. blood pressure _____

f. 182/80 _____

g. pulse _____

h. tachycardia _____

i. distended _____

j. edema _____

k. atherosclerosis _____

l. cardiovascular disease _____

m. hypertension _____

## EXERCISE 12-9  Spelling

*Circle any words that are spelled incorrectly in the list below.*

Then correct the spelling in the space provided.

1. anurysm _____

2. arhythmia _____

3. atherosclerosis _____

4. ischemia _____

5. thromboflebitis _____

6. vesoconstriction _____

7. chordae tendineae _____

8. coronery _____

9. sphygmomanometer _____

10. embolous _____

## Animations

Visit the companion website to view the videos on **Electrical Stimulation of the Heart** and **Ischemic and Hemorrhagic Strokes**.

## 12.11 Pronunciation and Spelling

*Listen, read, and study, so you can speak and write.*

1. Listen to each word on the audio file provided on the Student Companion Website.

2. Pronounce each word carefully.

3. Spell each word in the space provided.

| Word | Pronunciation | Spelling |
|------|---------------|----------|
| aneurysm | **AN**-yoo-riz-um | |
| angioplasty | **AN**-jee-oh-**plas**-tee | |
| aorta | ay-**OR**-tah | |
| arrhythmia | ah-**RITH**-mee-ah | |
| arteries | **AR**-ter-eez | |
| arterioles | ar-**TEER**-ee-ohlz | |
| arteriosclerosis | ar-**teer**-ee-oh-skleh-**ROH**-sis | |
| atheroma | **ath**-er-**OH**-mah | |
| atherosclerosis | **ath**-er-oh-skleh-**ROH**-sis | |
| atrioventricular | **ay**-tree-oh-ven-**TRICK**-yoo-lar | |
| bicuspid | bye-**KUS**-pid | |
| bradycardia | **brad**-ee-**KAR**-dee-uh | |
| capillaries | ka-**PILL**-ah-reez | |
| cardiologist | **kar**-dee-**OL**-oh-jist | |
| cardiomyopathy | **kar**-dee-oh-my-**OP**-ah-thee | |
| chordae tendineae | **KOR**-dee **TEN**-din-ee | |
| coronary | **KOR**-uh-**nehr**-ee | |
| electrocardiogram | ee-**leck**-troh-**KAR**-dee-oh-**gram** | |
| embolus | **EM**-boh-lus | |
| endocardium | **en**-doh-**KAR**-dee-um | |
| epicardium | **ep**-ih-**KAR**-dee-um | |
| fibrillation | **fib**-rih-**LAY**-shun | |

| Word | Pronunciation | Spelling |
|------|---------------|----------|
| infarction | in-FARK-shun | |
| ischemia | iss-KEE-me-ah | |
| myocardium | my-oh-KAR-dee-um | |
| palpitation | pal-pih-TAY-shun | |
| Purkinje | per-KIN-jee | |
| sphygmomanometer | sfig-moh-man-OM-eh-ter | |
| stethoscope | STETH-oh-skope | |
| tachycardia | tack-ee-KAR-dee-ah | |
| thrombophlebitis | throm-boh-fleh-BYE-tis | |
| thrombus | THROM-bus | |
| tricuspid | trigh-KUS-pid | |
| vasoconstriction | vas-oh-kon-STRICK-shun | |
| vasodilation | vas-oh-dye-LAY-shun | |
| veins | VAYNZ | |
| vena cava | VE-nah KAY-vah | |
| ventricle | VEN-trih-kul | |
| venules | VEN-yoolz | |

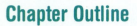

# CHAPTER 13

# Blood

## Chapter Outline

## Learning Objectives

*After studying this chapter and completing the review exercises, you should be able to:*

1. Name and describe the functions of the major components of blood.
2. Pronounce, spell, define, and write the medical terms related to the blood.
3. Describe common diseases of the blood.
4. Listen, read, and study so you can speak and write.

## Introduction

In the chapter on the skeletal system, you learned that blood cells are formed in the red bone marrow. In studying the cardiovascular system, you learned that blood carries oxygen and nutrients to the cells and carries away waste products. In this chapter, you will learn about the makeup of blood and its functions.

## 13.1  Major Components of Blood

PRACTICE FOR LEARNING: **Major Components of Blood**

Write the words below in the correct spaces in Figure 13-1. To help you, the number beside the word tells you where it goes on the figure. Be sure to pronounce each word as you write it. Repeat the pronunciation several times if you find the word hard to say.

1. plasma (**PLAZ**-mah)
2. formed elements
3. erythrocyte (eh-**RITH**-roh-sight)
4. thrombocyte (**THROM**-boh-sight)
5. basophil (**BAY**-soh-fill)
6. neutrophil (**NEW**-troh-fill)
7. eosinophil (ee-oh-**SIN**-oh-fill)
8. lymphocyte (**LIM**-foh-sight)
9. monocyte (**MON**-oh-sight)

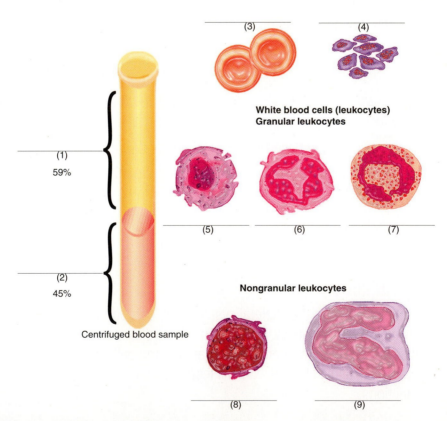

**Figure 13-1**  Formed elements of the blood.

## 13.2  Blood Composition

Whole blood is about 45% solid and 55% liquid, as illustrated in Figure 13-1. The solid portion is referred to as formed elements. Formed elements are produced in the bone marrow and consist of three types of blood cells: red blood cells (RBCs), white blood cells (WBCs), and platelets. RBCs are also called **erythrocytes**; WBCs are called **leukocytes**, and platelets are also called **thrombocytes**.

> **In Brief**
>
> Blood consists of formed elements and plasma.
>
> The liquid portion of blood is called plasma. Because plasma is more than 90% water, it is thin and almost colorless when it is separated from the blood cells.

## Formed Elements

Erythrocytes contain a protein called **hemoglobin** (**HEE**-moh-**gloh**-bin), abbreviated as Hgb. It has the ability to bind with oxygen and carbon dioxide. As erythrocytes circulate in the body, the hemoglobin in them transports oxygen to the organ cells and carries carbon dioxide away from the organ cells.

Leukocytes fight infections. They have the ability to move from the bloodstream into the site of infection in the tissues. New white blood cells replace old white cells that are destroyed in the fight against the infection. As illustrated in Figure 13-1, leukocytes are classified as either granular or nongranular. The granular leukocytes have a grain-like substance in the nucleus. They are further classified as either **eosinophils**, **basophils**, or **neutrophils**. The nongranular leukocytes are classified as either **monocytes** or **lymphocytes**.

Thrombocytes (platelets) initiate blood clotting when bleeding occurs. Platelets gather at the cut and combine with clotting factors in the plasma. This action causes a platelet plug to be formed where the vessel wall has been cut. The plug seals the cut to stop bleeding.

> **In Brief**
>
> **Formed elements**: erythrocytes, leukocytes, thrombocytes
>
> **Granular leukocytes**: basophils, neutrophils, and eosinophils
>
> **Nongranular leukocytes**: lymphocytes, monocytes
>
> **Erythrocytes** transport oxygen and carbon dioxide.
>
> **Leukocytes** fight infection.
>
> **Thrombocytes** are important in blood clotting.

Plasma carries many important solids. It transports proteins, fats, gases, salts, and hormones to their various places throughout the body and picks up waste materials from organ cells.

Proteins in the plasma function to maintain water balance in the blood. If too much water escapes from the blood and accumulates in the body tissues, it will cause pooling of water in body tissues. This is called **edema** (eh-**DEE**-mah).

Other proteins in plasma prevent excessive bleeding by making the blood clot. These proteins are called clotting factors. When clotting factors are removed from the plasma, the liquid that is left is called **serum** (**SEER**-um). In other words, serum is the clear fluid of plasma minus the clotting elements. Many blood tests are performed on serum.

---

**In Brief**    **Plasma** is the liquid portion of the blood.

**Serum** is plasma without the clotting elements.

---

## PRACTICE FOR LEARNING: **Blood Composition**

Choose the correct answer from those in parentheses.

1. Red blood cells are also known as (leukocytes/platelets/erythrocytes).
2. The liquid portion of the blood is called (plasma/serum).
3. Plasma minus the clotting factors is called (formed elements/serum/blood).
4. Accumulation of water in body tissue is called (anemia/edema/congestion).
5. Platelets are also called (leukocytes/thrombocytes/ erythrocytes).
6. The oxygen-carrying component of red blood cells is (plasma/serum/ hemoglobin).
7. The function of white blood cells is (blood clotting/fighting infections).
8. The function of thrombocytes is (blood clotting/fighting infections).

> Answers: 1. erythrocytes. 2. plasma. 3. serum. 4. edema. 5. thrombocytes.
> 6. hemoglobin. 7. fighting infections. 8. blood clotting.

## 13.3  Blood Types

The body's immune system produces **antibodies** (**AN**-tee-bah-deez) to protect it against invaders such as viruses and bacteria. Any substance that stimulates the body's immune response to produce antibodies is referred to as an **antigen** (**AN**-tih-jen). (Antigen is an abbreviation for the term "antibody generator.")

There are two proteins that may or may not be on the surface of red blood cells. These proteins are called antigens. The body reacts to them as if they were foreign bodies to be attacked, like viruses. In other words, antibodies are produced in response to these antigens. These proteins are referred to as type A and type B antigens. Blood is classified according to the presence or absence of these antigens. Type A blood has only type A antigens. Type B blood has only type B antigens. Type AB blood has both antigens. Type O blood has neither.

Persons who require a blood transfusion must receive the correct type of blood. If they receive blood that has an antigen that their blood does not recognize, antibodies will be formed because the antigen is seen as a foreign body. This reaction is called an antigen-antibody reaction.

The antigen-antibody reaction causes clumping of red blood cells and can be fatal. Blood must therefore be cross-matched before it is transfused into a patient.

There are several other blood antigens. The most important is the Rh antigen, which was first discovered by examining the blood of Rhesus monkeys. Most people are Rh positive (Rh+), meaning they have the Rh antigen. Those who lack it are Rh negative (Rh−).

**In Brief**

**Type A** blood has only A antigens.

**Type B** blood has only B antigens.

**Type AB** blood has both antigens.

**Type O** has neither antigen.

Most people are Rh positive—they have the Rh antigen.

## PRACTICE FOR LEARNING: Blood Types

Answer the following questions on the space provided.

**1.** Define antigen. _____
_____
_____

**2.** Name four blood types. _____
_____

**3.** What happens when a person is transfused with the wrong type of blood?
_____
_____

Answers: 1. any substance that stimulates the body's immune response to produce antibodies. 2. A, B, AB, O. 3. antigen-antibody reaction occurs, causing the red blood cells to clump.

## 13.4   New Roots, Suffixes, and Prefixes

Use these additional roots and suffixes when studying the terms in this chapter.

| ROOT | MEANING |
|------|---------|
| megal/o | large |
| norm/o | normal |
| poikil/o | variation; irregular |

| SUFFIX | MEANING |
|--------|---------|
| -lysis | destruction; breakdown; separation |
| -poietin | hormone regulating the production of blood cells |

## 13.5   Learning the Terms

### Roots

| ROOT chrom/o | | MEANING color |
|--------------|--------------|---------------|
| *Term* | *Term Analysis* | *Definition* |
| hyperchromia (high-per-**KROH**-mee-ah) | -ia = state of; condition hyper- = excessive | excessively pigmented (colored) red blood cells. The cause is high hemoglobin content |
| hypochromia (high-poh-**KROH**-mee-ah) | -ia = state of; condition hypo = below; deficient | underpigmented red blood cells. The cause is low hemoglobin content |
| normochromia (nor-moh-**KROH**-mee-ah) | -ia = state of; condition norm/o = normal | red blood cells that are normally pigmented |

| ROOT erythr/o | | MEANING red |
|---------------|--------------|-------------|
| *Term* | *Term Analysis* | *Definition* |
| erythropoietin (eh-**rith**-roh-**POY**-eh-tin) | -poietin = hormone regulating the production of blood cells | hormone in the kidney that stimulates the production of red blood cells in the bone marrow |

| ROOT hemat/o; hem/o | | MEANING blood |
| --- | --- | --- |
| Term | Term Analysis | Definition |
| hematologist (hee-mah-TOL-oh-jist) | -logist = specialist; one who studies | a specialist in the study of the blood, its disorders and treatment |
| hematology (hee-mah-TOL-oh-jee) | -logy = study of | study of blood, blood disorders, and their treatment |
| hemolysis (hee-MOL-ih-sis) | -lysis = breakdown; separation; destruction | breakdown of blood |

| ROOT leuk/o | | MEANING white |
| --- | --- | --- |
| Term | Term Analysis | Definition |
| leukocyte (LOO-koh-sight) | -cyte = cell | white blood cell |

| ROOT myel/o | | MEANING bone marrow (also spinal cord) |
| --- | --- | --- |
| Term | Term Analysis | Definition |
| myelogenous (my-eh-LOJ-en-us) | -genous = produced by | produced in the bone marrow |
| myelodysplastic syndrome (my-eh-loh-dis-PLAS-tick SIN-drohm) | -plastic = pertaining to development or formation dys- = poor; bad; abnormal syndrome = group of signs and symptoms that indicates a specific disease | poor development of the bone marrow results in a group of bone marrow disorders that is characterized by insufficient production of one or more types of blood cells |

| ROOT thromb/o | | MEANING clot |
| --- | --- | --- |
| Term | Term Analysis | Definition |
| thrombosis (throm-BOH-sis) | -osis = abnormal condition | abnormal condition of blood clots |
| thrombolysis (throm-BOL-ih-sis) | -lysis = destruction; breakdown; separation | breakdown of clots |

## Suffixes

| SUFFIX -blast | | MEANING immature; growing thing |
|---|---|---|
| Term | Term Analysis | Definition |
| hemocytoblast (hee-moh-SIGHT-oh-blast) | hem/o = blood cyt/o = cell | an immature blood cell that can develop into any type of mature blood cell. Also known as stem cells |
| megalocytoblast (meg-ah-loh-SIGHT-oh-blast) | megal/o = large cyt/o = cell | large immature cell |

| SUFFIX -cytosis | | MEANING condition of cells; slight increase in the number of cells |
|---|---|---|
| Term | Term Analysis | Definition |
| anisocytosis (an-eye-soh-sigh-TOH-sis) | anis/o = unequal | increased variation in the size of cells, especially red blood cells |
| leukocytosis (loo-koh-sigh-TOH-sis) | leuk/o = white | abnormal increase in the number of white blood cells |

**Note:** The increase in the number of white blood cells is not permanent. They are temporarily increased to fight an infection. After the infection has subsided, the number of white blood cells returns to normal. Compare with leukemia found in Section 13.6.

| | | |
|---|---|---|
| poikilocytosis (poy-kil-oh-sigh-TOH-sis) | poikil/o = variation; irregular | increased variation in the shape of cells, particularly red blood cells |

| SUFFIX -emia | | MEANING blood condition |
|---|---|---|
| Term | Term Analysis | Definition |
| anemia (ah-NEE-mee-ah) | an- = lack of; no; not | lack of red blood cells or hemoglobin content in the blood |
| erythremia (er-ih-THREE-mee-ah) | erythr/o = red | abnormal increase in the number of red blood cells |
| septicemia (sep-tih-SEE-me-ah) | septic/o = infection | microorganisms causing infection of the blood affecting the entire body; blood poisoning |

| SUFFIX -penia | | MEANING deficient; decrease |
|---|---|---|
| Term | Term Analysis | Definition |
| **erythrocytopenia** (eh-**rith**-roh-**sigh**-toh-**PEE**-nee-ah) | erythr/o = red cyt/o = cell | decrease in the number of red blood cells. Also known as **erythropenia** (eh-**rith**-roh-**PEE**-nee-**ah**) |
| **pancytopenia** (**pan**-sigh-toh-**PEE**-nee-ah) | pan- = all cyt/o = cell | decrease in the number of all blood cells |

| SUFFIX -poiesis | | MEANING production; manufacture; formation |
|---|---|---|
| Term | Term Analysis | Definition |
| **erythropoiesis** (eh-**rith**-roh-poy-**EE**-sis) | erythr/o = red | production of red blood cells |

| SUFFIX -stasis | | MEANING stopping; controlling |
|---|---|---|
| Term | Term Analysis | Definition |
| **hemostasis** (**hee**-moh-**STAY**-sis) | hem/o = blood | stopping of bleeding |

## 13.6 Pathology

### Anemia

Insufficient red blood cells and hemoglobin in the blood. The lack of hemoglobin makes the blood unable to carry enough oxygen to tissues. As a result, the patient becomes tired and pale. There are many different types of anemia. Some can be fatal, and others are benign. Common anemias are listed below.

### Aplastic

Aplastic anemia is a condition where the bone marrow fails to produce a sufficient amount of blood cells: erythrocytes, leukocytes, and thrombocytes. This results in pancytopenia, a deficiency of all cells.

### Iron Deficiency Anemia

Iron deficiency anemia is caused by inadequate iron absorption or increased iron requirement. Iron is necessary for the production of hemoglobin. Hemoglobin is necessary in red blood cells to transport oxygen to body tissues.

### Megaloblastic (**meg**-ah-loh-**BLAS**-tick) Anemia

Megaloblastic anemia is characterized by large immature red blood cells in the bone marrow instead of the normal biconcave disc shape. Most often this is due to the lack or ineffective use of Vitamin $B_{12}$ or folate (a B vitamin also known as folic acid).

### Pernicious (per-**NISH**-us) Anemia

Pernicious anemia is caused by the lack of vitamin $B_{12}$. Although Vitamin $B_{12}$ may be ingested in sufficient quantities, the intestine fails to absorb it.

### Sickle Cell

Sickle cell anemia is a hereditary condition where the red blood cells are sickle-shaped (crescent-shaped) rather than the typical biconcave disc shape. This abnormal shape reduces the ability of normal red blood cells to carry adequate oxygen to tissues.

## Hemophilia (**hee**-moh-**FEE**-lee-ah)

Hemophilia is a genetic condition characterized by a lack of clotting factors VIII and IX, which are necessary for blood to clot. The blood does not clot quickly and bleeding is prolonged. The patient can experience spontaneous or traumatic bleeding into skin, joints, or mouth. This can be fatal.

## Leukemia (loo-**KEE**-mee-ah)

Leukemia is a form of bone marrow cancer that results in a malignant increase in the number of white blood cells. The white blood cells eventually replace red blood cells, platelets, and normal functioning white blood cells. Oxygen delivery to tissues, blood clotting, and immunity are impaired as a result. Leukemic cells may metastasize to other organs such as the spleen, lymph nodes, and central nervous system.

## Multiple Myeloma (my-eh-**LOH**-mah)

This condition is a malignant neoplasm of the bone marrow. This results in bone destruction, as the tumor replaces bone.

## 13.7   Look-Alike and Sound-Alike Words

*Below is a list of look-alike and sound-alike words. Study the spelling and definitions of each set of words. Questions will follow in the Review Exercises.*

### TABLE 13-1   Look-Alike and Sound-Alike Words

| | |
|---|---|
| hemostasis | stoppage of blood |
| homeostasis | balanced yet varied state |
| leukopenia | deficiency of white blood cells |
| leukemia | malignant increase in the number of white blood cells |
| hyperchromic | excessively pigmented red blood cells |
| hypochromic | underpigmented red blood cells |
| myogenous | produced in muscle tissue |
| myelogenous | produced by bone marrow |
| erythremia | abnormal increase in the number of red blood cells |
| erythema | redness of the skin |

## 13.8   Review Exercises

### EXERCISE 13-1   Look-Alike and Sound-Alike

*Read the sentences carefully and circle the word in parentheses that correctly completes the meaning. Use Table 13-1 if it helps you.*

1. At the end of the operation, (**homeostasis/hemostasis**) was achieved by tying the blood vessels. The patient left the operating room in good condition.

2. In a certain type of anemia, there is underdevelopment of the bone marrow with associated (**leukemia/leukopenia**).

3. In iron deficiency anemia, the erythrocytes are less than their normal color, they are (**hyperchromic/hypochromic**).

4. Ms. Nussbaum was admitted with a diagnosis of acute (**myelogenous/myogenous**) leukemia.

5. Gaylene was admitted with (**erythremia/erythema**) to the entire body because of a rash due to a drug allergy.

## EXERCISE 13-2  Matching Word Parts with Meaning

*Match the word part in Column A with its meaning in Column B.*

| | Column A | Column B |
|---|---|---|
| _____ | **1.** hem/o | A. destruction |
| _____ | **2.** -lysis | B. condition of cells |
| _____ | **3.** -stasis | C. clot |
| _____ | **4.** -poiesis | D. blood |
| _____ | **5.** pan- | E. deficient |
| _____ | **6.** -penia | F. blood condition |
| _____ | **7.** thromb/o | G. stopping |
| _____ | **8.** -emia | H. all |
| _____ | **9.** -cytosis | I. production |
| _____ | **10.** -blast | J. immature |

## EXERCISE 13-3  Definitions—Anatomy and Pathology

*Define the following terms.*

1. **formed elements** _____

2. **plasma** _____

3. **hemophilia** _____

4. **edema** _____

5. **anemia** _____

6. **multiple myeloma** _____

7. **type A blood** _____

8. **hemoglobin** _____

9. **antibodies** _____

10. **antigens** _____

11. **leukemia** _____

12. **monocytes** _____

13. **platelets** _____

**14. serum** _____

**15. eosinophils** _____

## EXERCISE 13-4  Definitions—Learning the Terms

*Define the following terms.*

   **1. hematology** _____

   **2. myelogenous** _____

   **3. thrombosis** _____

   **4. thrombocyte** _____

   **5. thrombus** _____

   **6. hemocytoblast** _____

   **7. leukocytosis** _____

   **8. erythremia** _____

   **9. pancytopenia** _____

  **10. hemostasis** _____

  **11. anisocytosis** _____

  **12. poikilocytosis** _____

  **13. megalocytoblast** _____

  **14. myelodysplastic syndrome** _____

## EXERCISE 13-5  Spelling

*Circle any words that are spelled incorrectly in the list below. Then correct the spelling in the space provided.*

   **1.** cerum _____

   **2.** hemolysis _____

   **3.** plattelets _____

   **4.** myelogenous _____

   **5.** arithrocytes _____

**6.** leukopoiesis _____

**7.** hemostasis _____

**8.** hemopillia _____

**9.** adema _____

**10.** myeloma _____

## 13.9 Pronunciation and Spelling

**1.** Listen to each word on the audio file provided on the Student Companion Website.

**2.** Pronounce each word carefully.

**3.** Spell each word in the space provided.

| Word | Pronunciation | Spelling |
|---|---|---|
| anemia | ah-**NEE**-mee-ah | |
| antibodies | **AN**-tee-**bah**-deez | |
| anisocytosis | an-**eye**-soh-sigh-**TOH**-sis | |
| basophil | **BAY**-soh-fill | |
| edema | eh-**DEE**-mah | |
| eosinophil | **ee**-oh-**SIN**-oh-fill | |
| erythremia | **er**-ih-**THREE**-mee-ah | |
| erythrocyte | eh-**RITH**-roh-sight | |
| erythrocytopenia | eh-**rith**-roh-**sigh**-toh-**PEE**-nee-ah | |
| erythropoiesis | eh-**rith**-roh-poy-**EE**-sis | |
| hematology | **hee**-mah-**TOL**-oh-jee | |
| hemoglobin | **HEE**-moh-**gloh**-bin | |
| hemolysis | hee-**MOL**-ih-sis | |
| hemophilia | **hee**-moh-**FEE**-lee-ah | |
| hemostasis | **hee**-moh-**STAY**-sis | |
| leukemia | loo-**KEE**-mee-ah | |
| leukocytes | **LOO**-koh-sights | |
| leukocytosis | **loo**-koh-sigh-**TOH**-sis | |

| Word | Pronunciation | Spelling |
|------|--------------|----------|
| lymphocyte | **LIM**-foh-sight | |
| monocyte | **MON**-oh-sight | |
| myelodysplastic | **my**-eh-loh-dis-**PLAS**-tick | |
| myelogenous | **my**-eh-**LOJ**-en-us | |
| pancytopenia | **pan**-sigh-toh-**PEE**-nee-ah | |
| plasma | **PLAZ**-mah | |
| poikilocytosis | **poy**-kil-oh-sigh-**TOH**-sis | |
| serum | **SEER**-um | |
| thrombocyte | **THROM**-boh-sight | |
| thrombolysis | throm-**BOL**-ih-sis | |
| thrombosis | throm-**BOH**-sis | |

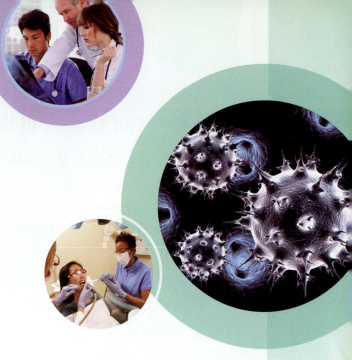

## CHAPTER 14

# Lymphatic and Immune Systems

## Chapter Outline

## Learning Objectives

*After studying this chapter and completing the review exercises, you should be able to:*

1. Locate and describe the organs of the lymphatic system.
2. Define terms relating to the immune system.
3. Pronounce, spell, define, and write the medical terms related to the lymphatic and immune systems.
4. Describe common diseases of the lymphatic and immune systems.
5. Listen, read, and study so you can speak and write.

## Introduction

The **lymphatic** (lim-**FAH**-tick) system is the body's other circulatory system. It works with the blood system to fight infection and disease, transport nutrients, and drain excess fluid from tissues.

## 14.1  Major Organs of the Lymphatic System

PRACTICE FOR LEARNING: **Major Organs of the Lymphatic System**

Write the words below in the correct spaces on Figure 14-1. To help you, the number beside the word tells you where it goes on the figure. Be sure to pronounce each word as you write it. Repeat the pronunciation several times if you find the word hard to say.

1. tonsils (**TON**-silz)
2. lymph vessels (**LIMF VESS**-elz)
3. thymus (**THIGH**-mus)
4. spleen (**SPLEEN**)
5. lymph nodes

## 14.2  Lymphatic System

As you saw in Figure 14-1, the lymphatic system consists of a vascular system, the lymph nodes, the thymus gland, the spleen, and the tonsils. The fluid traveling through the vascular system is called **lymph**.

The lymphatic system serves a number of important functions in the body. Of primary importance is the task of draining excess fluids away from body tissues and delivering them to the bloodstream. This system also transports nutrients to body tissues. Because of the presence of lymphocytes and monocytes, the lymphatic system also plays an important role in the body's defense against infection.

**In Brief**

**Parts of the lymphatic system**
vascular system, lymph,
lymph nodes, thymus gland, spleen

**Functions of the lymphatic system**
immunity,
drains excess fluid, carries nutrients

### Lymphatic Vessels

Look at Figure 14-2. You will see that the vascular system consists of three types of vessels: lymphatic capillaries, lymphatic vessels (lymphatics), and the right and left lymphatic ducts. (Left lymphatic duct is shown in Figure 14-3.)

The lymphatic capillaries are the smallest of these vessels. They are present in body tissues. The fluid in the body tissues is called interstitial (**in**-ter-**STISH**-al) fluid. Excess fluid and bacteria from body tissues seep into the lymphatic capillaries. Once inside the capillaries, the fluid is called lymph.

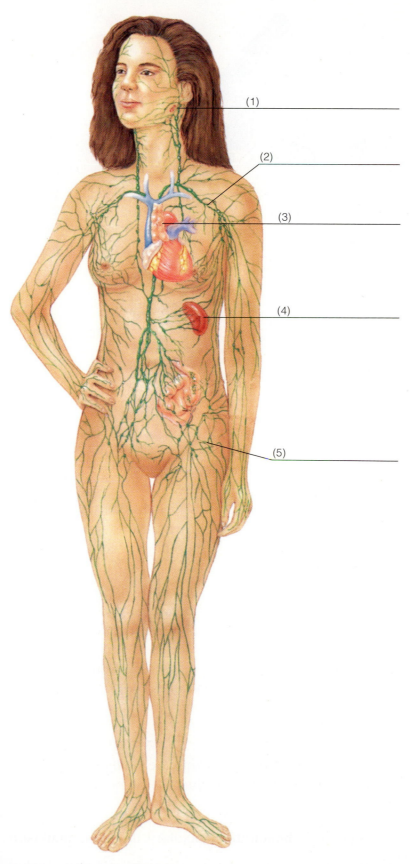

(1)

(2)

(3)

(4)

(5)

**Figure 14-1**  The lymphatic system.

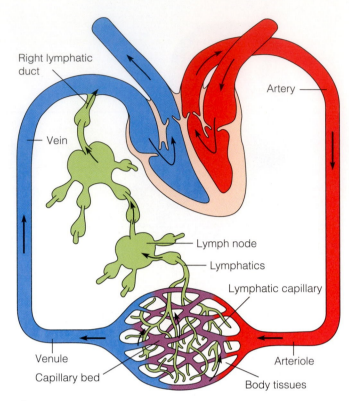

**Figure 14-2** Lymph vessels.

As illustrated in Figure 14-2, the lymph flows from the lymphatic capillaries, into larger vessels called lymphatics. The lymphatics ultimately drain into the largest vessels of the lymphatic system, called lymphatic ducts.

The two lymphatic ducts are shown in Figure 14-3. Lymph from the right side of the head, neck, and chest and from the right arm drains into the right lymphatic duct. Lymph from the rest of the body drains into the left lymphatic duct. Both of the lymphatic ducts drain into the bloodstream.

Lymph is cleaned by lymph nodes before it drains into the bloodstream. These nodes are located in clusters at various sites in the body. Look at Figure 14-3. You will see the principal clusters of nodes. They are called the cervical, submandibular, axillary, mediastinal, and inguinal nodes.

The lymph nodes act as filtration devices for lymph and contain a great number of white blood cells called **phagocytes** (**FAY**-goh-sights). Phagocytes (phag/o = to eat; -cyte = cell) eat bacteria.

---

**In Brief**

Lymph flows from the lymphatic capillaries ⟶ lymphatics ⟶ right and left lymphatic ducts ⟶ bloodstream

**Lymph node clusters**

cervical, submandibular, axillary, inguinal, mediastinal

**Lymph nodes** contain phagocytes that digest unwanted material.

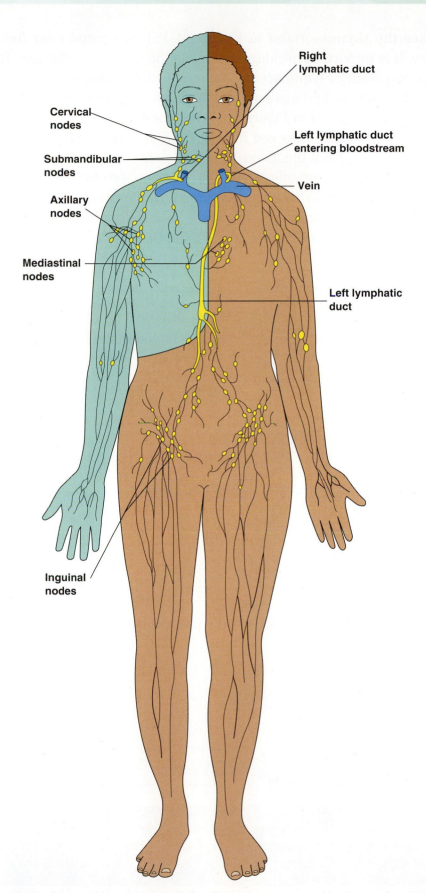

**Figure 14-3** Lymphatic ducts and lymph nodes. Notice the body areas served by the two lymphatic ducts.

You can see the **thymus gland** in Figure 14-1. It is located near the heart in the thoracic cavity. It is important because it protects the body from disease. It also plays a role in the development of lymphocytes. Remember from Chapter 13 that lymphocytes are white blood cells that fight against foreign substances such as viruses and bacteria.

The **spleen** is also shown in Figure 14-1. It is located in the left side of the abdominal cavity. It produces and stores red blood cells and gets rid of old red blood cells. It also eliminates bacteria from the blood.

Tonsils are made of lymphatic tissue. Three pairs are located in the throat. The **palatine** (**PAL**-ah-tine) tonsils are normally referred to simply as tonsils. The **pharyngeal** (far-**IN**-jee-al) tonsils are commonly called the **adenoids** (**AD**-eh-noids). The **lingual** (**LING**-gwal) tonsils are at the base of the tongue. Because of their location, they filter bacteria from food and air.

---

**In Brief**

The **thymus** is important in immunity.

The **spleen** stores and produces red blood cells, and gets rid of bacteria.

**Tonsils** filter bacteria.

---

PRACTICE FOR LEARNING: **Lymphatic System**

Write the answers to the following statements in the space provided.

**1.** Write the name of the fluid circulating through the lymphatic vessels.

_____

**2.** Write three functions of the lymphatic system.

_____

_____

_____

**3.** Lymph node clusters under the lower jaw are called

_____

**4.** The pharyngeal tonsils are commonly known as _____

**5.** List three functions of the spleen.

_____

_____

_____

**6.** Where is the thymus located? _____

> Answers: 1. lymph. 2. immunity, drains excess fluid, transports nutrients. 3. submandibular. 4. adenoids. 5. stores red blood cells; produces red blood cells; eliminates old red blood cells and bacteria. 6. near the heart in the thoracic cavity.

## 14.3 Immune System

The immune system is our protection against disease. This system includes the lymphoid organs (lymph nodes, spleen, and thymus). It also includes lymphocytes and antibodies. When a foreign substance, called an **antigen** (**AN**-tih-jen), invades the body, the immune response is turned on by two types of lymphocytes: T lymphocytes (T-cells) and B lymphocytes (B-cells).

T-cells recognize and kill cells that have been infected with a virus. They recognize and kill cancerous cells. T-cells are also known as killer or **cytotoxic** (**sigh**-toh-**TOCK**-sick) T-cells because of their function.

B-cells produce antibodies. These antibodies travel through the blood. They have the ability to attach to foreign cells, labeling them for destruction by phagocytes.

As mentioned in the previous chapter, antigen is a general term that refers to foreign substances such as bacteria and viruses, as well as to plant pollen and to red blood cells in transplanted tissues. Antigens stimulate the body's immune response to produce antibodies against substances not recognized by the body.

The specialized role of T-cells and antibodies in fighting antigens is made possible by the fact that each T-cell and each antibody binds to its own particular antigen-binding site.

---

**In Brief**

**Antigens**
foreign substance that stimulates the production of antibodies
**Antibodies** inactivate antigens.
**Lymphocytes** are important in the immune response.
Types of lymphocytes
T lymphocytes (T-cells)
B lymphocytes (B-cells)
**T cells** kill virus-infected cells and cancerous cells.
**B cells** produce antibodies.

---

### PRACTICE FOR LEARNING: Immune System

Underline the correct answer in each sentence.

**1.** (T-cells/B-cells) produce antibodies.

**2.** (T-cells/B-cells) recognize cells infected with a virus.

**3.** Lymphocytes are (red blood cells/white blood cells/platelets).

**4.** Bacteria, viruses, pollen, and dust are examples of (antibodies/antigens/immunity).

Answers: 1. B-cells. 2. T-cells. 3. white blood cells. 4. antigens.

## 14.4    New Roots, Suffixes, and Prefixes

Use these additional roots and suffixes when studying the terms in this chapter.

| ROOT | MEANING |
|------|---------|
| scint/i | spark |
| tox/o | poison |

| SUFFIX | MEANING |
|--------|---------|
| -edema | accumulation of fluid in body tissues; swelling |
| -kines | movement |
| -stitial | to place |

## 14.5    Learning the Terms

Following these steps will make it easier for you to learn medical terms:

1. Pronounce the term repeatedly until it is easy for you.
2. Write it down. Ensure the spelling is correct.
3. Also write the definition. If possible, relate the word to a word, thought, or picture that will help you remember it.
4. Analyze the term with the method taught in this text.

### Roots

| ROOT cyt/o | | MEANING cell |
|------------|--|--------------|
| *Term* | *Term Analysis* | *Definition* |
| cytokines (SIGH-toh-kighnz) | -kines = movement | proteins that signal cells to start the immune response. Examples are interferons and interleukins. |
| cytotoxic (sigh-toh-TOCK-sick) | -ic = pertaining to<br>tox/o = poison | pertaining to an agent that kills cells |

| ROOT immun/o | | MEANING immunity; safe |
| --- | --- | --- |
| Term | Term Analysis | Definition |
| immunodeficiency (im-yoo-no-dee-FISH-en-see) | deficiency = lacking | inadequate immune response |
| immunoglobulin (Ig) (im-yoo-noh-GLOB-yoo-lin) | globulin = protein | proteins that have the ability to attach to foreign cells, labeling them for destruction by phagocytes |
| immunology (im-yoo-NOL-oh-jee) | -logy = study of | study of the immune system |

| ROOT lymphaden/o | | MEANING lymph node |
| --- | --- | --- |
| Term | Term Analysis | Definition |
| lymphadenitis (lim-fad-eh-NIGH-tis) | -itis = inflammation | inflammation of the lymph nodes |
| lymphadenopathy (lim-fad-eh-NOP-ah-thee) | -pathy = disease | disease of the lymph nodes, especially enlargement of the lymph nodes |

| ROOT lymphangi/o | | MEANING lymph vessels |
| --- | --- | --- |
| Term | Term Analysis | Definition |
| lymphangitis (lim-fan-JIGH-tis) | -itis = inflammation | inflammation of the lymph vessels |

| ROOT lymph/o | | MEANING lymph |
| --- | --- | --- |
| Term | Term Analysis | Definition |
| lymphedema (lim-feh-DEE-mah) | -edema = accumulation of fluid in body tissues | accumulation of fluid in body tissues due to obstruction of lymphatic structures |
| lymphoid tissue (LIM-foyd) | -oid = resembling; pertaining to | resembling or pertaining to lymph tissue |

| Term | Term Analysis | Definition |
|------|---------------|------------|
| lymphoscintigraphy (lim-foh-sin-TIG-grah-fee) | -graphy = process of recording scint/i = spark | process of recording the lymphatic vessels or lymph nodes to produce images that detect metastatic tumors, lymphedema or lymph node blockage. A type of nuclear imaging process |

| ROOT splen/o | | MEANING spleen |
|--------------|--|-----------------|
| Term | Term Analysis | Definition |
| splenomegaly (splee-noh-MEG-ah-lee) | -megaly = enlargement | enlargement of the spleen |
| splenorrhagia (splee-noh-RAY-jee-ah) | -rrhagia = bursting forth | hemorrhage from the spleen |
| splenorrhaphy (splee-NOR-ah-fee) | -rrhaphy = suture | suture of the spleen |

| ROOT thym/o | | MEANING thymus gland |
|-------------|--|----------------------|
| Term | Term Analysis | Definition |
| thymectomy (thigh-MECK-toh-mee) | -ectomy = excision; surgical removal | excision of the thymus |

| ROOT tonsill/o | | MEANING tonsils |
|----------------|--|-----------------|
| Term | Term Analysis | Definition |
| tonsillectomy (ton-sih-LECK-toh-mee) | -ectomy = excision; surgical removal | excision of the tonsils |

## Suffixes

| SUFFIX -immune | | MEANING immunity; safe |
|---|---|---|
| Term | Term Analysis | Definition |
| autoimmune disease (aw-toh-ih-**MYOON**) | auto- = self | an immune response to one's own body tissue; destruction of one's cells by the immune system |

| SUFFIX -stitial | | MEANING to place |
|---|---|---|
| Term | Term Analysis | Definition |
| interstitial fluid (in-ter-**STISH**-al) | inter- = between | fluid placed between the tissue spaces |

## 14.6  Pathology

### Autoimmune Disease

Normally, the immune system attacks only foreign cells. In autoimmune disease, the immune system attacks the body's own cells instead of foreign cells. Examples are rheumatoid arthritis and multiple sclerosis.

### HIV and AIDS

Infection with the human immunodeficiency virus (HIV). This virus obstructs the body's ability to fight off disease-causing microorganisms such as bacteria, viruses, parasites, and fungi.

   With the appropriate drug treatment, a person can live with HIV for many years, functioning normally without major problems. Without the proper drug treatment, however, the disease progresses. The immune system becomes weakened and incapacitated. A diagnosis of **AIDS** (**AYDZ**) is given at this time. HIV infection and AIDS (acquired immunodeficiency syndrome) are the same disease. The label HIV is used when the disease is in its early stages. The label AIDS is used in the late stages of the disease.

## Hypersensitivity/Allergic Reactions

Abnormal inflammatory response or hypersensitivity to an allergen (any substance causing an allergic reaction such as pollen, dust, dander, and bee stings).

Allergic reactions occur when the body is exposed to a foreign substance that causes an immune response that is harmful to the body. The body's response can be mild or severe. It can include asthma, hay fever, hives (urticaria), allergic dermatitis, and allergic rhinitis. The most severe reaction is **anaphylactic** (**an**-ih-fih-**LACK**-tick) **shock**. This is an extreme reaction to the allergen, such as a bee sting. It can be fatal.

## Lymphoma

Lymphomas are tumors of lymphoid tissue. The major categories of malignant lymphoma are Hodgkin (**HOJ**-kin) disease and non-Hodgkin lymphoma. Although possessing similar names, these conditions have different characteristics. Hodgkin disease is diagnosed by the presence of **Reed-Sternberg** cells in the lymph nodes. In non-Hodgkin lymphoma, Reed-Sternberg cells are not present. Non-Hodgkin lymphoma is the more common condition.

## 14.7   Review Exercises

### EXERCISE 14-1   Matching Word Parts with Meaning

*Match the word part in Column A with its meaning in Column B.*

| | Column A | Column B |
|---|---|---|
| _____ | **1.** -edema | A. lymph vessel |
| _____ | **2.** -rrhaphy | B. bursting forth |
| _____ | **3.** -immune | C. self |
| _____ | **4.** lymphangi/o | D. between |
| _____ | **5.** lymphaden/o | E. accumulation of fluid in body tissues |
| _____ | **6.** -rrhagia | F. to place |
| _____ | **7.** auto- | G. lymph gland |
| _____ | **8.** inter- | H. enlargement |
| _____ | **9.** -stitial | I. suture |
| _____ | **10.** -megaly | J. safe |

## EXERCISE 14-2 Anatomy and Pathology

*Fill in the blanks with the most appropriate term listed below. Not all terms are used.*

| | | |
|---|---|---|
| allergen | HIV | spleen |
| allergy | Hodgkin disease | STI |
| anaphylactic shock | HPV | T-cells |
| B-cells | lymph nodes | thymus |
| edema | phagocytes | tonsils |

**1.** Structure that filters lymph of unwanted material _____

**2.** Leukocytes that eat unwanted material _____

**3.** Lymphoid organ that stores red blood cells _____

**4.** Structure in the throat that filters bacteria _____

**5.** White blood cells that kill cancerous cells _____

**6.** Cells that produce antibodies _____

**7.** Accumulation of fluid in body tissues _____

**8.** Any substance causing an allergic reaction _____

**9.** Extreme reaction to an allergen _____

**10.** Type of lymphoma _____

**11.** Microorganism causing AIDS _____

## EXERCISE 14-3 Fill in the Blank—Lymph Nodes

*Write the location of the following lymph nodes.*

a. **submandibular** _____

b. **axillary** _____

c. **inguinal** _____

d. **cervical** _____

## EXERCISE 14-4 Definitions—Learning the Terms

*Define the following terms.*

**1. immunodeficiency** _____

**2. lymphadenopathy** _____

3. **splenomegaly** _____

4. **lymphedema** _____

5. **interstitial fluid** _____

6. **immunoglobulins** _____

7. **cytotoxic** _____

8. **cytokines** _____

## EXERCISE 14-5  Building Medical Terms

*Build the medical words.*

1. study of the immune system _____

2. inflammation of the lymph glands _____

3. hemorrhage from the spleen _____

4. suture of the spleen _____

5. excision of the thymus _____

## EXERCISE 14-6  Spelling

*Circle any words that are spelled incorrectly in the list below. Then correct the spelling in the space provided.*

1. interstial fluid _____

2. lymphadenitis _____

3. imunology _____

4. tonsilectomy _____

5. thymectomy _____

## Animations

Visit the companion website to view the videos on **Lymph Nodes** and **Lymph**.

## 14.8 Pronunciation and Spelling

**1.** Listen to each word on the audio file provided on the Student Companion Website.

**2.** Pronounce each word carefully.

**3.** Spell each word in the space provided.

| Word | Pronunciation | Spelling |
|------|---------------|----------|
| adenoids | **AD**-eh-noids | |
| autoimmune | **aw**-toh-ih-**MYOON** | |
| anaphylactic | **an**-ih-fih-**LACK**-tick | |
| Hodgkin disease | **HOJ**-kin | |
| immunodeficiency | **im**-yoo-no-dee-**FISH**-en-see | |
| immunoglobulin | **im**-yoon-oh-**GLOB**-yoo-lin | |
| immunology | **im**-yoo-**NOL**-oh-jee | |
| interstitial | **in**-ter-**STISH**-al | |
| lymph | **LIMF** | |
| lymphadenitis | lim-**fad**-eh-**NIGH**-tis | |
| lymphadenopathy | lim-**fad**-eh-**NOP**-ah-thee | |
| lymphangitis | **lim**-fan-**JIGH**-tis | |
| lymphatic | lim-**FAH**-tick | |
| lymphedema | **lim**-feh-**DEE**-mah | |
| lymphocytes | **LIM**-foh-sights | |
| lymphoma | lim-**FOH**-mah | |
| lymphoscintigraphy | **lim**-foh-sin-**TIG**-grah-fee | |
| spleen | **SPLEEN** | |
| splenomegaly | **splee**-noh-**MEG**-ah-lee | |
| splenorrhagia | **splee**-noh-**RAY**-jee-ah | |
| thymectomy | thigh-**MECK**-toh-mee | |
| thymus | **THIGH**-mus | |
| tonsillectomy | **ton**-sih-**LECK**-toh-mee | |
| tonsils | **TON**-silz | |

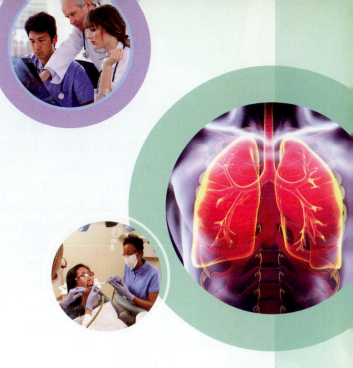

# Respiratory System

## Chapter Outline

## Learning Objectives

*After studying this chapter and completing the review exercises, you should be able to:*

1. Locate and describe the organs of the respiratory system.
2. Describe the functions of the respiratory structures.
3. Pronounce, spell, define, and write the medical terms related to the respiratory system.
4. Describe common diseases of the respiratory system.
5. Listen, read, and study so you can speak and write.

## Introduction

When you studied the cardiovascular system, you learned that blood travels to the lungs to pick up oxygen and give off wastes and carbon dioxide.

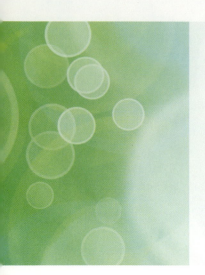

It then carries the oxygen to the body's cells and picks up more wastes and carbon dioxide. This chapter is about the respiratory system. It is responsible for the ongoing process of **respiration** (**res**-pih-**RAY**-shun). Respiration means taking in oxygen and giving off carbon dioxide.

The lungs get oxygen by breathing it in from the air. This is called inhalation. It is also called inspiration. The lungs get rid of the carbon dioxide by breathing out. This is called exhalation. It is also called expiration.

Various structures work together to make the passage of air into and out of the lungs possible. Together they are called the respiratory tract. As you will learn below, these structures are divided into two further categories: the upper respiratory tract (URT) and the lower respiratory tract (LRT).

## 15.1    Major Organs of the Respiratory System

**PRACTICE FOR LEARNING: Major Organs of the Respiratory System**

Write the words below in the correct spaces on Figure 15-1. To help you, the number beside the word tells you where it goes on the figure. Be sure to pronounce each word as you write it. Repeat the pronunciation several times if you find the word hard to say.

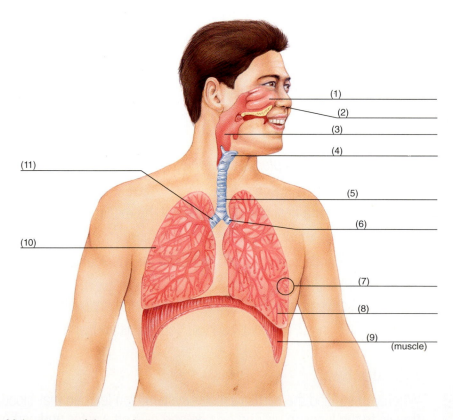

**Figure 15-1** Major organs of the respiratory system.

1. nasal cavity (**NAY**-zal)
2. nares (**NAH**-reez) (nostrils)
3. pharynx (**FAR**-inks)
4. larynx (**LAR**-inks)
5. trachea (**TRAY**-kee-ah)
6. left bronchus (**BRONG**-kus)
7. alveoli (al-**VEE**-oh-lye)
8. bronchiole (**BRONG**-kee-ohl)
9. diaphragm (**DYE**-ah-fram)
10. right lung
11. right bronchus (**BRONG**-kus)

## 15.2  Upper Respiratory Tract

**PRACTICE FOR LEARNING: Upper Respiratory Tract**

Write the words below in the correct spaces on Figure 15-2. To help you, the number beside the word tells you where it goes on the figure. Be sure to pronounce each word as you write it. Repeat the pronunciation several times if you find the word hard to say.

1. nasal cavity (**NAY**-zal)
2. epiglottis (**ep**-ih-**GLOT**-is)
3. vocal cords (**VOH**-kal **KORDZ**)
4. trachea (**TRAY**-kee-ah)
5. pharynx (**FAR**-inks)

The URT is illustrated in Figure 15-2. It includes the respiratory structures located outside the thoracic cavity. These are the nasal cavity, pharynx, larynx, and upper trachea. Mucous membrane lines the URT.

### Nasal Cavity

The nasal cavity is divided into right and left by a wall called the **nasal septum**. The nasal septum is part bone and part cartilage. Air enters the nasal cavity through the nares (nostrils). The hairs inside the nares filter out dust particles from the air as it is inhaled. These hairs are called **cilia** (**SIL**-ee-ah). The nasal cavity warms and moistens air. It is lined with nerve cells called **olfactory** (ol-**FACK**-toh-ree) **neurons** that provide us with our sense of smell. From the nares, the cavity extends to the pharynx.

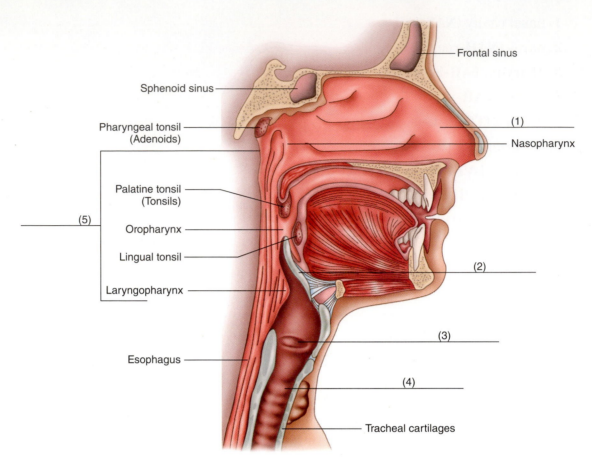

**Figure 15-2**  Structures of the Upper Respiratory Tract.

## Pharynx

As you can see in Figure 15-2, the pharynx is the throat. There are three sections to the pharynx: the **nasopharynx** (**nay**-zoh-**FAR**-inks), behind the nose; the **oropharynx** (**or**-oh-**FAR**-inks) behind the mouth; and the **laryngopharynx** (lah-**ring**-oh-**FAR**-inks) behind the larynx. The nasopharynx transports air only. The oropharynx and laryngo-pharynx transport air and food. The pharynx also contains the tonsils and adenoids, which function as part of the immune system as they fight off microorganisms that may be harmful to the body.

## Larynx

The larynx is the voice box. It consists of the vocal cords, the epiglottis, and the Adam's apple (thyroid cartilage).

The vocal cords are folds of mucous membrane. As air moves out of the lungs, it goes past the vocal cords. They vibrate and produce sound.

The epiglottis swings up and down like a lid. It covers the opening of the larynx dur-ing swallowing so that food from the pharynx does not go down the respiratory tract.

The Adam's apple is a large shield of cartilage that protects the inner structures. It is a bump that you can feel on the front of the neck.

| **In Brief** | **Nares** are the nostrils. |
| :--- | :--- |
| | **Pharynx** is the throat. |
| | **Larynx** is the voice box. |

PRACTICE FOR LEARNING: **Upper Respiratory Tract**

Fill in the blanks with the most appropriate answer.

1. Name the structure in the larynx that prevents food from entering the respiratory tract. _____

2. Write the function of the tonsils. _____

3. Write another name for nares. _____

4. Write the function of cilia. _____

> Answers: 1. epiglottis. 2. immunity. 3. nostrils. 4. filters out dust particles.

## 15.3  Lower Respiratory Tract

PRACTICE FOR LEARNING: **Lower Respiratory Tract**

Write the words below in the correct spaces on Figure 15-3. To help you, the number beside the word tells you where it goes on the figure. Be sure to pronounce each word as you write it. Repeat the pronunciation several times if you find the word hard to say.

1. trachea (**TRAY-**kee-ah)

2. primary bronchi (**BRONG-**keye)

3. bronchiole (**BRONG-**kee-ohl)

### Trachea, Bronchi, Bronchioles

The lower respiratory tract is illustrated in Figure 15-3. It includes the lower trachea, bronchi, and bronchioles. The trachea is the windpipe. It extends from the larynx to the **bronchi**. It is lined with mucous membrane and cilia, which filter the air.

The trachea branches into two tubes called the primary bronchi. Like the trachea, the primary bronchi (singular bronchus) (**BRONG-**ku**s**) are lined with mucous membrane and cilia. Each extends into a lung, and then branches into smaller and smaller bronchi. These small bronchi extend to tiny structures called bronchioles. The trachea and bronchi together form the tracheobronchial system. As you can see in Figure 15-3,

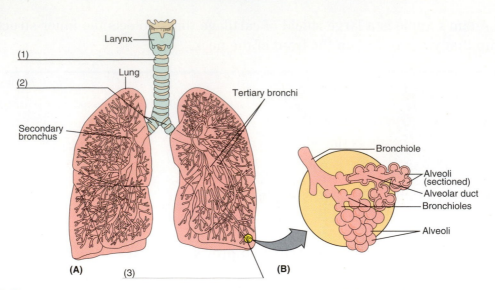

**Figure 15-3** Lower respiratory tract. A. Trachea, bronchi, and bronchioles. B. Bronchioles, alveolar duct, and alveoli.

the whole structure looks like an upside-down tree. As a result, it is often referred to as the tracheobronchial tree.

The tracheobronchial tree normally secretes mucus. This functions as a lubricant and protects against infection. When mucus and other matter are expelled from the trachea and the bronchus and through the mouth, it is called **sputum** (**SPYOO**-tum) or phlegm (**FLEM**). Laboratory examination of the sputum is helpful in diagnosing respiratory problems.

---

**In Brief**   **Trachea** is the windpipe.

**Trachea** branches into the primary bronchi, which eventually connect to bronchioles.

---

## Lungs and Alveoli

### PRACTICE FOR LEARNING: Lung

Write the words below in the correct spaces on Figure 15-4. To help you, the number beside the word tells you where it goes on the figure. Be sure to pronounce each word as you write it. Repeat the pronunciation several times if you find the word hard to say.

1. right superior lobe
2. right inferior lobe
3. right middle lobe
4. left inferior lobe
5. left superior lobe

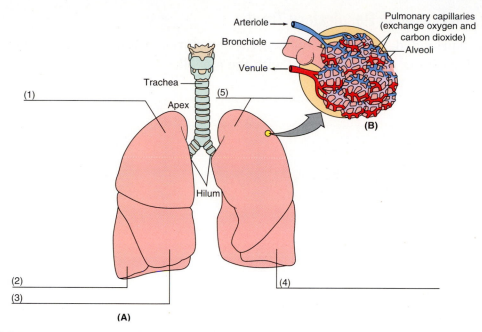

**Figure 15-4**  The lungs and alveoli. A. Structures of the lung. B. Pulmonary capillaries surrounding the alveoli.

The lungs lie in the thoracic cavity. The top of each lung is called the apex, and the bottom is the base. The right lung is divided into three lobes called the superior, middle, and inferior lobes. The left lung has no middle lobe (Figure 15-4A). Each lung is covered by a membrane called the **pleura** (**PLOOR**-ah).

Inside each lung are approximately 300 million **alveoli** (al-**VEE**-oh-lye) (Figure 15-3). They are like tiny balloons. When you inhale, the air goes down through the bronchioles and into the alveoli. They expand and fill up with air. The oxygen from the air is absorbed by the **pulmonary** (**PUL**-moh-ner-ee) **capillaries** that surround the alveoli (Figure 15-4B). The blood cells, specifically, the red blood cells, flowing through the capillaries take on the oxygen. The oxygenated blood continues on to the heart, to be pumped to the cells of the body. While the alveoli are giving off oxygen to the capillaries, they are also absorbing carbon dioxide from them. The carbon dioxide is expelled from the lungs during exhalation.

**In Brief**   **Right lung** has three lobes.

**Left lung** has two lobes.

**Alveoli** are responsible for gas exchange with the pulmonary capillaries.

**PRACTICE FOR LEARNING: Respiratory Tract**

In the space provided, name, in sequence, the structures through which air passes to the lungs. Start with the nasal cavity end with the alveoli.

_____

_____

_____

**Answer: nasal cavity, pharynx, larynx, trachea, bronchi, bronchioles, alveoli.**

## 15.4 | Paranasal Sinuses

**Paranasal** (**par**-ah-**NAY**-zal) **sinuses** (Figure 15-5) are hollow spaces in the skull bones. They are named after the bones in which they lie. There are four paranasal sinuses: frontal, ethmoid, sphenoid, and maxillary. They are lined with mucous membrane, which helps moisten and warm the air that is breathed in. The paranasal sinuses also help in producing voice sounds.

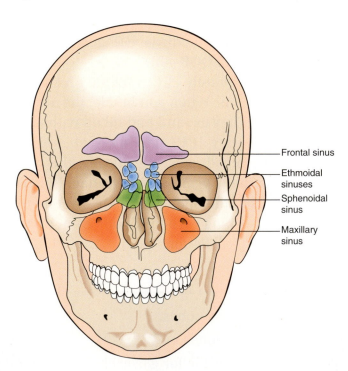

Frontal sinus

Ethmoidal sinuses

Sphenoidal sinus

Maxillary sinus

**Figure 15-5** Paranasal sinuses.

## 15.5  Pleural and Mediastinal Cavities

The thoracic cavity contains two smaller cavities called the **pleural** (**PLOOR**-al) and **mediastinal** (**me**-dee-as-**TYE**-nal) cavities (Figure 15-6). The mediastinal cavity is also known as the mediastinum (**mee**-dee-as-**TYE**-num).

As mentioned previously, the pleura surrounds the lungs. The pleura has an outer membrane and inner membrane. Between these two layers is an open space called the pleural cavity. This cavity is filled with fluid called pleural fluid. The fluid prevents friction between the two layers. The mediastinal cavity lies between the lungs and contains the heart, aorta, trachea, and esophagus.

**In Brief**  **Pleural cavity** surrounds the lungs.
**Mediastinal cavity** is between the lungs.

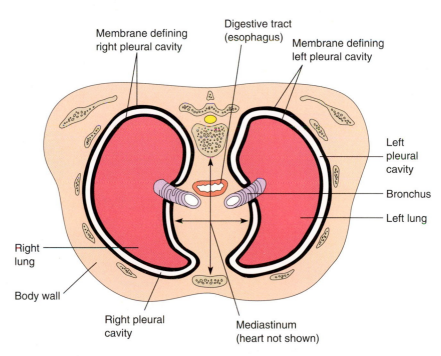

**Figure 15-6**  Mediastinal and pleural cavities.

PRACTICE FOR LEARNING: **Paranasal Sinuses, Pleural and Mediastinal Cavities**

Fill in the blanks with the most appropriate answer.

1. Write the functions of the paranasal sinuses.
   _____

2. Where is the pleural cavity?
   _____

**3.** Where is the mediastinal cavity?

_____

**4.** What does the pleural cavity contain?

_____

**5.** What organs are in the mediastinal cavity?

_____

> **Answers: 1.** warms and moistens air and aids in producing voice sounds. **2.** around the lungs. **3.** between the lungs. **4.** fluid. **5.** heart, aorta, trachea, and esophagus.

## 15.6  New Roots, Suffixes, and Prefixes

Use these additional roots, suffixes, and prefixes when studying the medical terms in this chapter.

| ROOT | MEANING |
|------|---------|
| atel/o | incomplete; imperfect |
| py/o | pus |

| SUFFIX | MEANING |
|--------|---------|
| -lytic | pertaining to destruction, separation, or breakdown |
| -or | person or thing that does something |

| PREFIX | MEANING |
|--------|---------|
| eu- | normal; good |
| oligo- | scanty; few |

## 15.7  Learning the Terms

Following these steps will make it easier for you to learn medical terms:

**1.** Pronounce the term repeatedly until it is easy for you.

**2.** Write it down. Ensure the spelling is correct.

**3.** Also write the definition. If possible, relate the word to a word, thought, or picture that will help you remember it.

**4.** Analyze the term with the method taught in this text.

## Roots

| ROOT adenoid/o | | MEANING adenoids |
|---|---|---|
| *Term* | *Term Analysis* | *Definition* |
| **adenoidectomy** (**ad**-eh-noid-**ECK**-toh-mee) | -ectomy = excision; surgical removal | excision of the adenoids |

| ROOT bronchi/o; bronch/o | | MEANING bronchus |
|---|---|---|
| *Term* | *Term Analysis* | *Definition* |
| **chronic bronchitis** (**KRAH**-nick brong-**KYE**-tis) | chronic = disease lasting over a long period of time  -itis = inflammation | inflammation of the bronchus lasting over a long period of time. Bronchitis is diagnosed as chronic when it lasts a total of three months in two consecutive years.  Compare with **acute bronchitis**. Acute refers to sudden onset and short duration. |
| **bronchorrhea** (brong-koh-**REE**-ah) | -rrhea = flow; discharge | bronchial discharge |
| **bronchodilator** (**brong**-koh-**DYE**-lay-tor) | -or = person or thing that does something  dilat/o = dilation; widening | drugs used to dilate the bronchus to relieve bronchospasm |
| **bronchospasm** (**BRONG**-koh-spazm) | -spasm = sudden, involuntary contraction | sudden, involuntary contraction of the bronchus |

| ROOT cost/o | | MEANING rib |
|---|---|---|
| *Term* | *Term Analysis* | *Definition* |
| **intercostal** (**in**-ter-**KOS**-tal) | -al = pertaining to  inter- = between | pertaining to between the ribs |
| **infracostal** (**in**-frah-**KOS**-tal) | -al = pertaining to  infra- = below | pertaining to below the ribs |

| ROOT laryng/o | | MEANING larynx; voice box |
|---|---|---|
| Term | Term Analysis | Definition |
| laryngotracheobronchitis (lah-**ring**-goh-**tray**-kee-oh-brong-**KYE**-tis) | -itis = inflammation<br>trache/o = trachea; windpipe | inflammation of the larynx and trachea. Also known as **croup** (**KROOP**).<br>Croup is a disease of infants and young children. |

| ROOT muc/o | | MEANING mucus (a sticky, thick secretion from mucous membrane) |
|---|---|---|
| Term | Term Analysis | Definition |
| mucolytic (**myoo**-koh-**LIH**-tick) | -lytic = pertaining to the breakdown or destruction | drugs used to break down thick mucus so it can be coughed up |

| ROOT nas/o (see also rhin/o) | | MEANING nose |
|---|---|---|
| Term | Term Analysis | Definition |
| nasopharyngeal (**nay**-zoh-far-**INN**-jee-al) | -eal = pertaining to<br>pharyng/o = pharynx; throat | pertaining to the nose and pharynx |

| ROOT ox/o | | MEANING oxygen |
|---|---|---|
| Term | Term Analysis | Definition |
| hypoxemia (**high**-pock-**SEE**-mee-ah) | -emia = blood condition<br>hypo- = below; abnormal decrease | abnormal decrease of oxygen levels in the blood |
| hypoxia (high-**POCK**-see-ah) | -ia = state of; condition<br>hypo- = deficient; abnormal decrease | deficiency of oxygen to tissues |

| ROOT<br>**pector/o (see also thorac/o)** | | MEANING<br>**chest** |
|---|---|---|
| *Term* | *Term Analysis* | *Definition* |
| **pectoral**<br>(**PECK-**toh-rahl) | -al = pertaining to | pertaining to the chest |

| ROOT<br>**pharyng/o** | | MEANING<br>**throat; pharynx** |
|---|---|---|
| *Term* | *Term Analysis* | *Definition* |
| **oropharyngeal**<br>(**or-**oh-far-**IN-**jee-al) | -eal = pertaining to<br>or/o = mouth | pertaining to the mouth and throat |

| ROOT<br>**phren/o** | | MEANING<br>**diaphragm** |
|---|---|---|
| *Term* | *Term Analysis* | *Definition* |
| **phrenic**<br>(**FREN-**ick) | -ic = pertaining to | pertaining to the diaphragm |

| ROOT<br>**pleur/o** | | MEANING<br>**pleura; pleural cavity** |
|---|---|---|
| *Term* | *Term Analysis* | *Definition* |
| **pleural effusion**<br>(**PLOOR-**al eh-**FYOO-**zhun) | -al = pertaining to<br>effusion = movement of fluid out of the blood vessels and into the tissues | movement of fluid out of the blood vessels into the pleural cavity |
| **pleuritis**<br>(ploor-**EYE-**tis) | -itis = inflammation | inflammation of the pleura; pleurisy |
| **pleurodynia**<br>(**ploor-**oh-**DIN-**ee-ah) | -dynia = pain | pain in the pleural cavity; pleuralgia |

| ROOT pneumon/o; pulmon/o | | MEANING lungs |
|---|---|---|
| *Term* | *Term Analysis* | *Definition* |
| pneumococcus (**noo**-moh-**KOCK**-us) | -coccus = berry-shaped bacteria | berry-shaped bacteria attacking the lungs and other parts of the body. Illnesses can include: pneumonia, meningitis, middle ear infections, and septicemia. Plural form is pneumococci. |
| pulmonary edema (**PUL**-moh-ner-ee eh-**DEE**-mah) | -ary = pertaining to edema = accumulation of fluid in body tissues | accumulation of fluid in the lung tissue |

| ROOT rhin/o | | MEANING nose |
|---|---|---|
| *Term* | *Term Analysis* | *Definition* |
| otorhinolaryngology (oh-toh-**rye**-noh-**lar**-in-**GOL**-oh-jee) | -logy = study of ot/o = ear laryng/o = voice box; larynx | the study of the ears, nose, and throat. Abbreviated **ENT**. |
| rhinorrhea (rih-noh-**REE**-ah) | -rrhea = discharge | discharge from the nose; runny nose |
| rhinoplasty (**RYE**-noh-**plas**-tee) | -plasty = surgical reconstruction; surgical repair | surgical repair of the nose; plastic surgery on the nose for cosmetic or reconstructive purposes; a nose job |

| ROOT spir/o | | MEANING breathing |
|---|---|---|
| *Term* | *Term Analysis* | *Definition* |
| spirometry (spye-**ROM**-eh-tree) | -metry = process of measuring | process of measuring airflow and volume into and out of lungs |

| ROOT steth/o | | MEANING chest |
|---|---|---|
| *Term* | *Term Analysis* | *Definition* |
| stethoscope (**STETH**-oh-skope) | -scope = instrument used to examine | instrument used to listen to chest sounds |

| ROOT thorac/o | | MEANING chest |
|---|---|---|
| Term | Term Analysis | Definition |
| **thoracocentesis** (**thoh**-rah-koh-sen-**TEE**-sis) | -centesis = surgical puncture | surgical puncture to remove fluid from the pleural cavity (Figure 15-7). Also known as thoracentesis (**thor**-ah-sen-**TEE**-sis) and pleurocentesis (**ploor**-oh-sen-**TEE**-sis) |

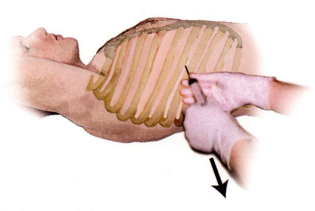

**Figure 15-7** Thoracocentesis.

| | | |
|---|---|---|
| **thoracotomy** (**thor**-ah-**KOT**-oh-mee) | -tomy = process of cutting | process of cutting into the chest |

| ROOT tonsill/o | | MEANING tonsils |
|---|---|---|
| Term | Term Analysis | Definition |
| **tonsillectomy** (**ton**-sih-**LECK**-toh-mee) | -ectomy = surgical excision; removal | excision of the tonsils<br><br>When the tonsils are removed with the adenoids, the operation is tonsillectomy and adenoidectomy (T&A). |
| **tonsillitis** (**ton**-sih-**LYE**-tis) | -itis = inflammation | inflammation of the tonsils |

| ROOT trache/o | | MEANING trachea; windpipe |
|---|---|---|
| Term | Term Analysis | Definition |
| **endotracheal** (**en**-doh-**TRAY**-kee-al) | -eal = pertaining to endo- = within | pertaining to within the trachea |
| **tracheostomy** (**tray**-kee-**OS**-toh-mee) | -stomy = new opening | new opening into the trachea is created through the neck and a tube is inserted to assist breathing. The tracheostomy tube may be temporary or permanent (Figure 15-8). |

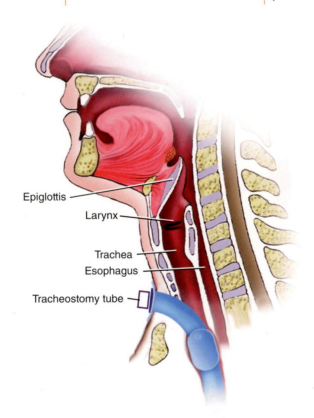

Epiglottis

Larynx

Trachea

Esophagus

Tracheostomy tube

**Figure 15-8** Tracheostomy.

| **tracheotomy** (**tray**-kee-**OT**-oh-mee) | -tomy = process of cutting | process of cutting into the trachea (Figure 15-9) |
|---|---|---|

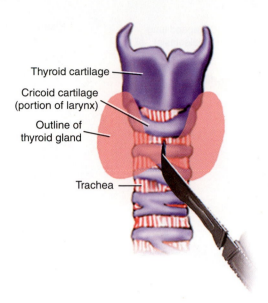

**Figure 15-9** Tracheotomy.

## Suffixes

| SUFFIX -capnia | | MEANING carbon dioxide |
|---|---|---|
| *Term* | *Term Analysis* | *Definition* |
| hypercapnia (**high**-per-**KAP**-nee-ah) | hyper- = excessive; above normal | excessive levels of carbon dioxide in the blood |

| SUFFIX -ectasis | | MEANING dilation; stretching; widening |
|---|---|---|
| *Term* | *Term Analysis* | *Definition* |
| atelectasis (**at**-eh-**LECK**-tah-sis) | atel/o = incomplete; imperfect | incomplete expansion of the lung; collapsed lung (Figure 15-10). If this condition happens in a newborn, it is called **hyaline** (**HIGH**-ah-leen) **membrane disease**. |

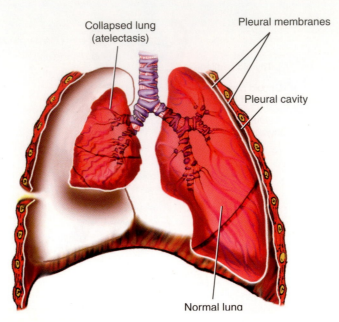

**Figure 15-10**  Atelectasis of right lung (collapsed lung).

| Term | Term Analysis | Definition |
|---|---|---|
| **bronchiectasis** (**brong**-kee-**ECK**-tah-sis) | bronchi/o = bronchus | dilation or widening of the bronchus (Figure 15-11) |

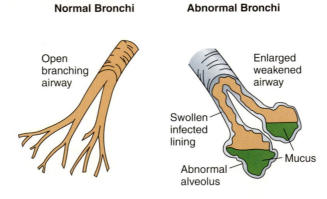

**Figure 15-11**  In bronchiectasis, the bronchi loses its elasticity and widens. Mucus accumulates in the alveoli, making breathing difficult.

| SUFFIX -phonia | | MEANING voice | |
|---|---|---|
| Term | Term Analysis | Definition |
| **aphonia** (ah-**FOH**-nee-ah) | a- = no; not; lack of | loss of voice |
| **dysphonia** (dis-**FOH**-nee-ah) | dys- = difficult; bad; painful | difficulty in speaking |

| SUFFIX -pnea | | MEANING breathing |
|---|---|---|
| Term | Term Analysis | Definition |
| apnea (**AP**-nee-ah) | a- = no; not; lack of | no breathing (Figure 15-12D) |
| bradypnea (**brad**-ip-**NEE**-ah) | brady- = slow | slow breathing (Figure 15-12C) |
| dyspnea (**DISP**-nee-ah) | dys- = painful; difficult; bad | painful breathing |
| eupnea (yoop-**NEE**-ah) | eu- = normal; good | normal breathing (Figure 15-12A) |
| hyperpnea (**high**-perp-**NEE**-ah) | hyper- = abnormal increase; excessive | abnormal increase in depth and rate of breathing (Figure 15-12E) |
| oligopnea (**ol**-ih-gop-**NEE**-ah) | oligo- = scanty; few | infrequent breathing |
| orthopnea (**or**-thop-**NEE**-ah) | ortho- = straight | difficulty breathing except in the upright position |
| tachypnea (**tack**-ip-**NEE**-ah) | tachy- = fast | fast breathing (Figure 15-12B) |

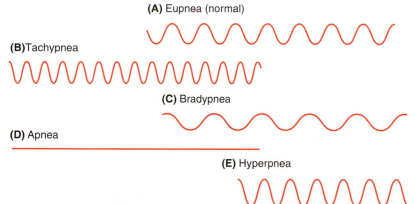

**(A)** Eupnea (normal)

**(B)** Tachypnea

**(C)** Bradypnea

**(D)** Apnea

**(E)** Hyperpnea

**Figure 15-12**  Breathing patterns.

| SUFFIX -ptysis | | MEANING spitting |
|---|---|---|
| Term | Term Analysis | Definition |
| hemoptysis (hee-**MOP**-tih-sis) | hem/o = blood | spitting up of blood |

| SUFFIX -sphyxia | | MEANING pulse |
|---|---|---|
| *Term* | *Term Analysis* | *Definition* |
| asphyxia (as-**FICK**-see-ah) | a- = no; not; lack of | lack of oxygen to body tissues; can interfere with respiration and eventually lead to a loss of pulse |

| SUFFIX -thorax | | MEANING chest |
|---|---|---|
| *Term* | *Term Analysis* | *Definition* |
| hemothorax (**hee**-moh-**THOR**-acks) | hem/o = blood | blood in the pleural cavity |
| hydrothorax (**high**-droh-**THOR**-acks) | hydr/o = water | fluid in the pleural cavity |
| pneumothorax (**noo**-moh-**THOR**-acks) | pneum/o = air | collection of air in the pleural cavity (Figure 15-13) |
| pyothorax (**pye**-oh-**THOR**-acks) | py/o = pus | pus in the pleural cavity (Figure 15-13); **empyema** (**em**-pye-**EE**-mah) |

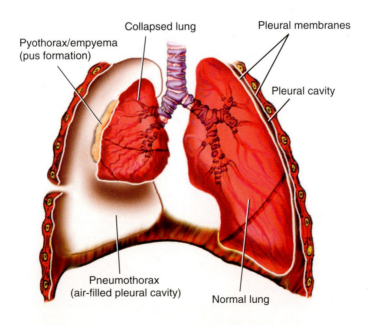

Collapsed lung

Pleural membranes

Pyothorax/empyema (pus formation)

Pleural cavity

Pneumothorax (air-filled pleural cavity)

Normal lung

**Figure 15-13** Pneumothorax and pyothorax. External pressure from air or pus causes the lung to collapse.

## 15.8 Pathology

### Allergic rhinitis (rye-**NYE**-tis)

This condition is an allergic response to inhaled allergens (foreign substances). It is characterized by rhinorrhea, ophthalmorrhea, nasal pruritus (itchiness), and congestion. Also includes hay fever and seasonal rhinitis due to the inhalation of pollen and molds.

### Asthma (**AZ**-mah)

A bronchospasm that results in airway obstruction (Figure 15-14). Inhaled allergens, such as chemicals, pollen, dust, or mold, can irritate the airways. This can cause bronchospasm, which obstructs the airways and makes breathing difficult.

Although the bronchospasm can be reversed with the proper drug treatment, prolonged spasm of the bronchus can be fatal.

### Bronchogenic Carcinoma

Malignant neoplasm of the lung arising from the bronchus or bronchioles.

Cigarette smoking is the cause of most lung cancers. Other factors may be radiation exposure and inhalation of carcinogenic agents such as asbestos.

Treatment includes surgery to remove the tumor. Radiotherapy and chemotherapy are also used to kill cancer cells.

### Chronic Obstructive Pulmonary Disease (COPD)

COPD is a chronic disease of the respiratory tract that obstructs air flow to the lungs and body tissues. The diagnosis is given to the patient when they have two or more of the

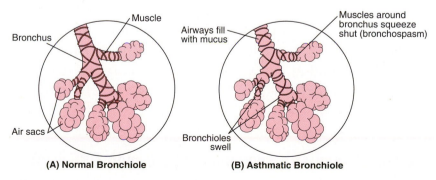

**Figure 15-14** Asthma. A. Normal bronchiole: muscles are relaxed and the airways are open. B. Asthmatic bronchiole: muscles tighten and airways fill with mucus.

following chronic conditions: chronic bronchitis, asthma, and emphysema (described below). Over time, these conditions weaken the lung, making breathing difficult.

### Cystic Fibrosis (**SIS**-tick fye-**BROH**-sis)

Cystic fibrosis (CF) is a genetic disease involving the lungs, pancreas, and sweat glands. The abnormal secretion of thick gel-like mucus from these organs causes damage to the lung, nutritional deficiency, and sweat gland abnormalities.

### Deviated Nasal Septum (**NAY**-zal **SEP**-tum)

This condition is a shift of the nasal septum away from the midline, usually caused by trauma.

### Emphysema (**em**-fih-**SEE**-mah)

Emphysema involves loss of elasticity and overexpansion (dilation) of the alveoli. Once this happens, they do not return to their normal size and the air becomes trapped in them. This obstructs the passage of oxygen from the lungs into body tissues. This leads to eventual destruction of the alveoli and loss of pulmonary function. Cigarette smoking is a major risk factor.

### Epistaxis (ep-ih-**STACK**-sis)

Bleeding from the nostrils or nosebleed. Trauma to the nose is the usual cause, although a dry climate can also cause bleeding. As for diseases, upper respiratory tract infection, allergies, drug intake, and blood disorders are common causes.

### Pneumoconiosis (**new**-moh-**koh**-nee-**OH**-sis), Black Lung

Accumulation of dust particles in the lung from long exposure and inhalation of irritants, often from an occupational environment. The numerous types of pneumoconioses are named for the type of dust inhaled. **Silicosis** (**sill**-ih-**KOH**-sis) is caused by the inhalation of silica dust found in quartz and sand. **Anthracosis** (an-thrah-**KOH**-sis) is caused by the inhalation of coal dust. It is also known as **black lung disease**. Asbestosis is caused by the inhalation of asbestos.

### Pneumonia (noo-**MOH**-nee-ah); Pneumonitis (noo-mon-**EYE**-tiss)

Pneumonia is inflammation of the lung caused by infection. As the condition progresses, the effects of the inflammatory process cause the lung to become solid. This is called **consolidation** (kon-**sol**-ih-**DAY**-shun). This hinders the exchange of oxygen and carbon

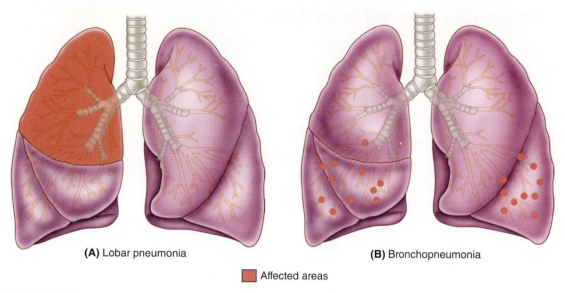

**(A)** Lobar pneumonia      **(B)** Bronchopneumonia

■ Affected areas

**Figure 15-15** Two types of pneumonia. A. Lobar pneumonia results in consolidation of a lobe of the lung. B. In bronchopneumonia there is consolidation around the bronchioles.

dioxide between blood vessels. Following a regime of antibiotic therapy, the pneumonia resolves, and the consolidation disappears. This is called **resolution**.

Pneumonia is described by the type of infectious material or the location of the pneumonia (Figure 15-15). For example, streptococcus pneumonia is caused by streptococcus bacteria, while lobar pneumonia is pneumonia affecting a lobe of the lung. **Aspiration pneumonia** does not describe the infectious material or location of the pneumonia. Aspiration pneumonia is caused by the intake (aspiration) of food, liquid, or vomit into the lung.

## Tuberculosis (too-**ber**-kyoo-**LOH**-sis)

Tuberculosis (TB) is caused by the **Mycobacterium** (**my**-koh-back-**TEER**-ee-um) **tuberculosis** bacteria, which is carried through the air and inhaled into the lungs. Most often TB is seen in patients with a weakened immune system caused by conditions such as AIDS.

## 15.9 Look-Alike and Sound-Alike Words

*Below is a list of look-alike and sound-alike words. Study the spelling and definitions of each set of words. Questions will follow in the Review Exercises.*

## TABLE 15-1 Look-Alike and Sound-Alike

| | |
|---|---|
| breath | (BREHTH) air taken into the lungs (noun) |
| breathe | (BREETH) to take air into the lungs (verb) |
| expiration | to breathe out from the lung |
| inspiration | to draw air into the lungs |
| perfusion | to pour through (to perfuse blood through blood vessels) |
| profusion | abundance; excess |
| hoarse | harsh and rough in sound |
| horse | a four-legged, hoofed animal |
| course | sequence of events |
| coarse | rough; abrasive |
| intracostal | within the ribs |
| intercostal | between the ribs |
| infracostal | below the ribs |
| mucous (adjective) | pertaining to mucus. Mucous (adjective) describes membrane (noun). For example mucous membrane. |
| mucus (noun) | thick, sticky substance secreted from mucous membrane |
| rales | abnormal crackling sound heard on respiration |
| rails | a bar extending from one support to another to form a railing or guardrail |

## 15.10 Review Exercises

### EXERCISE 15-1 Look-Alike and Sound-Alike Words

*Read the sentences carefully and circle the word in parentheses that correctly completes the meaning. Use Table 15-1 if it helps you.*

1. On examination there was decreased (**breath/breathe**) sounds in the lower third of the right lung.

2. The patient has recurring pain when he tries to (**breath/breathe**).

3. (**Inspiratory/Expiratory**) wheezing was noted when the patient took a deep (**breath/breathe**).

4. The head injury caused a (**perfusion/profusion**) of blood.

5. The lung scan showed normal (**profusion/perfusion**) of blood through the lungs.

6. The child was seen two days ago, and at that time had a barky cough and sounded (**hoarse/horse**).

7. The disease took its normal (**course/coarse**), and the patient was discharged seven days following admission.

8. Chest x-ray showed the lung tissue to be (**course/coarse**) and granular.

9. Lungs were noted to have (**rails/rales**) at the left base with decreased (**breath/breathe**) sounds.

10. Place the (**rales/rails**) in the upright position.

11. The patient was seen in the emergency room coughing up (**mucous/mucus**) and vomiting blood.

12. On examination, the (**mucus/mucous**) membrane showed redness and scarring.

## EXERCISE 15-2 Matching Word Parts with Meaning

*Match the word part in Column A with its meaning in Column B.*

| | Column A | Column B |
|---|---|---|
| _____ | **1.** ox/o | A. pertaining to |
| _____ | **2.** -ectasis | B. diaphragm |
| _____ | **3.** pector/o | C. voice |
| _____ | **4.** phren/o | D. straight |
| _____ | **5.** oligo- | E. normal |
| _____ | **6.** pulmon/o | F. nose |
| _____ | **7.** rhin/o | G. oxygen |
| _____ | **8.** -ar | H. dilation |
| _____ | **9.** eu- | I. chest |
| _____ | **10.** ortho- | J. few; scanty |
| _____ | **11.** -phonia | K. lung |
| _____ | **12.** -pnea | L. pulse |
| _____ | **13.** -sphyxia | M. breathing |

## EXERCISE 15-3  Matching—Anatomy

*Match the structure in Column A with its description in Column B.*

| | Column A | Column B |
|---|---|---|
| _____ | **1.** cilia | A. exchanges oxygen and carbon dioxide |
| _____ | **2.** olfactory neurons | B. prevents food from entering the respiratory tract |
| _____ | **3.** pharynx | C. nostrils |
| _____ | **4.** paranasal sinuses | D. mucus and other matter ejected from the mouth |
| _____ | **5.** larynx | E. throat |
| _____ | **6.** alveoli | F. filters out dust particles |
| _____ | **7.** trachea | G. voice box |
| _____ | **8.** sputum | H. windpipe |
| _____ | **9.** epiglottis | I. warms and moistens air |
| _____ | **10.** nares | J. sense of smell |

## EXERCISE 15-4  Pathology

*Select the disease from the list below that best fits its description that follows.*

pneumoconiosis _____

asthma _____

atelectasis _____

tuberculosis _____

croup _____

emphysema _____

pleurisy _____

pneumonia _____

bronchiectasis _____

cystic fibrosis _____

**1.** Bronchospasm resulting in airway obstruction _____

**2.** Overexpansion of the alveoli _____

**3.** Inflammation of the pleura _____

**4.** Widening of the bronchi traps mucus in the bronchial tubes, causing obstructed airflow _____

**5.** Inflammation of the lung _____

**6.** Inflammation of the larynx, trachea, and bronchus in young children

_____

**7.** Incomplete expansion of the alveoli _____

**8.** A genetic disease involving the lungs, pancreas, and sweat glands

_____

**9.** Caused by a type of *Mycobacterium* _____

**10.** Accumulation of dust particles in the lungs _____

## EXERCISE 15-5  Labeling—Respiratory Tract

*Using the body structures listed below, label Figure 15-16. Write your answer in the numbered spaces provided below, or if you prefer, on the diagram.*

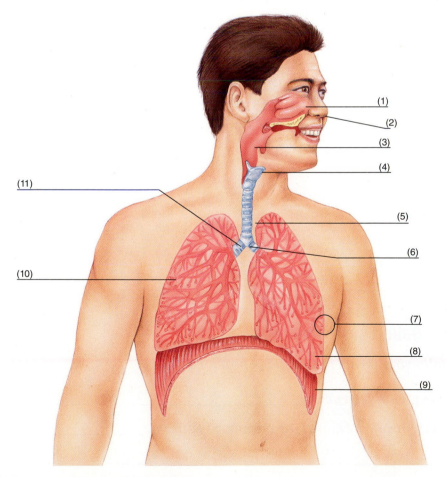

**Figure 15-16** Structures of the respiratory system.

alveoli _____

bronchiole _____

diaphragm _____

larynx _____

left bronchus _____

nares _____

nasal cavity _____

pharynx _____

right bronchus _____

right lung _____

trachea _____

1. _____

2. _____

3. _____

4. _____

5. _____

6. _____

7. _____

8. _____

9. _____

10. _____

11. _____

## EXERCISE 15-6  Definitions—Anatomy

*Define the following terms in the space provided.*

1. **upper respiratory tract** _____

2. **paranasal sinuses**. Name four paranasal sinuses. _____

_____

_____

3. olfactory neurons _____

4. mediastinum _____

5. nasal septum _____

6. nares _____

7. pulmonary capillaries _____

8. alveoli _____

9. mucous _____

10. mucus _____

## EXERCISE 15-7 Definitions—Learning the Terms

*Define the following terms.*

1. bronchodilator _____

2. mucolytic _____

3. phrenic _____

4. pulmonary edema _____

5. otorhinolaryngology _____

6. rhinorrhea _____

7. stethoscope _____

8. thoracotomy _____

9. aphonia _____

10. dysphonia _____

11. orthopnea _____

12. bradypnea _____

13. hemoptysis _____

14. asphyxia _____

15. nasopharyngeal _____

16. eupnea _____

17. oligopnea _____

18. tonsillitis _____

## EXERCISE 15-8  Building Medical Words

*I. Use the suffix -pnea to build medical words for the following definitions.*

**a.** fast breathing _____

**b.** breathing only in the upright position _____

**c.** no breathing _____

**d.** slow breathing _____

**e.** infrequent breathing _____

**f.** abnormal increase in depth and rate of breathing

_____

**g.** difficult breathing _____

**h.** normal breathing _____

*II. Use rhin/o to build medical words for the following definitions.*

**a.** discharge from the nose _____

**b.** surgical reconstruction of the nose _____

*III. Use trache/o to build medical words for the following definitions.*

**a.** new opening into the trachea _____

**b.** process of cutting into the trachea _____

**c.** pertaining to within the trachea _____

*IV. Use -thorax to build medical words for the following definitions.*

**a.** blood in the pleural cavity _____

**b.** pus in the pleural cavity _____

**c.** water in the pleural cavity _____

**d.** air in the pleural cavity _____

## EXERCISE 15-9  Definitions in Context

*Define the bolded terms in context. Use your medical dictionary if necessary.*

This 64-year-old female with advanced **COPD** was admitted to the hospital with a five-day history of increased **dyspnea** to the point that she was **SOB** (had shortness of breath) at rest.

There was evidence of right **inferior lobe pneumonia** on x-ray. Laboratory tests including **hemoglobin** and white blood cell count were normal. **Sputum** taken from the **oropharynx** was examined for growth of **streptococci** and **staphylococci**.

    **a.** COPD _____

    **b.** dyspnea _____

    **c.** SOB _____

    **d.** inferior lobe pneumonia _____

    **e.** hemoglobin _____

    **f.** sputum _____

    **g.** oropharynx _____

    **h.** streptococci _____

    **i.** staphylococci _____

## EXERCISE 15-10  Spelling

*Circle any words that are spelled incorrectly in the list below. Then correct the spelling in the space provided.*

  **1.** diaphram _____

  **2.** epiglottis _____

  **3.** dispnea _____

  **4.** plurisy _____

  **5.** mediastinum _____

  **6.** stethoscope _____

  **7.** tackypnea _____

  **8.** emphysema _____

  **9.** plural cavity _____

**10.** asphixia _____

## Animations

Visit the companion website to view the videos on **Respiration Safeguards**, **Bronchial Structures**, and **Asthma**.

## 15.11  Pronunciation and Spelling

1. Listen to each word on the audio file provided on the Student Companion Website.

2. Pronounce each word carefully.

3. Spell each word in the space provided.

| Word | Pronunciation | Spelling |
|------|---------------|----------|
| adenoidectomy | **ad**-eh-noid-**ECK**-toh-mee | |
| alveoli | al-**VEE**-oh-lye | |
| asthma | **AZ**-mah | |
| atelectasis | **at**-eh-**LECK**-tah-sis | |
| bradypnea | **brad**-ip-**NEE**-ah | |
| bronchiectasis | **brong**-kee-**ECK**-tah-sis | |
| bronchiole | **BRONG**-kee-ohl | |
| bronchitis | brong-**KYE**-tis | |
| bronchodilator | **brong**-koh-**DYE**-lay-tor | |
| bronchus | **BRONG**-kus | |
| cilia | **SIL**-ee-ah | |
| croup | **KROOP** | |
| diaphragm | **DYE**-ah-fram | |
| dysphonia | dis-**FOH**-nee-ah | |
| emphysema | **em**-fih-**SEE**-mah | |
| empyema | **em**-pye-**EE**-mah | |
| endotracheal | **en**-doh-**TRAY**-kee-al | |
| epiglottis | **ep**-ih-**GLOT**-is | |
| eupnea | yoop-**NEE**-ah | |
| hemothorax | **hee**-moh-**THOR**-acks | |
| hydrothorax | **high**-droh-**THOR**-acks | |
| hyperpnea | **high**-perp-**NEE**-ah | |
| hypoxia | high-**POCK**-see-ah | |
| laryngotracheobronchitis | lah-**ring**-goh-**tray**-kee-oh-brong-**KYE**-tis | |
| mediastinal | **me**-dee-as-**TYE**-nal | |
| larynx | **LAR**-inks | |

| Word | Pronunciation | Spelling |
|------|---------------|----------|
| mucolytic | **myoo**-koh-**LIH**-tick | |
| nares | **NAH**-reez | |
| olfactory | ol-**FACK**-toh-ree | |
| oligopnea | **ol**-ih-**GOP**-nee-ah | |
| orthopnea | **or**-thop-**NEE**-ah | |
| otorhinolaryngology | **oh**-toh-**rye**-noh-**lar**-in-**GOL**-oh-jee | |
| pharynx | **FAR**-inks | |
| pleura | **PLOOR**-al | |
| pleurisy | **PLOOR**-ih-see | |
| pneumonia | noo-**MOH**-nee-ah | |
| stethoscope | **STETH**-oh-skope | |
| tonsillectomy | **ton**-sih-**LECK**-toh-mee | |
| trachea | **TRAY**-kee-ah | |
| tracheostomy | **tray**-kee-**OS**-toh-mee | |

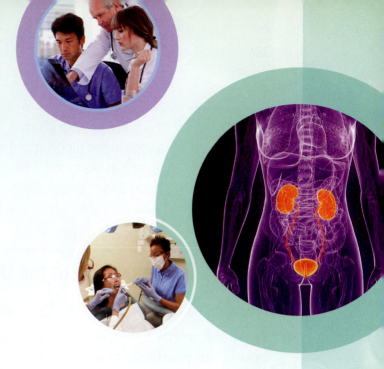

# CHAPTER 16

# Urinary System

## Chapter Outline

## Learning Objectives

*After studying this chapter and completing the review exercises, you should be able to:*

1.  Name and locate the organs of the urinary system.
2.  Describe the structure and functions of the kidney, ureters, bladder, and urethra.
3.  Describe how the kidneys produce urine.
4.  Pronounce, spell, define, and write the medical terms related to the urinary system.
5.  Describe common diseases of the urinary system.
6.  Listen, read, and study so you can speak and write.

## Introduction

In previous chapters you learned that when the blood delivers oxygen to the cells, it also picks up carbon dioxide and other waste products. Through the process of respiration, the carbon dioxide goes from the blood into the alveoli in the lungs. It is then exhaled from the body. The other waste products remain in the blood. The urinary system filters these waste products from the blood and excretes them from the body.

## 16.1 Major Organs of the Urinary System

### PRACTICE FOR LEARNING: Major Organs of the Urinary System

Write the words below in the correct spaces on Figure 16-1. To help you, the number beside the word tells you where it goes on the figure. Be sure to pronounce each word as you write it. Repeat the pronunciation several times if you find the word hard to say.

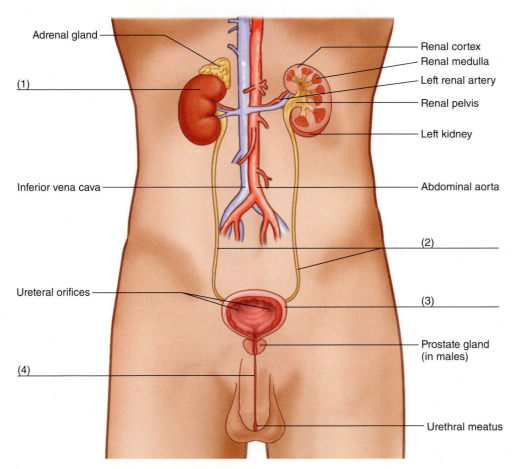

Adrenal gland

(1)

Renal cortex
Renal medulla
Left renal artery
Renal pelvis

Left kidney

Inferior vena cava

Abdominal aorta

(2)

Ureteral orifices

(3)

Prostate gland
(in males)

(4)

Urethral meatus

**Figure 16-1** Major organs of the urinary system.

1. **right** kidney (**KID**-nee)

2. ureters (yoo-**REE**-terz)

3. urinary bladder (**YOO**-rih-**nar**-ee **BLAH**-der)

4. urethra (yoo-**REE**-thrah)

The urinary system is illustrated in Figure 16-1. It consists of two kidneys, two tubes called ureters, a sac called the urinary bladder, and another tube called the urethra.

## 16.2  Structure and Function of the Urinary System

### Kidneys

The kidneys are each shaped like a bean. They are about the size of your fist. They are located at the back of the abdomen, one on each side of the lumbar vertebrae. The kidneys filter the blood to remove waste products. These waste products combine with water to form **urine** (**YOO**-rin). Urine flows out of the kidneys into the **renal pelvis** (**REE**-nal **PEL**-vis), which is the dilated portion of the ureter.

The kidneys also maintain a proper balance of electrolytes, water, and acids within body fluids. Electrolytes, such as sodium ($NA^+$), potassium ($K^+$), and calcium ($Ca^+$), are important to muscle and nerve function. When the level of these electrolytes is too high, the kidney secretes them into the urine. When the body needs these products, they are held back in the body fluid.

### Ureters, Bladder, and Urethra

As you can see in Figure 16-1, the ureters are long, narrow tubes that connect the kidneys to a sac called the urinary bladder. Urine constantly flows through the ureters to the urinary bladder. The urine enters the bladder through ureteral orifices (**OR**-ih-fis-ez) in the wall of the urinary bladder. Orifice means opening. The bladder stores urine. When the bladder is full, the urine is squeezed out into the urethra. This act of emptying the bladder is called **voiding**, **urination**, or **micturition** (**mick**-too-**RIH**-shun). This action is regulated by the nervous system. Any dysfunction of the urinary bladder due to disease of the nervous system is called **neurogenic** (**noor**-oh-**JEN**-ick) **bladder**.

The urethra (Figure 16-1) carries urine out of the body. In females, the urethra is about 1.6 inches (4.1 cm) long. In males, it is approximately 8 inches (20.3 cm), running through the penis. In the male, the urethra also serves as part of the reproductive system for the transport of sperm. The external opening of the urethra is called the **urinary meatus** (mee-**AY**-tuss).

**In Brief**

**Kidneys**

Filter blood, remove waste products

Urine moves from the kidneys ⟶ ureters ⟶ urinary bladder ⟶ urethra ⟶ out of the body

**Electrolytes**

sodium, potassium, calcium

**Function**

muscle and nerve function

PRACTICE FOR LEARNING: **Kidneys, Ureters, Bladder, and Urethra**

Choose the correct answer from the choices in parentheses.

1. The (bladder/ureter/urethra) is a long, narrow tube extending from the kidney for the passage of urine.
2. Urine is stored in the (ureter/urethra/bladder/kidney).
3. The (kidneys/ureters/bladder/urethra) filter waste products from the blood.
4. All blood goes to the (kidneys/ureters/bladder/urethra).
5. The (kidneys/ureters/bladder/urethra) is (are) part of the male reproductive system.

Answers: 1. ureter. 2. bladder. 3. kidneys. 4. kidneys. 5. urethra.

## 16.3  Urine Production in the Kidney

Inside each kidney, there are approximately one million **nephrons** (**NEF**-ronz) (Figure 16-2). These microscopic structures are responsible for filtering the blood and producing urine. Using your finger on Figure 16-2B, follow the path that blood flows through the kidneys. Start at the **glomerulus** (gloh-**MER**-yoo-luss), the first part of the nephron. It filters the blood of waste products and unnecessary nutrients. The filtered blood continues through the blood vessels returning to the heart. The unwanted material combines with water to form urine. The urine travels the length of the nephron and is excreted through the **collecting ducts**, ureters, and urethra to the outside of the body. Notice the blood vessels around the nephron. These are called the **peritubular capillaries**. The close proximity of the vessels to the nephron allows waste products and nutrients to move easily between the two.

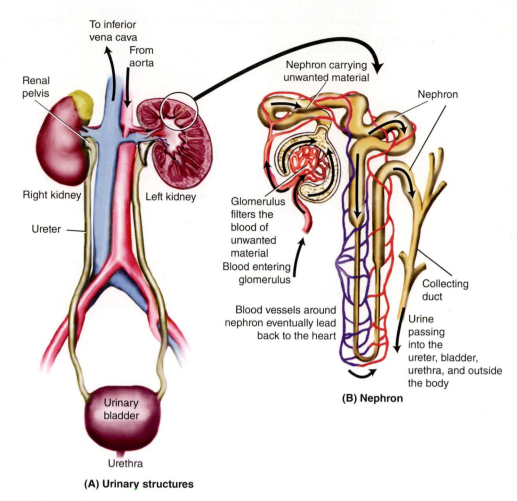

To inferior
vena cava

From
aorta

Renal
pelvis

Right kidney

Left kidney

Ureter

Urinary
bladder

Urethra

**(A) Urinary structures**

Nephron carrying
unwanted material

Nephron

Glomerulus
filters the
blood of
unwanted
material

Blood entering
glomerulus

Blood vessels around
nephron eventually lead
back to the heart

Collecting
duct

Urine
passing
into the
ureter, bladder,
urethra, and outside
the body

**(B) Nephron**

**Figure 16-2** The nephron.

| In Brief | The **nephron** filters unwanted material from the blood. |
|---|---|
| | Filtered (cleaned) blood remains inside the blood vessels and returns to the heart. |
| | The unwanted material stays in the nephron and is excreted as urine. |

## 16.4 New Roots, Suffixes, and Prefixes

Use these additional roots when studying the medical terms in this chapter.

| ROOT | MEANING |
|---|---|
| noct/o | night |
| urin/o | urine |

## 16.5 | Learning the Terms

Following these steps will make it easier for you to learn medical terms:

1. Pronounce the term repeatedly until it is easy for you.
2. Write it down. Ensure the spelling is correct.
3. Also write the definition. If possible, relate the word to a word, thought, or picture that will help you remember it.
4. Analyze the term with the method taught in this text.

### Roots

| ROOT<br>cyst/o (see also vesic/o) | | MEANING<br>bladder; cyst (closed sac or cavity filled with fluid) |
|---|---|---|
| *Term* | *Term Analysis* | *Definition* |
| **cystitis**<br>(sis-**TYE**-tis) | -itis = inflammation | inflammation of the bladder |
| **cystocele**<br>(**SIS**-toh-seel) | -cele = hernia; **protrusion or displacement of an organ** | displacement of the bladder against the vaginal wall |
| **cystopexy**<br>(**SIS**-toh-**peck**-see) | -pexy = surgical fixation | surgical fixation of the bladder to the abdominal wall |
| **cystoscopy**<br>(sis-**TOS**-koh-pee) | -scopy = process of visually examining | process of visually examining the bladder (Figure 16-3). |

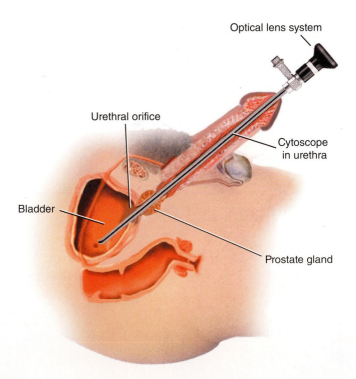

**Figure 16-3** Cystoscopy.

| Term | Term Analysis | Definition |
|------|---------------|------------|
| **polycystic kidneys** (**pol**-ee-**SIS**-tick) | -ic = pertaining to<br>poly- = many<br>In this term, the root cyst/o = cyst | cysts gradually replace normal renal tissue. With the replacement of normal renal tissue with many cysts, the kidney is unable to function, resulting in renal failure. (Figure 16-4) |

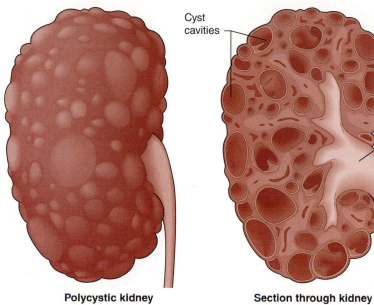

**Polycystic kidney**          **Section through kidney**

**Figure 16-4**  Polycystic kidneys.

| ROOT<br>glomerul/o | | MEANING<br>glomerulus (portion of the nephron that filters blood) | |
|---|---|---|---|
| Term | Term Analysis | Definition | |
| **glomerulonephritis** (gloh-**mer**-yoo-loh-neh-**FRY**-tis) | -itis = inflammation<br>nephr/o = kidney | inflammation of the glomerulus and kidney; Bright disease | |

| ROOT<br>meat/o | | MEANING<br>meatus (opening at the tip of the urethra) | |
|---|---|---|---|
| Term | Term Analysis | Definition | |
| **meatotomy** (**mee**-ah-**TOT**-oh-mee) | -tomy = process of cutting | process of cutting into the urinary meatus (to widen the meatus) | |

| ROOT<br>nephr/o (see also ren/o) | | MEANING<br>kidney |
|---|---|---|
| *Term* | *Term Analysis* | *Definition* |
| **hydronephrosis**<br>(**high**-droh-neh-**FROH**-sis) | -osis = abnormal condition<br>hydr/o = water | accumulation of urine in the renal pelvis. This abnormality is due to a blockage of urine flowing through the ureters. This blockage is caused by a kidney stone or a stricture (narrowing) of the ureter. (Figure 16-5) |

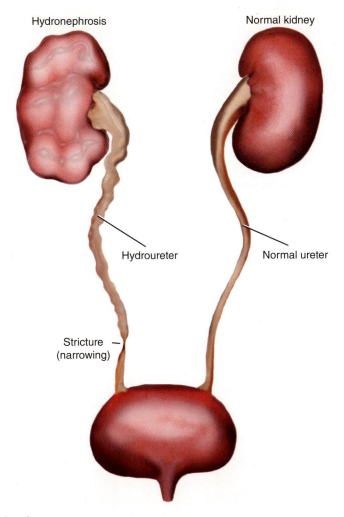

Hydronephrosis

Normal kidney

Hydroureter

Normal ureter

Stricture (narrowing)

**Figure 16-5** Hydronephrosis.

| | | |
|---|---|---|
| **nephrolithiasis**<br>(**nef**-roh-lih-**THIGH**-ah-sis) | -iasis = abnormal condition<br>lith/o = stones | kidney stones, also known as renal calculi (Figure 16-6) |

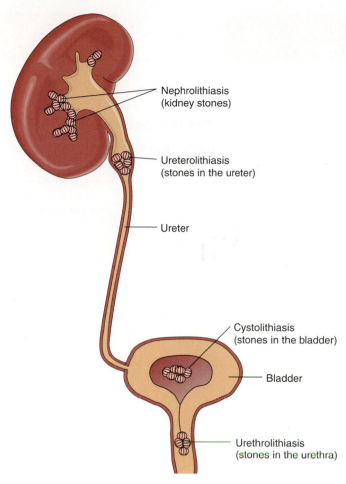

Nephrolithiasis
(kidney stones)

Ureterolithiasis
(stones in the ureter)

Ureter

Cystolithiasis
(stones in the bladder)

Bladder

Urethrolithiasis
(stones in the urethra)

**Figure 16-6**  Stones along the urinary tract.

| ROOT **pyel/o** | | MEANING **renal pelvis; kidney pelvis** |
|---|---|---|
| *Term* | *Term Analysis* | *Definition* |
| **intravenous pyelogram (IVP)** (**in**-trah-**VEE**-nus **PYE**-eh-loh-gram) | -ous = pertaining to<br>intra- = within<br>ven/o = vein<br>-gram = record | an x-ray of the kidneys and ureters following administration of a contrast medium. A contrast medium highlights internal structures to improve visibility. |
| **pyelonephritis** (**pye**-eh-loh-neh-**FRY**-tis) | -itis = inflammation<br>nephr/o = kidney | inflammation of the renal pelvis and kidney because of a urinary tract infection that spreads to the kidneys |

| ROOT ren/o | | MEANING kidney |
|---|---|---|
| *Term* | *Term Analysis* | *Definition* |
| renal hypoplasia (**REE**-nal **high**-poh-**PLAY**-zee-ah) | -al = pertaining to<br>-plasia = formation; development<br>hypo- = under; below normal; deficient | underdeveloped kidney |

| ROOT ureter/o | | MEANING ureter |
|---|---|---|
| *Term* | *Term Analysis* | *Definition* |
| ureteral (yoo-**REE**-ter-al) | -al = pertaining to | pertaining to the ureter |
| ureterectasis (yoo-**ree**-ter-**ECK**-tah-sis) | -ectasis = dilation; stretching; widening | dilation of ureter |
| ureterorrhagia (yoo-**ree**-ter-oh-**RAY**-jee-ah) | -rrhagia = hemorrhage; bursting forth | bleeding from the ureter |

| ROOT urethr/o | | MEANING urethra |
|---|---|---|
| *Term* | *Term Analysis* | *Definition* |
| transurethral (**tranz**-yoo-**REE**-thral) | -al = pertaining to<br>trans- = through; across | pertaining to something moving through the urethra |
| urethropexy (yoo-**REE**-throh-**peck**-see) | -pexy = surgical fixation | surgical fixation of the urethra to nearby tissue |
| urethrostenosis (yoo-**ree**-troh-steh-**NOH**-sis) | -stenosis = narrowing | narrowing of the urethra |

| ROOT ur/o | | MEANING urinary tract; urine; urination |
|---|---|---|
| *Term* | *Term Analysis* | *Definition* |
| uremia (yoo-**REE**-mee-ah) | -emia = blood condition | accumulation of waste products in the blood; also known as azotemia (**az**-oh-**TEE**-mee-ah). A toxic state when kidney failure causes the buildup of wastes in the blood. |

| Term | Term Analysis | Definition |
|------|--------------|-----------|
| **urologist** (yoo-**ROL**-ah-jist) | -logist = specialist | specialist in the study of the urinary system in females and the urinary and reproductive systems in males |
| **urogram** (**YOO**-roh-gram) | -gram = record | x-ray of the urinary tract (Figure 16-7) |

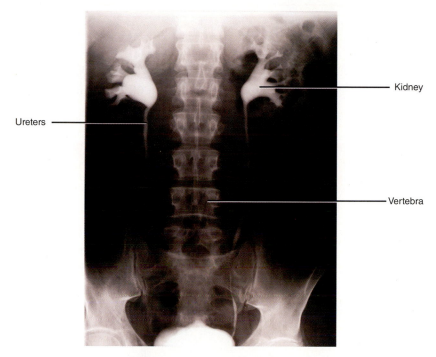

Ureters

Kidney

Vertebra

**Figure 16-7** An excretory urogram showing the kidneys and ureters.

| ROOT **vesic/o** | | MEANING **bladder** | |
|------------------|--|---------------------|--|
| Term | Term Analysis | Definition |
| **vesical** (**VES**-ih-kal) | -al = pertaining to | pertaining to the bladder |
| **vesicovaginal fistula** (**vess**-ih-koh-**VAH**-jih-nal **FISS**-tyoo-lah) | -al = pertaining to vagin/o = vagina fistula = abnormal passage | abnormal passage between the bladder and vagina allowing constant involuntary flow of urine from the bladder to the vagina (Figure 16-8) |

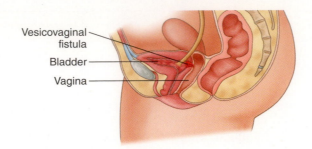

**Figure 16-8** A vesicovaginal fistula results in the abnormal flow of urine from bladder into vagina.

**Helping You Remember** Do not confuse vesic**al** with vesi**cle**. *Vesical* means "pertaining to the bladder." *Vesicle* means a "small sac containing liquid; a blister."

| SUFFIX -lysis | | MEANING separation; breakdown; destruction |
|---|---|---|
| Term | Term Analysis | Definition |
| dialysis (dye-**AL**-ih-sis) | dia- = through; complete | mechanical replacement of kidney function when the kidney is not working (Figure 16-9); hemodialysis (**hee**-moh-dye-**AL**-ih-sis) |

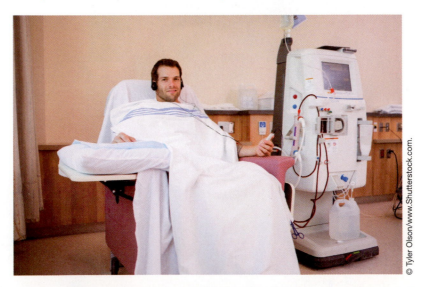

© Tyler Olson/www.Shutterstock.com.

**Figure 16-9** Hemodialysis. Mechanical replacement of kidney function when the kidney is not working. Once the patient's blood has been filtered, it is returned to the patient's body.

| urinalysis (**yoo**-rih-**NAL**-ih-sis) | urin/o = urine ana- = apart | laboratory analysis of urine |

| SUFFIX -tripsy | | MEANING crushing |
| --- | --- | --- |
| Term | Term Analysis | Definition |
| lithotripsy (LITH-oh-trip-see) | lith/o = stone; calculus | crushing of kidney stones tiny enough to be eliminated without surgical removal. Extracorporeal (ex-trah-kor-por-ee-al) shock wave lithotripsy uses ultrasound to crush the stones, which are then passed into the urine. Extracorporeal means outside the body (Figure 16-10). |

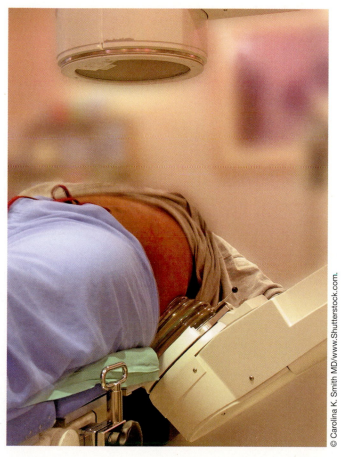

© Carolina K. Smith MD/www.Shutterstock.com.

Figure 16-10 Extracorporeal shockwave lithotripsy uses ultrasound to destroy kidney stones.

| SUFFIX -uria | | MEANING urine; urination |
|---|---|---|
| Term | Term Analysis | Definition |
| anuria (ah-**NOO**-ree-ah) | an- = no; not; lack of | no urine formation; also known as **suppression** (suh-**PRESH**-un) |
| dysuria (dis-**YOO**-ree-ah) | dys- = painful; bad; difficult | painful urination |
| hematuria (**hem**-ah-**TOO**-ree-ah) | hemat/o = blood | blood in the urine |
| nocturia (nock-**TOO**-ree-ah) | noct/o = night | frequent urination at night |
| oliguria (**ol**-ih-**GOO**-ree-ah) | oligo- = scanty; deficient; few | decreased urination |
| polyuria (**pol**-ee-**YOO**-ree-ah) | poly- = many | excretion of large amounts of urine |
| pyuria (pye-**YOO**-ree-ah) | py/o = pus | pus in the urine |

## Prefixes

| PREFIX in- | | MEANING no; not |
|---|---|---|
| Term | Term Analysis | Definition |
| incontinence (in-**KON**-tih-nens) | continence = to stop | no control over excretory functions such as urination or feces |

## 16.6   Pathology

### Nephrotic (neh-**FROT**-ick) Syndrome

A group of conditions involving damaged glomeruli and abnormal protein filtration.

Under normal circumstances the glomeruli filter waste products and excess water from the blood. When the glomeruli are damaged, protein is filtered when it should not be. This condition may result in **hyperproteinuria** (**high**-per-**proh**-tee-**NOOR**-ee-ah), excessive protein in the urine and **hypoproteinemia** (**high**-poh-**proh**-tee-**NEE**-mee-ah), decreased protein in the blood because the protein is being excreted in the urine. Edema, which is the abnormal accumulation of water in body tissues, can also be a problem.

## Renal Failure

Loss of kidney function. **Acute renal failure** comes on suddenly and is of short duration. **Chronic renal failure** comes on gradually and is of long duration. **End-stage renal disease** (ESRD) is the final stage of renal failure. Without adequate filtration, the waste products build up in the blood and death occurs because of uremia.

## Voiding Disorders

### Urinary Incontinence (in-**KON**-tih-nens)

Involuntary outflow of urine. Stress incontinence occurs when there is pressure on the bladder from coughing or laughing. Urge incontinence is the inability to stop the flow of urine once the urge has been felt.

### Urinary Retention

Inability of the bladder to empty completely during urination. If urine needs to be removed from the bladder before an effective treatment has been established, **catheterization** (**kath**-eh-ter-eye-**ZAY**-shun) may be done. This involves the insertion of a flexible tube (catheter) into the bladder to withdraw urine. The catheter is placed through the urethra and into the bladder (Figure 16-11A, and 11B).

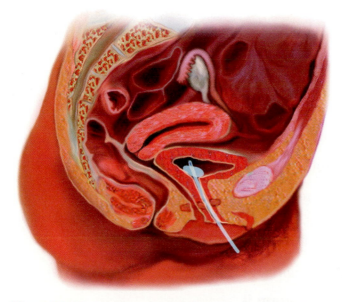

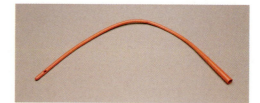

**Figure 16-11**  Catheterization. A. Catheter is placed in the bladder to drain urine. B. Catheter.

## 16.7   Look-Alike and Sound-Alike Words

*Below is a list of look-alike and sound-alike words. Study the spelling and definitions of each set of words. Questions will follow in the Review Exercises.*

### TABLE 16-1   Look-Alike and Sound-Alike Words

| | |
|---|---|
| **anuresis** | retention of urine in the bladder |
| **enuresis** | bedwetting at night |
| **creatine** | an amino acid found in tissues, especially muscles |
| **creatinine** | waste product excreted in the urine; elevated in kidney disease |
| **ureteral** | pertaining to the ureter |
| **urethral** | pertaining to the urethra |
| **vesical (adjective)** | pertaining to the bladder |
| **vesicle (noun)** | blister |

## 16.8   Review Exercises

### EXERCISE 16-1   Look-Alike and Sound-Alike Words

*Read the sentences carefully and circle the word in parentheses that correctly completes the meaning. Use Table 16-1 if it helps you.*

1. The patient complains of severe (**anuresis/enuresis**) to the point that he was wearing pads at night.

2. Mr. Chavez was admitted with glomerulonephritis. His laboratory tests showed abnormal levels of urinary (**creatine/creatinine**).

3. This woman has had three previous attacks of right (**urethral/ureteral**) pain.

4. Repeat cystoscopies resulted in multiple (**vesicals/vesicles**) in the bladder.

5. After elevation of the (**vesical/vesicle**) neck, incontinence stopped.

### EXERCISE 16-2   Matching Word Parts with Meaning

*Match the word part in Column A with its meaning in Column B.*

| | Column A | Column B |
|---|---|---|
| _____ | 1. dia- | A. opening at the tip of the urethra |
| _____ | 2. -plasia | B. kidney |

| | Column A | Column B |
|---|---|---|
| _____ | **3.** py/o | C. pus |
| _____ | **4.** pyel/o | D. stone |
| _____ | **5.** vesic/o | E. night |
| _____ | **6.** meat/o | F. through; complete |
| _____ | **7.** noct/o | G. bladder |
| _____ | **8.** lith/o | H. scanty |
| _____ | **9.** oligo- | I. formation; development |
| _____ | **10.** nephr/o | J. renal pelvis |

### EXERCISE 16-3  Labeling—Urinary Tract

*Using the body structures listed below, label Figure 16-12. Write your answer in the numbered spaces provided below, or if you prefer, on the diagram.*

kidney

_____

ureter

_____

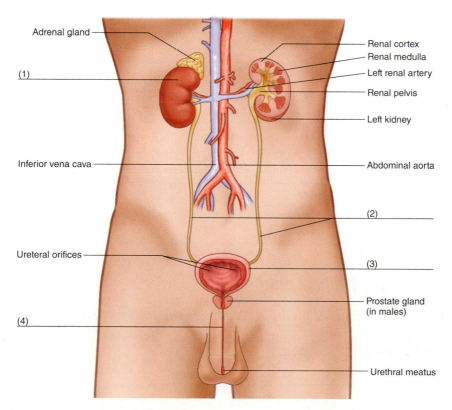

**Figure 16-12**  Major organs of the urinary system.

urethra _____

urinary bladder _____

    **1.** _____

    **2.** _____

    **3.** _____

    **4.** _____

## EXERCISE 16-4   Definitions—Learning the Terms

*Define the following terms.*

    **1. cystoscope** _____

    **2. meatotomy** _____

    **3. urethropexy** _____

    **4. renal hypoplasia** _____

    **5. dialysis** _____

    **6. urethral** _____

    **7. azotemia** _____

    **8. anuria** _____

    **9. dysuria** _____

  **10. suppression** _____

  **11. polyuria** _____

  **12. pyuria** _____

  **13. urologist** _____

## EXERCISE 16-5   Building Medical Words

*I. Use the suffix -uria to build medical words for the following definitions.*

    **a.** no urine formation _____

    **b.** painful urination _____

    **c.** blood in the urine _____

    **d.** frequent urination at night _____

  **e.** decreased (infrequent) urination _____

  **f.** pus in the urine _____

  **g.** excretion of large amounts of urine _____

*II. Use the combining form cyst/o to build medical words for the following definitions.*

  **a.** inflammation of the bladder _____

  **b.** instrument used to visually examine the inside of the bladder

  _____

## EXERCISE 16-6  Definitions—Pathology

*Define the following diseases.*

 **1.** polycystic kidneys

_____

_____

 **2.** incontinence

_____

_____

 **3.** nephrolithiasis

_____

_____

 **4.** renal failure

_____

_____

 **5.** pyelonephritis

_____

_____

 **6.** urinary retention

_____

_____

**7.** nephrotic syndrome

_____

_____

**8.** neurogenic bladder

_____

_____

**9.** ureterorrhagia

_____

_____

**10.** nephroptosis

_____

_____

### EXERCISE 16-7  Definitions in Context

_Define the bolded terms in the spaces provided. Use your medical dictionary if necessary._

ADMISSION DIAGNOSIS: RIGHT HYDROURETER AND HYDRONEPHROSIS

HISTORY OF PRESENT ILLNESS

A 65-year-old man was admitted with abdominal pain. He had been having this pain off and on for the past two years. On admission, he was found to have **renal calculi**. A **urography** was performed that showed poor function on the right with a **hypoplastic** scarred kidney. The patient therefore underwent a **cystoscopy** and **MRI**, revealing a poorly positioned right kidney with a **stricture** involving the **distal** one-third of the ureter. The patient was admitted at this time for consideration of **nephrectomy**.

a. **hydronephrosis** _____

b. **renal calculi** _____

c. **urography** _____

d. **hypoplastic kidney** _____

e. **cystoscopy** _____

f. **MRI** _____

g. **stricture** _____

h. **distal** _____

i. **nephrectomy** _____

## EXERCISE 16-8 Spelling

*Circle any words that are spelled incorrectly in the list below. Then correct the spelling in the space provided.*

**1.** glomairulus _____

**2.** cistitis _____

**3.** retention _____

**4.** urineation _____

**5.** nephrolithiasis _____

**6.** dialisis _____

**7.** vesical _____

**8.** incontinance _____

**9.** cathaterization _____

**10.** excretion _____

## Animations

Visit the companion website to view the video on **Cystoscopy**.

## 16.9 Pronunciation and Spelling

**1.** Listen to each word on the audio file provided on the Student Companion Website.

**2.** Pronounce each word carefully.

**3.** Spell each word in the space provided.

| Word | Pronunciation | Spelling |
|------|---------------|----------|
| **anuria** | ah-**NOO**-ree-ah | |
| **bladder** | **BLAH**-der | |
| **catheterization** | **kath**-eh-ter-eye-**ZAY**-shun | |
| **cystitis** | sis-**TYE**-tis | |

| Word | Pronunciation | Spelling |
|------|---------------|----------|
| cystoscope | **SIS-**toh-skope | |
| dialysis | dye-**AL-**ih-sis | |
| dysuria | dis-**YOO-**ree-ah | |
| glomerulonephritis | glow-**mer-**yoo-loh-neh-**FRY-**tis | |
| glomerulus | gloh-**MER-**yoo-luss | |
| hematuria | **hem-**ah-**TOO-**ree-ah | |
| hydronephrosis | **high-**droh-neh-**FROH-**sis | |
| incontinence | in-**KON-**tih-nens | |
| intravenous pyelogram | **in-**trah-**VEE-**nus **PYE-**eh-loh-gram | |
| kidney | **KID-**nee | |
| meatotomy | **mee-**ah-**TOT-**oh-mee | |
| meatus | me-**AY-**tuss | |
| micturition | **mick-**too-**RIH-**shun | |
| nephrolithiasis | **nef-**roh-lith-**THIGH-**ah-sis | |
| nephrotic | neh-**FROT-**ick | |
| nocturia | nock-**TOO-**ree-ah | |
| oliguria | **ol-**ih-**GOO-**ree-ah | |
| polycystic | **pol-**ee-**SIS-**tick | |
| polyuria | **pol-**ee-**YOO-**ree-ah | |
| pyuria | pye-**YOO-**ree-ah | |
| renal hypoplasia | **REE-**nal **high-**poh-**PLAY-**zee-ah | |
| transurethral | **tranz-**yoo-**REE-**thral | |
| uremia | yoo-**REE-**mee-ah | |
| ureter | yoo-**REE-**ter | |
| ureteral | yoo-**REE-**ter-al | |
| ureterectasis | yoo-**ree-**ter-**ECK-**tah-sis | |
| urethra | yoo-**REE-**thrah | |
| urinalysis | **yoo-**rih-**NAL-**ih-sis | |
| urologist | yoo-**ROL-**ah-jist | |

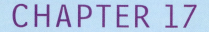

## CHAPTER 17

# Male Reproductive System

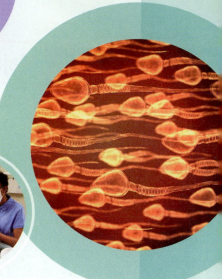

## Chapter Outline

## Learning Objectives

*After studying this chapter and completing the review exercises, you should be able to:*

1. Name and locate the organs of the male reproductive system.
2. Describe the structures and functions of the male reproductive system.
3. Pronounce, spell, define, and write the medical terms related to the male reproductive system.
4. Describe common diseases of the male reproductive system.
5. Listen, read, and study so you can speak and write.

## Introduction

The male reproductive system performs three basic tasks. The first is to manufacture sperm that carries the genetic code of the male. The second is to produce the hormone **testosterone** (tess-**TOSS**-ter-ohn). The third is to deliver sperm and semen out of the male's body.

## 17.1  Major Organs of the Male Reproductive System

**PRACTICE FOR LEARNING: Major Organs of the Male Reproductive System**

Write the words below in the correct spaces on Figure 17-1. To help you, the number beside the word tells you where it goes on the figure. Be sure to pronounce each word as you write it. Repeat the pronunciation several times if you find the word hard to say.

1. vas deferens (**VASS DEF**-er-enz)
2. penis (**PEE**-nis)
3. glans penis (**GLANZ**)
4. testis (**TEST**-tis)
5. scrotum (**SKROH**-tum)
6. epididymis (**ep**-ih-**DID**-ih-mis)
7. bulbourethral gland (**bul**-boh-yoo-**REE**-thral **GLAND**)
8. prostate (**PROSS**-tayt)
9. ejaculatory duct (ee-**JACK**-yoo-lah-**tor**-ee **DUCT**)
10. seminal vesicle (**SEM**-ih-nal **VESS**-ih-kul)

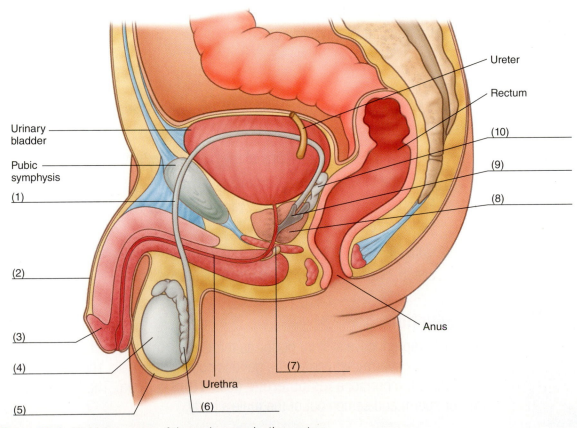

**Figure 17-1**  (A) Major organs of the male reproductive system.

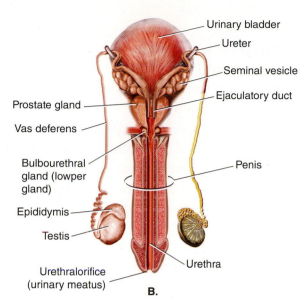

Urinary bladder

Ureter

Seminal vesicle

Ejaculatory duct

Prostate gland

Vas deferens

Bulbourethral
gland (lowper
gland)

Penis

Epididymis

Testis

Urethra

Urethralorifice
(urinary meatus)

B.

**Figure 17-1** (B) The testicles and vas deferens are bilateral.

## 17.2 Structure and Function of the Male Reproductive System

Sperm is produced in the testes (**TESS**-tees) (singular testis). The testes are also called the **testicles** (**TESS**-tih-kulz). The sperm is mixed with **semen** (**SEE**-men). Semen is a fluid produced by specific male reproductive organs and then delivered out of the body through the reproductive tract. The other components of the male reproductive system are the accessory reproductive organs and **external genitalia** (**jen**-ih-**TAIL**-ee-yah). The entire male reproductive system is illustrated in Figure 17-1.

### Testes

The testes are located in an external skin sac called the **scrotum** (**SKROH**-tum). The production of sperm is called **spermatogenesis** (**sper**-mah-toh-**JEN**-eh-sis). The testes also produce the hormone **testosterone**. It is essential for spermatogenesis and for the development of secondary male gender characteristics such as facial hair, muscularity, and voice change at puberty.

### Epididymis, Vas Deferens, Seminal Vesicle, and Ejaculatory Duct

Using your finger, trace the entire reproductive tract on Figure 17-1B. It begins with the **epididymis** (**ep**-ih-**DID**-ih-mis), which is a coiled tube on the superior surface of each testicle. Sperm are stored there. The epididymis leads into a duct called the ductus deferens or vas deferens. This duct encircles the urinary bladder and joins with the duct of the seminal vesicle to form the ejaculatory duct. This duct joins the urethra, which passes through a hole in the prostate gland.

## Accessory Organs

The accessory organs can also be seen in Figure 17-1. They are the seminal vesicles, the prostate gland, and bulbourethral glands, which are also called **Cowper** (**KOW**-per) **glands**. The accessory organs secrete substances that together form the fluid in which sperm is ejaculated, called **semen**. This substance nourishes and protects sperm.

The prostate is the largest of the accessory organs. The prostate is located just inferior to the bladder. It is a doughnut-shaped gland with a hole in the middle through which the urethra passes. It secretes a milky substance that forms about 50% of the semen. The secretion contains enzymes, nutrients for sperm mobility, and prostate-specific antigen (PSA). PSA testing may be used as an indicator of prostatic cancer.

## External Genitalia

The scrotum and the penis are the external genitalia. The scrotum is the sac that holds the testicles. The penis is a sex organ used to deliver sperm into the female. The end of the penis is called the **glans penis**. It contains the opening for urination and ejaculation, called the **urethral orifice** (yoo-**REE**-thral **OR**-ih-fis). The urethral orifice is also called the urinary **meatus** (**mee-AY**-tuss). The glans is covered with loose skin called the foreskin or **prepuce** (**PREE**-pyoos). This skin may be removed by a surgical process called **circumcision** (**ser**-kum-**SIZH**-un).

---

**In Brief**

**Male reproductive organs**

**Testes:** produces sperm and testosterone

**Epididymis:** stores sperm

**Vas deferens, ejaculatory duct, urethra:** transport sperm

**Accessory organs** seminal vesicles, prostate, and bulbourethral glands

**Function:** secretes semen to protect and nourish sperm

**External genitalia** scrotum and penis

**Scrotum:** holds the testicles

**Penis:** delivers sperm to female

---

PRACTICE FOR LEARNING: **Male Reproductive Structure and Function**

**1.** Write the function for the following structures:

    **a.** testicles _____

    **b.** epididymis _____

   **c.** vas deferens _____

   **d.** seminal vesicles, prostate gland, and bulbourethral glands
   _____

2. From the list of words below, complete sentences a, b, c, and d. Not all terms are used.

   Cowper

   epididymis

   glans penis

   prepuce

   scrotum

   testicles

   urethral orifice

   ductus deferens

   **a.** The end of the penis is called the _____.

   **b.** The urinary meatus is also known as the _____.

   **c.** The glans penis is covered with loose skin called
   _____.

   **d.** A sac containing the testicles is _____.

   **e.** Another name for bulbourethral gland is _____.

   **Answers: 1. a. produce sperm and testosterone. b. stores sperm. c. transports sperm. d. all of these structures secrete fluid that together form semen. 2. a. glans penis. b. urethral orifice. c. prepuce. d. scrotum. e. Cowper.**

## 17.3  New Roots, Suffixes, and Prefixes

Use these additional roots and suffixes when studying the terms in this chapter.

| ROOT | MEANING |
| --- | --- |
| crypt/o | hidden |
| varic/o | varicose vein |

| SUFFIX | MEANING |
|---|---|
| -cidal | to kill |
| -genesis | production; formation |
| -ism | condition; process |
| -pause | stopping |

## 17.4   Learning the Terms

Following these steps will make it easier for you to learn medical terms:

1. Pronounce the term repeatedly until it is easy for you.
2. Write it down. Ensure the spelling is correct.
3. Also write the definition. If possible, relate the term to a word, thought, or picture that will help you remember it.
4. Analyze the term with the method taught in this text.

### Roots

| ROOT andr/o | | MEANING male |
|---|---|---|
| Term | Term Analysis | Definition |
| androgenic (an-droh-JEN-ick) | -genic = producing | producing masculinizing effects |
| andropause (AN-droh-pawz) | -pause = stopping | decrease of the male hormone testosterone. May be referred to as male menopause |

| ROOT balan/o | | MEANING glans penis |
|---|---|---|
| Term | Term Analysis | Definition |
| balanorrhea (bal-an-oh-REE-ah) | -rrhea = flow; discharge | discharge from the glans penis |

| ROOT<br>mast/o | | MEANING<br>breast |
| --- | --- | --- |
| *Term* | *Term Analysis* | *Definition* |
| **gynecomastia**<br>(**gye**-neh-koh-**MAS**-tee-ah) | -ia = condition<br>gynec/o = woman | abnormal enlargement of the male breast |

| ROOT<br>orchid/o; orchi/o (see also testicul/o) | | MEANING<br>testicle; testis |
| --- | --- | --- |
| *Term* | *Term Analysis* | *Definition* |
| **cryptorchidism**<br>(krip-**TOR**-kih-**diz**-um) | -ism = process<br>crypt/o = hidden | undescended testicles (Figure 17-2). |

**Note:** During fetal development, one or both testicles may fail to descend into the scrotum, remaining instead in the abdominal cavity. If not treated, this condition results in sterility.

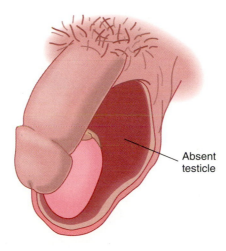

— Absent testicle

**Figure 17-2**  Cryptorchidism.

| **orchidectomy**<br>(**or**-kih-**DECK**-tah-mee) | -ectomy = excision; surgical removal | surgical removal of both testicles; castration |
| --- | --- | --- |
| **orchidopexy**<br>(**OR**-kid-oh-**peck**-see) | -pexy = surgical fixation | surgical fixation of the testicle into the scrotum; treatment for cryptorchidism |
| **orchitis**<br>(or-**KYE**-tis) | -itis = inflammation | inflammation of the testicle |

| ROOT prostat/o | | MEANING prostate |
|---|---|---|
| *Term* | *Term Analysis* | *Definition* |
| **prostatitis** (**pross**-tah-**TYE**-tis) | -itis inflammation | inflammation of the prostate |
| **transurethral prostatectomy (TUP)** (**tranz**-yoo-**REE**-thral **pros**-teh-**TECK**- teh-mee) | -al = pertaining to trans- = through; across -ectomy = excision; surgical removal | partial excision of the prostate using a **resectoscope** (ree-**SECK**-toh-skohp) passed through the urethra. Unwanted prostatic tissue is removed by dissection. It is also known as transurethral resection of the prostate (TURP) (Figure 17-3). See benign prostatic hypertrophy in Section 17.5 that follows. |

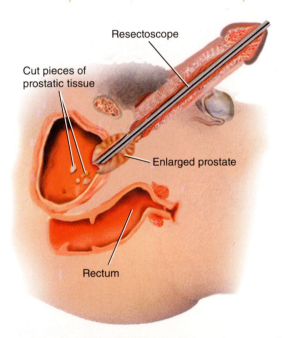

Resectoscope

Cut pieces of prostatic tissue

Enlarged prostate

Rectum

**Figure 17-3** Transurethral resection of prostate (TURP); also known as transurethral prostatectomy.

**Helping You Remember**   Do not confuse prostate, a male reproductive gland, with prostrate, meaning "stretched out on the ground."

| ROOT sperm/o; spermat/o | | MEANING spermatozoa; sperm; seminal fluid |
|---|---|---|
| Term | Term Analysis | Definition |
| aspermatogenesis (ay-**sper**-mah-toh-**JEN**-eh-sis) | -genesis = production; formation a- = no; not; lack of | no production of spermatozoa |
| **Note:** The singular of spermatozoa is spermatozoon. | | |
| hematospermia (**hee**-mah-toh-**SPER**-mee-ah) | -ia = condition hemat/o = blood | condition of blood in the seminal fluid |
| oligospermia (**ol**-ih-goh-**SPER**-mee-ah) | -ia = condition oligo- = deficient; scanty; few | deficient number of spermatozoa |
| spermatocidal (**sper**-mah-toh-**SYE**-dal) | -cidal = to kill | to kill or destroy spermatozoa; spermicidal |

| ROOT testicul/o | | MEANING testicle; testis |
|---|---|---|
| Term | Term Analysis | Definition |
| testicular (tes-**TICK**-yoo-lar) | -ar = pertaining to | pertaining to the testicle |

| ROOT vas/o | | MEANING vessel; vas deferens |
|---|---|---|
| Term | Term Analysis | Definition |
| vasectomy (vah-**SECK**-toh-mee) | -ectomy = excision; surgical removal | excision of the vas deferens or a portion of it (Figure 17-4) |

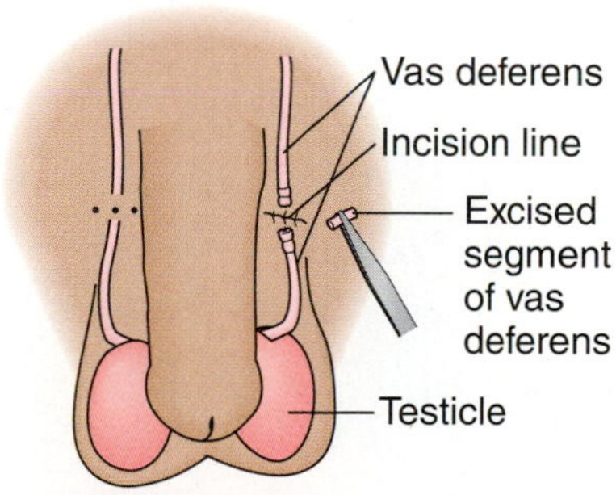

**Figure 17-4** Vasectomy.

| | | |
|---|---|---|
| vasovasostomy (**vay**-soh-vah-**ZOSS**-toh-mee) | -stomy = new opening vas/o = vas deferens | a vasectomy reversal; reattachment of two ends of the vas deferens that were previously separated. |

## Suffixes

| SUFFIX<br>-cele | | MEANING<br>hernia; protrusion; displacement |
|---|---|---|
| *Term* | *Term Analysis* | *Definition* |
| **hematocele**<br>(**HEE**-mah-toh-**seel**) | hemat/o = blood | accumulation of blood around the testicles |
| **hydrocele**<br>(**HIGH-**droh-seel) | hydr/o = water | accumulation of fluid around the testicles (Figure 17-5) |

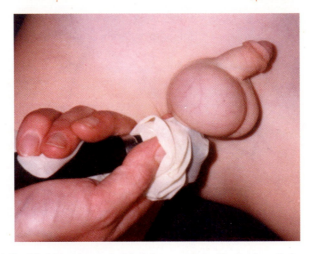

**Figure 17-5**  Hydrocele. A flashlight is shown behind the scrotum. If a hydrocele is present, a red glow will show up in the scrotum because the light will pass through it. If a tumor is present, no glow will show up.

**Note:** Hematocle can be used generally to describe any effusion of blood into a body cavity. Likewise, hydrocele can be used to describe the accumulation of fluid in any body cavity.

| **varicocele**<br>(**VAR**-ih-koh-**seel**) | varic/o = varicose veins; dilated, twisted veins | dilation of the testicular veins inside the scrotum (Figure 17-6) |
|---|---|---|

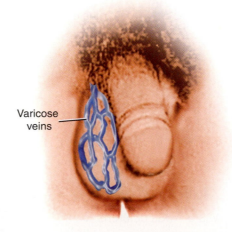

Varicose
veins

**Figure 17-6**  Varicocele.

| SUFFIX -potence | | MEANING power |
|---|---|---|
| Term | Term Analysis | Definition |
| impotence (**IM**-poh-tens) | in- = no; not | inability to achieve or maintain an erection |

> **Helping You Remember**  The prefix "in-" changes to "im-" in the word "impotence" because the suffix starts with "p."

| SUFFIX -spadias | | MEANING opening; split |
|---|---|---|
| Term | Term Analysis | Definition |
| epispadias (**ep**-ih-**SPAY**-dee-as) | epi- = on; upon; above | congenital opening of the meatus on the dorsum (top side) of the penis (Figure 17-7A) |
| hypospadias (**high**-poh-**SPAY**-dee-as) | hypo- = under | congenital opening of the urinary meatus on the ventral side (underside) of the penis; (Figure 17-7B) |

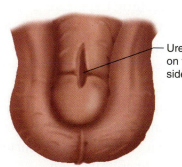
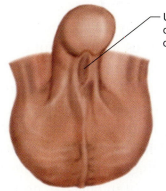

Urethra opens on the upper side of the penis

Urethra opens on the underside of the penis

**Figure 17-7**  A. Epispadias. B. Hypospadias.

## Prefixes

| PREFIX circum- | | MEANING around |
|---|---|---|
| *Term* | *Term Analysis* | *Definition* |
| circumcision (ser-kum-**SIZH**-un) | -ion = process<br>cis/o = to cut | removal of the prepuce or foreskin (Figure 17-8) |

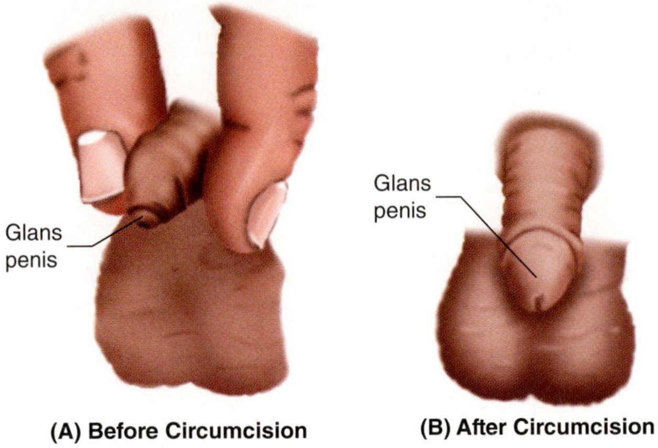

Glans penis

Glans penis

**(A) Before Circumcision**       **(B) After Circumcision**

**Figure 17-8**  Circumcision.

## 17.5  Pathology

### Benign Prostatic Hypertrophy

Benign prostatic hypertrophy (BPH) is also known as benign prostatic hyperplasia. This condition is a noncancerous enlargement of the prostate. The urethra goes through an opening in the prostate very much like a straw would go through a doughnut hole. If the prostate enlarges, it squeezes the urethra and obstructs the flow of urine (Figure 17-9). This causes urinary retention.

This condition frequently occurs in men over 60 years of age. Transurethral resection of the prostate (TURP) is a commonly performed treatment (Figure 17-3). Excess prostatic tissue obstructing the flow of urine is removed using a resectoscope inserted through the urethra. This is an effective procedure but requires hospitalization.

In recent years, alternative procedures have been developed to **ablate** (destroy) the obstructing prostatic tissue. The surgery is called ablation (ab-**LAY**-shun). The tissue is ablated using heat, laser, electricity, or microwaves. The removal of tissue unblocks the flow of urine. These procedures are considered **minimally invasive surgery**. This means the operation is less extensive with fewer and smaller incisions. The hospital stay is shorter, and there is less chance for complications.

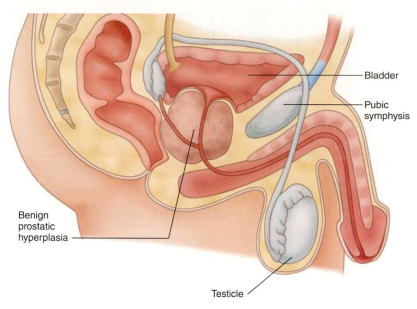

Bladder

Pubic symphysis

Benign prostatic hyperplasia

Testicle

**Figure 17-9** Benign prostatic hypertrophy.

## Carcinoma of the Prostate

Malignant tumor of the prostate is one of the most common types of cancer in men. A digital rectal examination (DRE) is helpful in detecting early prostatic cancer. A normal prostate feels solid and smooth. A cancerous prostate is described as **indurated** (**IN**-doo-**rayt**-ed) meaning hard. **Prostatic-specific antigen** (**PSA**) is a laboratory test that measures the level of PSA in the blood. PSA is a protein produced by the prostate gland. An elevated PSA may indicate prostatic cancer.

## Phimosis (fih-**MOH**-sis)

Tightened foreskin that cannot be pulled back. Secretions can accumulate between the foreskin and the penis, causing inflammation. May lead to penile cancer. Circumcision is the method of treatment.

## Sexually Transmitted Infection (STI)

Sexually transmitted infections, are also known as **venereal** (veh-**NEER**-ee-al) disease (VD) or sexually transmitted disease (STD). They occur in both men and women. A list of the most common STDs is found in Section 18.6 (the pathology section on the Female Reproductive System).

## Testicular Cancer

Malignant tumor of the testicles. It is most common in men between the ages of 15 and 40. When treated early, the cancer is curable.

## 17.6 Look-Alike and Sound-Alike Words

*Below is a list of look-alike and sound-alike words. Study the spelling and definitions of each set of words. Questions will follow in the Review Exercises.*

### TABLE 17-1 Look-Alike and Sound-Alike Words

| | |
|---|---|
| prostate | male reproductive gland |
| prostrate | stretched out on the ground |
| glans | refers to glans penis (end of the penis) |
| glands | a group of cells whose function is the production and secretion of a particular substance |
| hyperplastic | pertaining to an abnormal increase in the number of cells in tissues |
| hypoplastic | pertaining to an underdevelopment of an organ or tissue |

## 17.7 Review Exercises

### EXERCISE 17-1 Look-Alike and Sound-Alike Words

*Read the sentences carefully and circle the word in parentheses that correctly completes the meaning. Use Table 17-1 if it helps you.*

1. Physical examination at the time of admission revealed the (**prostrate/prostate**) to be smooth, benign, and enlarged.

2. The patient was found (**prostrate/prostate**) outside his apartment having suffered an apparent heart attack.

3. The (**glans/glands**) were swollen and there was evidence of lymphadenopathy.

4. Examination of the patient's testicle revealed the gland to be approximately twice its normal size. The (**hyperplastic/hypoplastic**) testicle was noted three months ago.

### EXERCISE 17-2 Matching Word Parts with Their Meaning

*Match the word part in Column A with the meaning in Column B.*

| | Column A | Column B |
|---|---|---|
| _____ | **1.** orchid/o | A. male |
| _____ | **2.** hemat/o | B. glans penis |

| | Column A | Column B |
|---|---|---|
| _____ | **3.** varic/o | C. power |
| _____ | **4.** -potence | D. opening |
| _____ | **5.** crypt/o | E. hernia |
| _____ | **6.** andr/o | F. around |
| _____ | **7.** -spadias | G. blood |
| _____ | **8.** circum- | H. dilated, twisted veins |
| _____ | **9.** -cele | I. hidden |
| _____ | **10.** balan/o | J. testicle |

## EXERCISE 17-3 Definitions—Anatomy, Physiology, and Pathology

*In the space provided, write the medical term that is described below.*

**1.** structure producing sperm and testosterone _____

**2.** structure that stores sperm _____

**3.** three structures that secrete substances to nourish sperm

_____, _____,

_____

**4.** the medical term meaning sperm production _____

**5.** structure that encases the testicles _____

**6.** noncancerous enlargement of the prostate _____

**7.** tightened foreskin that cannot be pulled back _____

**8.** another term for foreskin _____

## EXERCISE 17-4 Learning the Terms

*Define the following medical words.*

**1. androgenic** _____

**2. balanorrhea** _____

**3. cryptorchidism** _____

**4. aspermatogenesis** _____

**5. vasectomy** _____

**6. transurethral** _____

7. impotence _____

8. hypospadias _____

9. circumcision _____

10. congenital _____

## EXERCISE 17-5  Building Medical Words

*Write the medical word for the following definitions.*

a. accumulation of fluid around the testicle _____

b. surgical fixation of the testicle _____

c. deficient number of spermatozoa _____

d. pertaining to the testicle _____

e. accumulation of blood around the testicles _____

f. dilation of testicular veins inside the scrotum _____

g. opening of the urinary meatus on the underside of the penis

_____

h. inflammation of the testicle _____

i. to kill or destroy spermatozoa _____

j. producing masculinizing effects _____

## EXERCISE 17-6  Labeling—Male Reproductive System

*Using the body structures listed below, label Figure 17-10. Write your answer in the numbered spaces provided below, or if you prefer, on the diagram.*

bulbourethral gland _____

ejaculatory duct _____

epididymis _____

glans penis _____

penis _____

prostate _____

scrotum _____

seminal vesicle _____

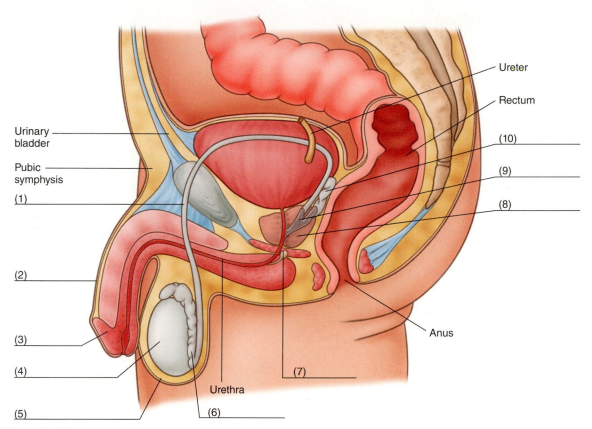

**Figure 17-10** Major organs of the male reproductive system.

testis _____

vas deferens _____

1. _____

2. _____

3. _____

4. _____

5. _____

6. _____

7. _____

8. _____

9. _____

10. _____

## EXERCISE 17-7  Spelling

*Circle any words that are spelled incorrectly in the list below. Then correct the spelling in the space provided.*

1. prostratic _____

2. ressection _____

3. injurated _____

4. epididmus _____

5. seminal vesical _____

6. balanorhea _____

7. cryptorchidism _____

8. impotance _____

9. genitalia _____

10. orifce _____

## Animations

Visit the companion website to view the video on **Male Reproductive System.**

## 17.8  Pronunciation and Spelling

1. Listen to each word on the audio file provided on the Student Companion Website.

2. Pronounce each word carefully.

3. Spell each word in the space provided.

| Word | Pronunciation | Spelling |
|---|---|---|
| **androgenic** | an-droh-**JEN**-ick | |
| **aspermatogenesis** | ay-**sper**-mah-toh-**JEN**-eh-sis | |
| **balanorrhea** | **bal**-an-oh-**REE**-ah | |
| **benign prostatic hypertrophy** | be-**NINE** proh-**STAT**-ick **HIGH**-per-troh-fee | |
| **circumcision** | **ser**-kum-**SIZH**-un | |

| Word | Pronunciation | Spelling |
|------|---------------|----------|
| cryptorchidism | krip-**TOR**-kih-**diz**-um | |
| epididymis | **ep**-ih-**DID**-ih-mis | |
| glans penis | **GLANZ PEE**-nis | |
| hematocele | **HEE**-mah-toh-**seel** | |
| hypospadias | **high**-poh-**SPAY**-dee-as | |
| impotence | **IM**-poh-tens | |
| oligospermia | **ol**-ih-goh-**SPER**-mee-ah | |
| orchidopexy | **OR**-kid-oh-**peck**-see | |
| orchitis | or-**KYE**-tis | |
| prostate | **PROSS**-tayt | |
| prostatitis | **pross**-tah-**TYE**-tis | |
| semen | **SEE**-men | |
| scrotum | **SKROH**-tum | |
| spermatogenesis | **sper**-mah-toh-**JEN**-eh-sis | |
| testicles | **TESS**-tih-kulz | |
| testicular | tes-**TICK**-yoo-lar | |
| testes | **TESS**-teez | |
| testosterone | tess-**TOSS**-ter-ohn | |
| varicocele | **VAR**-ih-koh-**seel** | |
| vas deferens | **VASS DEF**-er-enz | |
| vasectomy | vah-**SECK**-toh-mee | |

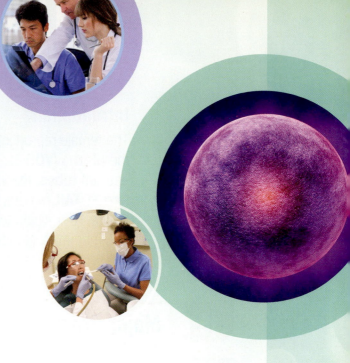

# Female Reproductive System

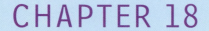

## Chapter Outline

## Learning Objectives

*After studying this chapter and completing the review exercises, you should be able to:*

1. Name and locate the organs of the female reproductive system.
2. Describe the structures and functions of the female reproductive system.
3. Define terms related to obstetrics.
4. Pronounce, spell, define, and write the medical terms related to the female reproductive system.
5. Describe common diseases of the female reproductive system.
6. Listen, read, and study so you can speak and write.

## Introduction

The female reproductive system consists of the **ovaries** (**OH**-vah-reez), the **uterus** (**YOO**-ter-us), the **uterine** or **fallopian** (fah-**LOH**-pee-an) **tubes**, the **vagina** (vah-**JIGH**-nah), the external **genitalia** (**jen**-ih-**TAIL**-ee-ah), and the **mammary** (**MAM**-ah-ree) **glands**. Figure 18-1 illustrates these structures (except for the external genitalia and mammary glands).

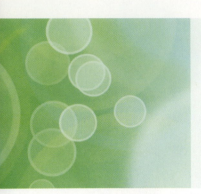

## 18.1  Major Organs of the Female Reproductive System

**PRACTICE FOR LEARNING: Major Organs of the Female Reproductive System**

Write the words below in the correct spaces on Figure 18-1. (Some urinary structures are also included.) To help you, the number beside the word tells you where it goes on the figure. Be sure to pronounce each word as you write it. Repeat the pronunciation several times if you find the word hard to say.

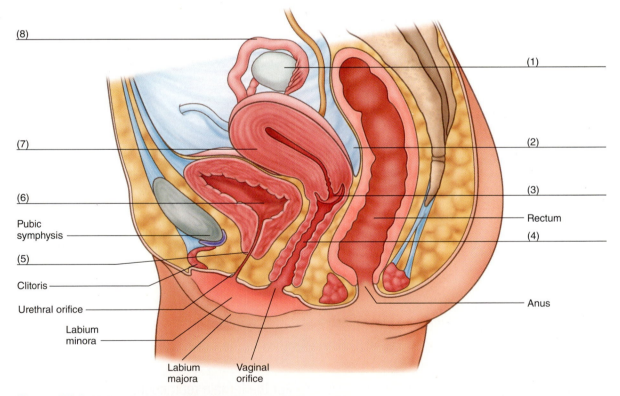

**Figure 18-1**  Major structures of the female reproductive system.

1. ovary (**OH**-vah-ree)

2. rectouterine pouch (**reck**-toh-**YOO**-ter-in **POWCH**)

3. cervix uteri (**SER**-vicks **YOO**-ter-eye)

4. vagina (vah-**JIGH**-nah)

5. urethra (yoo-**REE**-thra)

6. urinary bladder (**YOO**-rih-**nar**-ee **BLAH**-der)

7. uterus (**YOO**-ter-us)

8. fallopian tubes (fal-**LOH**-pee-an **TOOBZ**)

## 18.2   Structure and Function of the Female Reproductive System

### Ovaries

The ovaries are almond-shaped glands. They are located in the pelvic cavity. There is one on each side of the uterus. They are held in place by ligaments. The ovaries discharge the egg or **ovum** (**OH**-vum) (plural ova) and produce various hormones.

The ovaries of a newborn female contain a lifetime supply of immature eggs. Each egg is housed within a small sac called a follicle. Egg release from the follicle begins at puberty, which is the age at which sexual reproduction is possible. One egg is released into the pelvic cavity approximately every 28 days, and slowly makes its way to the fallopian tubes, also known as uterine tubes. This alternates from ovary to ovary each time. The process is called **ovulation** (**ov**-yoo-**LAY**-shun).

The ovaries release the hormones **estrogen** (**ES**-troh-jen) and **progesterone** (pro-**JES**-teh-rohn). Estrogen helps develop the secondary female characteristics such as the breasts and pubic hair. Progesterone stimulates the growth of blood vessels in the uterus. Estrogen also stimulates the thickening of the uterine lining to prepare for the implantation of a fertilized egg. If no fertilization takes place, this buildup of tissue is sloughed (**SLUFT**) off (discharged) in a process called **menstruation** (**men**-stroo-**AY**-shun) or **menses** (**MEN**-seez). Sometime between the ages of 45 and 55, all of the eggs either have been discharged or have degenerated. The reproductive cycle then ceases, and the woman is in **menopause** (**MEN**-oh-pawz).

### Fallopian Tubes

The fallopian tubes are shown in Figure 18-2. They link the ovaries and the uterus. The distal end of each tube is equipped with tiny finger-like projections called **fimbriae** (**FIM**-bree-ee). They sweep back and forth, creating waves in the fluid surrounding the ovary. The waves pull an ovum into the tube, and it is then transported to the uterus.

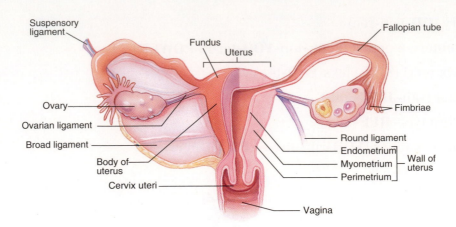

**Figure 18-2** Uterus, fallopian tubes, ovaries, and related structures.

Fertilization is the union of the ovum and sperm. Sperm enters the female reproductive tract following ejaculation by the male. Fertilization usually takes place inside the fallopian tube. If the ovum is fertilized, it begins to grow into a **fetus** (**FEE**-tus), the name given to the unborn baby. If it is not fertilized, the ovum breaks down within 24 hours after ovulation.

## Uterus

The uterus is a muscular, thick-walled organ. It is shaped like an inverted pear and is held in place in the pelvic cavity by ligaments (Figure 18-2 ). The superior, rounded portion of the uterus is called the **fundus** (**FUN**-dus). The middle portion is the body. The inferior portion is the **cervix uteri** (**SER**-vicks **YOO**-ter-eye), which projects into the vagina.

Inside the uterus is a hollow space in which the fetus develops. This space is enclosed by three walls: the **endometrium** (**en**-doh-**MEE**-tree-um), **myometrium** (**my**-oh-**MEE**-tree-um), and **perimetrium** (**per**-ih-**MEE**-tree-um). The endometrium is sloughed off during menstruation. The myometrium is the muscular wall. The perimetrium is the outermost wall.

In Figure 18-1, you can see the lowest point of the abdominal cavity. It is called the **rectouterine pouch**. It is also called the cul-de-sac of Douglas (**kuhl**-deh-sack of **DUG**-lass). It lies between the uterus and the rectum.

The uterine tubes, ovaries, and the ligaments holding the uterus in place are collectively called the **adnexa** (ad-**NECK**-sah).

## Vagina

The vagina can be seen in Figure 18-2. It is a muscular tube leading from the cervix uteri to the exterior. It is approximately 6 inches (15 cm) long and is lined with mucous membrane.

The vagina accepts the penis of the male during intercourse (coitus) (**KOY**-tuss). It is also called the birth canal.

> **In Brief**
>
> **Ovaries**
>
> discharge ova and produce estrogen and progesterone
>
> **Estrogen**
>
> important in the development of female secondary sex characteristics
>
> also thickens the uterine lining
>
> **Progesterone**
>
> stimulates the growth of blood vessels in the endometrium
>
> **Fallopian tubes**
>
> transport the egg to the uterus
>
> **Uterus**
>
> houses and protects the developing fetus
>
> **Vagina**
>
> birth canal; accepts the penis during coitus

## External Genitalia

The external genitalia, or **vulva** (**VUL**-vah), are illustrated in Figure 18-3.

The area from the vulva to the anus is called the **perineum** (**per**-ih-**NEE**-um).

The other parts of the external genitalia are the clitoris (**KLIT**-eh-riss) or (klih-**TOR**-iss), **labium majora** (**LAY**-bee-um mah-**JOR**-ah), **labium minora** (mih-**NOR**-ah), and **mons pubis** (**MONZ PYOO**-bis). Also included are **Bartholin** (**BAR**-toh-lin) **glands**. They secrete lubricants for intercourse.

> **In Brief**
>
> **External genitalia**
>
> consist of the clitoris, labium majora, labium minora, mons pubis, Bartholin glands, and perineum

## Breasts

### PRACTICE FOR LEARNING: The Breasts

Write the words below in the correct spaces on Figure 18-4. To help you, the number beside the word tells you where it goes on the figure. Be sure to pronounce each word as you write it. Repeat the pronunciation several times if you find the word hard to say.

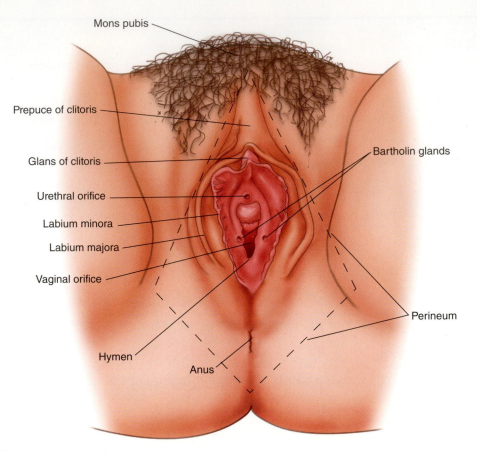

**Figure 18-3** External genitalia.

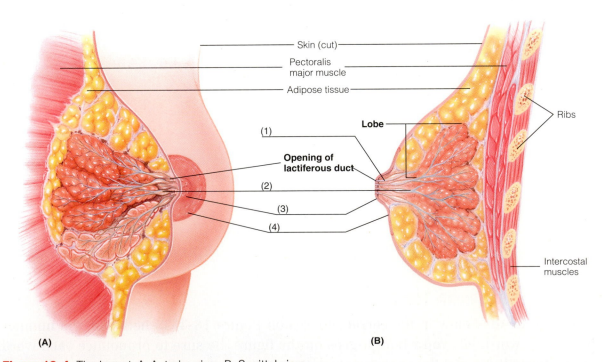

**Figure 18-4** The breast. A. Anterior view. B. Sagittal view.

1. lactiferous ducts (lack-**TIF**-er-us **DUKTS**)
2. lactiferous sinus (lack-**TIF**-er-us **SIGH**-nus)
3. nipple (**NIH**-pul)
4. areola (ah-**REE**-oh-lah)

Figure 18-4 illustrates the structures of the breast or mammary gland. The nipple is surrounded by a darker ring of skin called the **areola** (ah-**REE**-oh-lah).

The mammary glands produce milk after childbirth. Each gland consists of a number of **lobes** (**LOHBZ**), which contain many little sacs (lobules) that secrete milk. The milk is stored in **lactiferous** (lack-**TIF**-er-us) **sinuses**. It travels through the lacterifous (milk) ducts to tiny openings in the nipple. Oils produced by glands in the areola help minimize drying out of the skin around the nipple due to breastfeeding.

## PRACTICE FOR LEARNING: Female Reproductive Organs

Write the structure responsible for the functions listed below.

1. holds the fetus during pregnancy _____
2. lubricates the vagina for intercourse _____
3. acts as the birth canal _____
4. transports the egg to the uterus _____
5. secretes estrogen and progesterone _____
6. ovulation _____

> Answers: 1. uterus. 2. Bartholin gland. 3. vagina. 4. fallopian tubes/uterine tubes. 5. ovaries. 6. ovaries.

## PRACTICE FOR LEARNING: Female Reproductive Organs

Match the structure in column A with its location in Column B. A letter can be used more than once.

| | Column A | Column B |
|---|---|---|
| _____ | 1. cul-de-sac of Douglas | A. abdominal cavity |
| _____ | 2. Bartholin gland | B. breast |
| _____ | 3. areola | C. external genitalia |
| _____ | 4. ovary | D. fallopian tube |
| _____ | 5. fundus | E. pelvic cavity |
| _____ | 6. fimbriae | F. uterus |
| _____ | 7. cervix | |

> Answers: 1. A. 2. C. 3. B. 4. E. 5. F/E (uterus which is located in the pelvic cavity). 6. D/E (fallopian tube which is located in the pelvic cavity). 7. F/E (uterus which is located in the pelvic cavity).

## 18.3 Obstetrics

**Obstetrics** (ob-**STET**-ricks) is the branch of medicine dealing with pregnancy, childbirth, and the postpartum period. Childbirth is also known as **parturition** (par-tyoo-**RISH**-un). The postpartum period is also known as the **puerperium** (pyoo-er-**PEER**-ee-um). The specialist is called an **obstetrician** (ob-steh-**TRIH**-shun). **Gynecology** (gye-neh-**KOL**-eh-jee) is the medical-surgical specialty dealing with the female reproductive system in the nonpregnant state. The two specialities are combined and named Obstetrics and Gynecology. They are often abbreviated OB/GYN.

### Pregnancy

Conception or fertilization takes place in the fallopian tube. The fertilized egg is called the **zygote** (**ZYE**-goht). It implants in the wall of the uterus. The zygote is referred to as the embryo (**EM**-bree-oh) after the second week of pregnancy. After the eighth week, it is called the fetus (**FEE**-tus). Full development takes about 40 weeks. This is called the **gestation** (jess-**TAY**-shun) **period**.

At the beginning of pregnancy, the **placenta** develops and attaches high up on the uterine wall. The placenta is an organ. It allows for the exchange of nutrients and waste products between mother and developing embryo. This exchange is made possible by the **umbilical** (um-**BILL**-ih-kahl) **cord**, the lifeline between mother and baby.

The placenta is made up of the **chorion** (**KOR**-ee-on) and the **amnion** (**am**-nee-on). The chorion is the outermost layer. The amnion is the innermost layer (Figure 18-5). The embryo (and later the fetus) is encased within the amnion. The amnion is filled with **amniotic fluid**, which protects the embryo.

The placenta secretes a hormone called **human chorionic gonadotrophin** (**kor**-ee-**ON**-ick **goh**-nah-doh-**TROH**-fin). The abbreviation is **HCG**. A pregnancy test looks for the presence of HCG. When it is detected, pregnancy is confirmed.

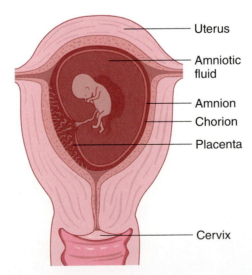

Uterus

Amniotic fluid

Amnion

Chorion

Placenta

Cervix

**Figure 18-5** Placenta. Chorion is the outer layer. Amnion is the inner layer. Within the amniotic cavity the fetus floats while developing.

Fetal abnormalities are detected by two diagnostic procedures: **amniocentesis** (**am**-nee-oh-sen-**TEE**-sis) and **chorionic** (**kor**-ee-**ON**-ick) **villius sampling** (CVS) (Figure 18-6). With amniocentesis, amniotic fluid is withdrawn from the amniotic sac during 15 to 18 weeks' gestation. In CVS, placental tissue is removed during 9 to 11 weeks' gestation. In both procedures, certain genetic and chromosomal abnormalities such as Down Syndrome can be detected through examination of the amnitoic fluid and placental tissue.

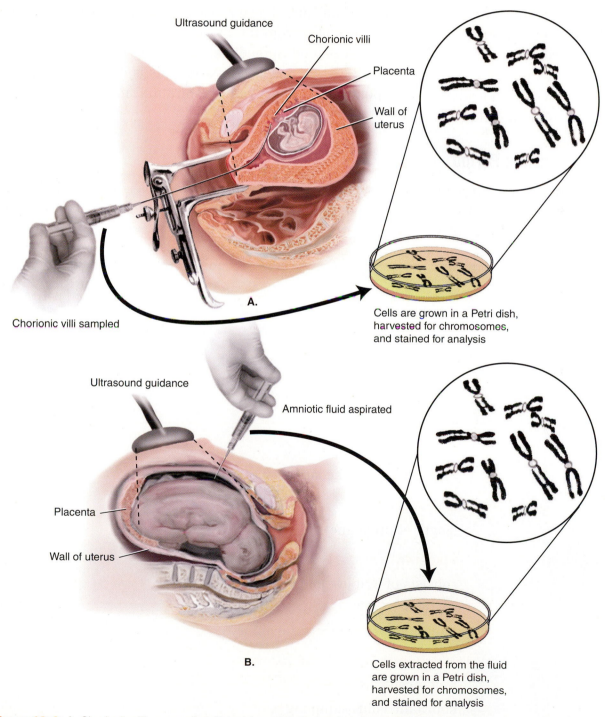

Ultrasound guidance

Chorionic villi

Placenta

Wall of uterus

**A.**

Chorionic villi sampled

Cells are grown in a Petri dish, harvested for chromosomes, and stained for analysis

Ultrasound guidance

Amniotic fluid aspirated

Placenta

Wall of uterus

**B.**

Cells extracted from the fluid are grown in a Petri dish, harvested for chromosomes, and stained for analysis

**Figure 18-6** A. Chorionic villus sampling (9 to 11 weeks). B. Amniocentesis (15 to 18 weeks).

## Childbirth

At the end of the gestation period, the birth process begins. It is called parturition. The uterine muscles begin to contract and the uterus expands. This marks the beginning of labor. Occasionally, the contractions stop. This is called **uterine inertia** (**YOO**-ter-in in-**ER**-shee-ah). Ultimately, the contractions move the infant through the cervix and vagina. Normal delivery is head first. If the baby is turned around with the buttocks first, it is called a **breech** (**BREECH**) delivery. A **cesarean** (seh-**ZER**-ee-an) section (**CS**) may have to be performed. This involves removal of the baby through an incision in the abdomen and uterus.

After delivery, the placenta is expelled from the uterus. It is called the **afterbirth**. The condition of the newborn is evaluated immediately following delivery and again after 15 minutes. A rating called an **Apgar score** is made. This is done by evaluating each of the following on a 2-point scale: heart rate, respiration, muscle tone, reflex response, and color. The highest rating is 10.

## Postpartum Period

The **postpartum period** follows childbirth. It lasts for 6 to 8 weeks. It is also known as the puerperium. During this period, the uterus returns to normal size. This process is called **involution** (**in**-voh-**LOO**-shun).

---

**In Brief**

**Parturition**
childbirth

**Puerperium**
postpartum period

**Zygote**
fertilized egg

**Embryo**
zygote after the second week of pregnancy

**Gestation**
length of pregnancy

**Placenta**
consists of amnion and chorion
secretes HCG
amniotic fluid protects the embryo

**Diagnostic Procedures**
amniocentesis
chorionic villus sampling

**PRACTICE FOR LEARNING: Obstetrics**

Choose the correct answer from the choices given.

1. The postpartum period is also known as _____.

   postnatal period     parturition     involution     puerperium

2. The fertilized egg is called _____.

   embyro     fetus     zygote     baby

3. The organ responsible for nourishing the fetus and removing waste products is the _____.

   uterus     ovaries     placenta     mammary glands

4. An Apgar score represents the _____.

   condition of the newborn     condition of the mother     dilation of the cervix

5. Human chorionic gonadotrophin is secreted by the

   _____.

   uterus     ovaries     placenta     mammary glands

> Answers: 1. puerperium. 2. zygote. 3. placenta. 4. condition of newborn. 5. placenta.

## 18.4  New Roots, Suffixes, and Prefixes

Use these additional roots, suffixes, and prefixes when studying the medical words in this chapter.

| ROOT | MEANING |
|------|---------|
| flex/o | bend |
| men/o | month; menses; menstruation |
| tub/o | tube |
| versi/o | turning; tilting; tipping |

| SUFFIX | MEANING |
|--------|---------|
| -an | pertaining to |
| -arche | beginning |
| -ine | pertaining to |

| PREFIX | MEANING |
|--------|---------|
| multi- | many |
| nulli- | none |
| primi- | first |

## 18.5   Learning the Terms

Following these steps will make it easier for you to learn medical terms:

1. Pronounce the term repeatedly until it is easy for you.
2. Write it down. Ensure the spelling is correct.
3. Also write the definition. If possible, relate the word to a word, thought, or picture that will help you remember it.
4. Analyze the term with the method taught in this text.

### Terms Pertaining to the Female Reproductive System

#### Roots

| ROOT<br>cervic/o | MEANING<br>cervix; cervix uteri; neck of the uterus | |
|------------------|------------------|------------------|
| *Term* | *Term Analysis* | *Definition* |
| **cervicitis**<br>(**ser**-vih-**SIGH**-tis) | -itis = inflammation | inflammation of the cervix |
| **cervical dysplasia**<br>(**SER**-vih-kal dis-**PLAY**-see-ah) | -al = pertaining to<br><br>-plasia = development; formation<br><br>dys- = abnormal; bad; difficult | abnormal cellular development on the surface of the cervix uteri, indicating precancerous changes in its cells |
| **cervical polyp**<br>(**SER**-vih-kal **POL**-up) | -al = pertaining to<br><br>polyp = protruding balloon-like neoplasm attached to the mucous membrane by a thin stalk. A type of skin lesion. | abnormal growth extending from the mucous membrane of the cervix uteri (Figure 18-7); usually benign but can turn cancerous |

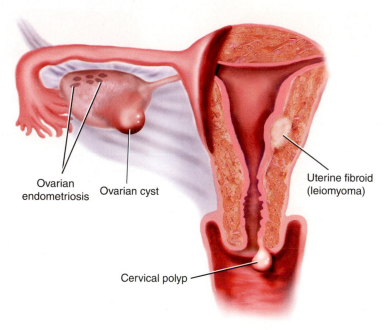

Ovarian endometriosis   Ovarian cyst

Uterine fibroid (leiomyoma)

Cervical polyp

**Figure 18-7** Cervical polyp, endometriosis, ovarian cyst, and uterine fibroid.

| ROOT colp/o (see also vagin/o) | | MEANING vagina |
|---|---|---|
| Term | Term Analysis | Definition |
| colpopexy (kol-poh-PECK-see) | -pexy = surgical fixation | surgical fixation of the vagina to a surrounding structure |
| colporrhaphy (kohl-POR-ah-fee) | -rrhaphy = suture | suturing of the vagina |

| ROOT episi/o | | MEANING vulva; external genitalia |
|---|---|---|
| Term | Term Analysis | Definition |
| episiotomy (eh-piz-ee-OT-oh-mee) | -tomy = process of cutting | surgical incision into the perineum. This enlarges the vaginal orifice and prevents tearing of the tissues as the infant moves out of the uterus. |
| episiorrhaphy (eh-piz-ee-OR-ah-fee) | -rrhaphy = suture | suturing of the vulva and perineum for repair of an episiotomy or laceration |

| ROOT fibr/o | | MEANING fibers; fibrous tissue |
|---|---|---|
| Term | Term Analysis | Definition |
| **fibroadenoma** (**fye**-broh-**ad**-eh-**NOH**-mah) | -oma = mass, tumor aden/o = gland | abnormal masses in the breast that are round, firm, and rubbery; involves the fibrous connective tissue in a gland. |

| ROOT galact/o | | MEANING milk |
|---|---|---|
| Term | Term Analysis | Definition |
| **galactorrhea** (geh-**lack**-toh-**REE**-ah) | -rrhea = flow or discharge | spontaneous flow of breast milk in a woman who is not breastfeeding |

| ROOT gynec/o | | MEANING woman |
|---|---|---|
| Term | Term Analysis | Definition |
| **gynecologist** (**gye**-neh-**KOL**-eh-jist) | -logist = specialist | specialist in the study of diseases and treatment of the female genital tract |

| ROOT hyster/o (see also metr/o and uter/o) | | MEANING uterus |
|---|---|---|
| Term | Term Analysis | Definition |
| **hysterectomy** (**hiss**-ter-**ECK**-toh-mee) | -ectomy = excision; surgical removal | surgical removal of the uterus (Figure 18-8) |

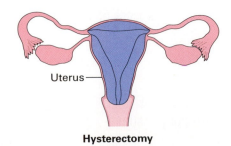

Uterus

**Hysterectomy**

**Figure 18-8**  Hysterectomy.

| Term | Term Analysis | Definition |
|---|---|---|
| hysterosalpingography (**hiss**-tehr-oh-**sal**-ping-**GOG**-rah-fee) | -graphy = process of recording; producing images salping/o = fallopian tubes | x-ray of the uterus and fallopian tubes following injection of a contrast medium |

| ROOT labi/o | | MEANING lips |
|---|---|---|
| Term | Term Analysis | Definition |
| labial (**LAY**-bee-al) | -al = pertaining to | pertaining to lips |

| ROOT lact/o | | MEANING milk |
|---|---|---|
| Term | Term Analysis | Definition |
| lactogenesis (**lack**-toh-**JEN**-ih-sis) | -genesis = production; formation | production and secretion of milk from the breast |

| ROOT ligati/o | | MEANING binding; tying |
|---|---|---|
| Term | Term Analysis | Definition |
| tubal ligation (**TOO**-bal lye-**GAY**-shun) | -ion = process -al = pertaining to tub/o = tube; fallopian tube | female sterilization by blocking the fallopian tubes. This prevents the sperm from fertilizing the egg. If no fertilization occurs, the woman cannot become pregnant. The tubes can be blocked by cutting and ligating (tying), clamping, cauterization (burning), or a combination of these procedures (Figure 18-9). |

**Note:** A tubal ligation does not involve removal of the uterus or any other organs. Menstruation continues.

Fallopian tube

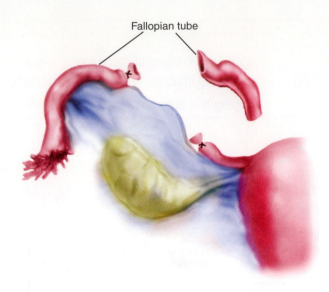

**Figure 18-9** Tubal ligation.

| ROOT mamm/o; mast/o | | MEANING breast |
|---|---|---|
| *Term* | *Term Analysis* | *Definition* |
| **mammary** (**MAM**-ah-ree) | -ary = pertaining to | pertaining to the breast |
| **mastectomy** (mas-**TECK**-toh-mee) | -ectomy = excision; surgical removal | surgical removal of the breast |
| **mastopexy** (**MAS**-toh-**peck**-see) | -pexy = surgical fixation | surgical fixation of the breast |

**Note:** Mastopexy is a type of plastic surgery performed on drooping breasts to improve their look and form.

| ROOT men/o | | MEANING menses; menstruation; month |
|---|---|---|
| *Term* | *Term Analysis* | *Definition* |
| **amenorrhea** (ah-**men**-oh-**REE**-ah) | -rrhea = discharge; flow  a- = no; not | no menstruation |
| **dysmenorrhea** (**dis**-men-oh-**REE**-ah) | -rrhea = discharge; flow  dys- = painful; difficult; bad | painful menstruation |
| **menarche** (men-**AR**-kee) | -arche = beginning | beginning of menstrual function |
| **menorrhea** (**men**-oh-**REE**-ah) | -rrhea = discharge; flow | normal menstruation |
| **menorrhagia** (**men**-oh-**RAY**-jee-ah) | -rrhagia = bursting forth; abnormal bleeding | excessive uterine bleeding during menstruation |

| ROOT metr/o | | MEANING uterus |
|---|---|---|
| Term | Term Analysis | Definition |
| metrorrhagia (meh-troh-RAY-jee-ah) | -rrhagia = bursting forth; abnormal bleeding | abnormal uterine bleeding at times other than at the regular menstrual period |
| menometrorrhagia (men-oh-met-roh-RAY-jee-ah) | -rrhagia = bursting forth; abnormal bleeding | excessive bleeding during menses and at irregular intervals between periods |

| ROOT oophor/o (see also ovari/o) | | MEANING ovary |
|---|---|---|
| Term | Term Analysis | Definition |
| oophororrhagia (oh-off-oh-RAY-jee-ah) | -rrhagia = bursting forth; abnormal bleeding | hemorrhaging from the ovary |

| ROOT ovari/o | | MEANING ovary |
|---|---|---|
| Term | Term Analysis | Definition |
| ovarian cyst (oh-VAR-ree-an SIST) | -an = pertaining to cyst = closed sac or cavity containing fluid, semifluid, or solid material | abnormal cystic growth on the ovary (see Figure 18-7) |
| ovariorrhexis (oh-var-ee-oh-RECK-sis) | -rrhexis = rupture | ruptured ovary |

| ROOT perine/o | | MEANING perineum (area between the vagina and the anus) |
|---|---|---|
| Term | Term Analysis | Definition |
| perineorrhaphy (per-ih-nee-OR-ah-fee) | -rrhaphy = suture | suturing of the perineum following laceration of the area during delivery of the fetus |

| ROOT salping/o (see also -salpinx) | | MEANING fallopian tube; uterine tube |
|---|---|---|
| Term | Term Analysis | Definition |
| salpingo-oophorectomy (sal-**ping**-goh-oh-**off**-oh -**RECK**-toh-mee) | -ectomy = excision; surgical removal<br>oophor/o = ovary | surgical removal of the fallopian tubes and ovaries |

| ROOT uter/o | | MEANING uterus |
|---|---|---|
| Term | Term Analysis | Definition |
| intrauterine (**in**-trah-**YOO**-ter-in) | -ine = pertaining to<br>intra- = within | pertaining to within the uterus |
| uterine fibroids (**YOO**-ter-in **FYE**-broidz) | -ine = pertaining to<br>fibroid = type of benign tumor | a benign tumor of the uterine muscle (see Figure 18-7); also known as fibroid, myoma, or fibromyoma (figh-broh-my-OH-mah) |
| uterovesical (**yoo**-ter-oh-**VES**-ih-kal) | -al = pertaining to<br>vesic/o = bladder | pertaining to the uterus and bladder |

| ROOT vagin/o | | MEANING vagina |
|---|---|---|
| Term | Term Analysis | Definition |
| vaginomycosis (**vaj**-ih-noh-mye-**KOH**-sis) | -osis = abnormal condition<br>myc/o = fungus | fungal infection of the vagina |

| ROOT vulv/o | | MEANING vulva; external genitalia; pudendum |
|---|---|---|
| Term | Term Analysis | Definition |
| vulvorectal (**vul**-voh-**RECK**-tal) | -al = pertaining to<br>rect/o = rectum | pertaining to the vulva and rectum |

| SUFFIX -cele | | MEANING hernia; protrusion; displacement |
|---|---|---|
| *Term* | *Term Analysis* | *Definition* |
| **cystocele** (**SIS**-toh-seel) | cyst/o = bladder | protrusion of the bladder into the vaginal wall (Figure 18-10A and 18-10B) |

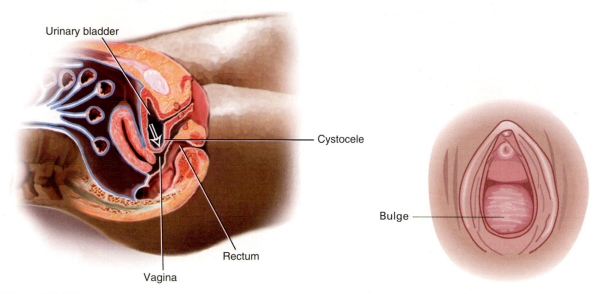

**Figure 18-10**  A. Cystocele, lateral view. Notice the protrusion of the bladder into the vaginal wall. B. Bulging of vaginal wall, characteristic of a cystocele.

| | | |
|---|---|---|
| **rectocele** (**RECK**-toh-seel) | rect/o = rectum | protrusion of the rectum into the vaginal wall (Figure 18-11) |

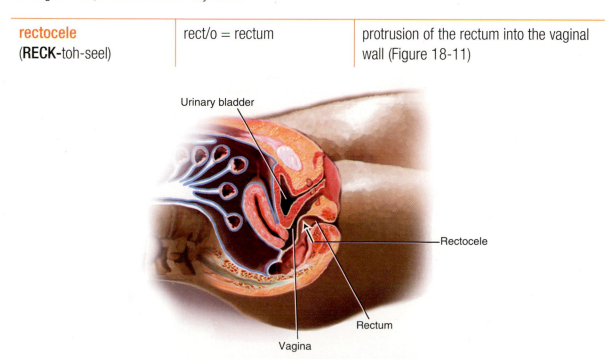

**Figure 18-11**  Retrocele. Notice the protrusion of the rectum into the vaginal wall.

## Suffixes

| SUFFIX -salpinx | | MEANING fallopian tube; uterine tube |
|---|---|---|
| Term | Term Analysis | Definition |
| hydrosalpinx (**high**-dro-**SAL**-pinks) | hydr/o = water | accumulation of a watery fluid in the fallopian tube |

| PREFIX ante- | | MEANING before |
|---|---|---|
| Term | Term Analysis | Definition |
| anteflexion (**an**-tee-**FLECK**-shun) | -ion = process flex/o = bending | bending forward of a part of an organ; normal position of the uterus (Figure 18-12A) |
| anteversion (**an**-tee-**VER**-zhun) | -ion = process versi/o = tilting; tipping | tilting forward of an organ or part of an organ; forward tilting of the uterus over the bladder (Figure 18-12B ); normal position of the uterus. |

| PREFIX retro- | | MEANING back; behind |
|---|---|---|
| Term | Term Analysis | Definition |
| retroflexion (**ret**-roh-**FLECK**-shun) | -ion = process flex/o = bending | bending back of a part of an organ. Abnormal position of the uterus (Figure 18-12C) |
| retroversion (**ret**-roh-**VER**-zhun) | -ion = process versi/o = tilting; tipping | tilting backward of an organ or part of an organ. Abnormal position of the uterus. (Figure 18-12D) |

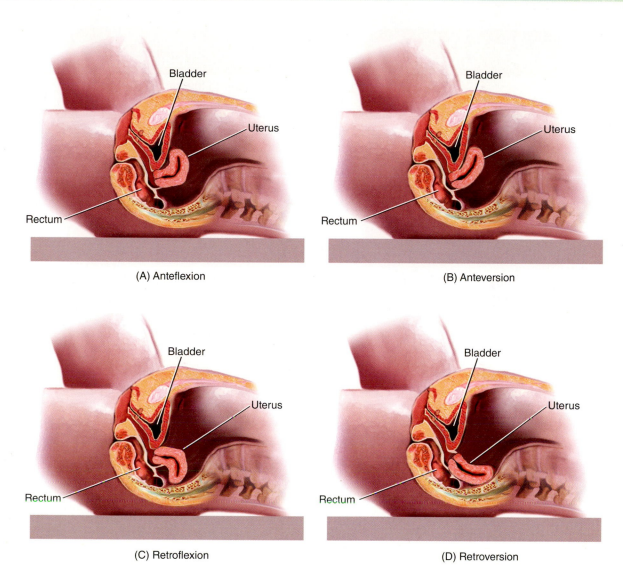

**Figure 18-12** Uterine positions. A. Anteflexion. B. Anteversion. C. Retroflexion. D. Retroversion. Anteflexion and anteversion are normal uterine positions.

# Terms Pertaining to Obstetrics

## Roots

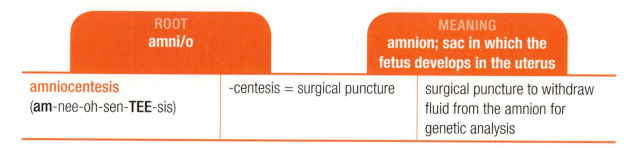

| ROOT<br>amni/o | | MEANING<br>amnion; sac in which the<br>fetus develops in the uterus |
|---|---|---|
| **amniocentesis**<br>(**am**-nee-oh-sen-**TEE**-sis) | -centesis = surgical puncture | surgical puncture to withdraw fluid from the amnion for genetic analysis |

| ROOT nat/o | | MEANING birth |
|---|---|---|
| postnatal (pohst-**NAY**-tal) | -al = pertaining to<br>post- = after | pertaining to the period after birth of the newborn |
| prenatal (pree-**NAY**-tal) | -al = pertaining to<br>pre- = before | pertaining to before birth (referring to the fetus); antenatal |

| ROOT top/o | | MEANING place |
|---|---|---|
| ectopic pregnancy (eck-**TOP**-ick **PREG**-nan-see) | -ic = pertaining to<br>ec- = out | pregnancy occurring in a place other than the uterus, such as the fallopian tube |

## Suffixes

| SUFFIX -gravida | | MEANING pregnancy |
|---|---|---|
| multigravida (**mul**-tih-**GRAV**-ih-dah) | multi- = multiple | a woman who has been pregnant two or more times (written gravida II, gravida III, gravida IV, etc., or GI, GII, GIII, GIV, etc.) |
| nulligravida (**nul**-ih-**GRAV**-ih-dah) | nulli- = none | a woman who has never been pregnant |
| primigravida (**prih**-mih-**GRAV**-ih-dah) | primi- = first | a woman who is pregnant for the first time |

| SUFFIX -para | | MEANING to bear; give birth |
|---|---|---|
| multipara (mul-**TIP**-ah-rah) | multi- = multiple | a woman who has given birth to two or more viable infants. Viable means that the fetus can live on its own outside the uterus. Written para II, para III, etc., or PII, PIII, etc. |
| nullipara (nul-**LIP**-ah-rah) | nulli- = none | a woman who has never given birth to a viable infant |
| primipara (prye-**MIP**-ah-rah) | primi- = first | a woman who has given birth to a viable infant for the first time (written para I or P1) |

| SUFFIX -partum | | MEANING labor; delivery; childbirth |
| --- | --- | --- |
| antepartum (an-tee-PAR-tum) | ante- = before | before birth (referring to the mother) |
| postpartum (pohst-PAR-tum) | post- = after | after birth (referring to the mother) |

## 18.6 Pathology

### Diseases Relating to the Female Reproductive System

#### Breast Cancer

Breast cancer is a malignant tumor of the breast. If left untreated, the cancer can metastasize. This means that it spreads to the surrounding breast tissue, to the lymph nodes, and then to other parts of the body through the blood and lymph. Breast cancer is described in stages ranging from 0 to IV depending upon the size of the tumor, the lymph node involvement, and degree of **metastasis**. In stage 0, the tumor is small, there is no lymph node involvement, and no metastasis. In stage IV, there is lymph node involvement, and the tumor has spread to distant organs. Stages I to III are varying degrees of severity between stages 0 and IV.

The exact cause is unknown. Breast cancer is associated with several risk factors: family history, high estrogen levels, age, alcohol consumption, and obesity. Two breast cancer genes have been identified, **BRCA1** and **BRCA2**. Inheritance of either one of these genes can increase the chance of breast cancer, although cancer is not inevitable.

Treatment includes surgical removal of the tumor by **lumpectomy** (lump-**ECK**-toh-mee). The cancerous tissue is removed, but the remainder of the breast tissue is left intact. At the same time, lymph nodes are checked to see if the cancer has spread beyond the breast. This is followed by **radiation therapy** (radiotherapy) to kill cancer cells.

Another surgical procedure is **mastectomy**, the surgical removal of the breast. This involves excising the entire breast. The axillary lymph nodes may or may not be removed. Mastectomy is followed by chemotherapy and radiation therapy. If the mastectomy also includes removal of the pectoral muscles and axillary lymph nodes, it is called **radical mastectomy**.

#### Cervical Cancer

Cervical cancer involves the infiltration of cancer cells into the neck of the uterus. A sexually transmitted infection, **human papillomavirus** (**pap**-ih-**LOH**-mah-**vye**-rus) (**HPV**) causes most cases of cervical cancer.

### Endometriosis (**en**-doh-**mee**-tree-**OH**-sis)

Endometrial tissue found at sites other than the uterus (Figure 18-7). The ectopic (out of place) endometrial tissue finds its way into the pelvic cavity by moving out of the uterus and through the open fallopian tubes. Other abnormal sites where the endometrium can be found include the ovaries, tubes, and abdominal cavity.

### Uterine (Endometrial) Cancer

Endometrial cancer is a malignant tumor of the endometrium, which lines the uterus. Uterine cancer is the most common cancer of the reproductive organs. The exact cause is unknown. A combination of surgery, radiation therapy, hormonal therapy, and chemotherapy is the most common treatment. A **total abdominal hysterectomy** (TAH) is done. In some cases, a total abdominal hysterectomy with **bilateral salpingo-oophorectomy** (BSO) is necessary. The abbreviation then becomes TAH-BSO. If the cancer is spreading, a **radical hysterectomy** may be performed. This includes removal of the nearby lymph nodes.

### Uterine Prolapse

Protrusion or displacement of the uterus through the vaginal canal. There are three stages (degrees) of prolapse, depending on how far into the vaginal canal the uterus has fallen. First degree: The uterus projects into the vaginal canal but not into the **introitus** (in-**TROH**-ih-tuss) (entrance to the vagina). Second degree: The uterus projects further into the vaginal canal up to the introitus. Third degree: The uterus and cervix project through the introitus. This stage is also known as **procidentia** (**proh**-sih-**DEN**-shah). These are illustrated in Figure 18-13.

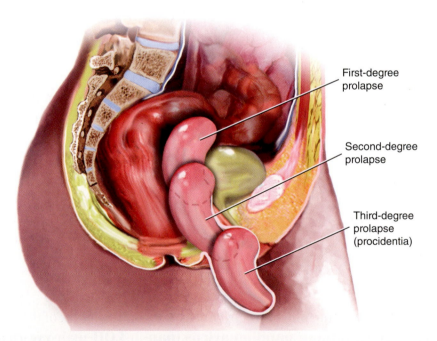

First-degree prolapse

Second-degree prolapse

Third-degree prolapse (procidentia)

**Figure 18-13**  Uterine prolapse. First degree: The cervix projects into the vaginal canal but does not project into the introitus (entrance to the vagina). Second degree: The uterus projects further into the vaginal canal up into the introitus. Third degree: The uterus and cervix project through the introitus. This stage is also known as procidentia (**proh**-sih-**DEN**-shah).

## Sexually Transmitted Infections (STIs)

STIs, also known as venereal disease (VD) and sexually transmitted disease (STD), include any disease that has been transmitted through any type of sexual activity, including vaginal, oral, and anal sex.

The most common types of STIs are:

- acquired immunodeficiency syndrome (AIDS) caused by human immunodeficiency virus (HIV)
- chlamydia (klah-**MID**-ee-ah), caused by *Chlamydia trachomatis* (klah-**MID**-ee-ah tray-koh-**MAH**-tiss)
- genital herpes (**JEN**-ih-tahl **HER**-peez), caused by the herpes simplex virus (Figure 18-14)
- genital warts caused by the human papillomavirus (Figure 18-15)
- gonorrhea (**gon**-oh-**REE**-ah) caused by *Neisseria* (nigh-**SEE**-ree-ah) *gonorrhoeae*
- human immunodeficiency virus infection. If left untreated HIV infection will lead to AIDS.
- syphilis (**SIF**-ih-lis) caused by *Treponema pallidum* (**trep**-oh-**NEE**-mah **PAL**-ih-dum)
- trichomoniasis (**trick**-oh-mon-**EYE**-ah-sis) caused by *Trichomonas vaginalis*

In the early stages of these diseases, the patient is often asymptomatic (there are no symptoms). The patient may therefore spread the disease to other persons without knowing it. If left untreated, permanent damage to the reproductive organs may result.

# Conditions Relating to Obstetrics

## Abortion

Abortion is the termination of pregnancy before the embryo or fetus is viable. A **spontaneous abortion** is also known as a **miscarriage** and occurs because of an abnormality or genetic disorder. A **therapeutic abortion** or **induced abortion** is performed intentionally by drug intake or by mechanical means. An operation called **dilation and curettage** (**kyoo**-reh-**TAZH**) (D&C) may be performed. This involves the widening

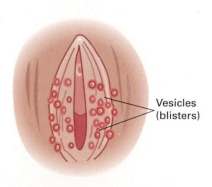

Vesicles
(blisters)

**Figure 18-14**  Genital herpes.

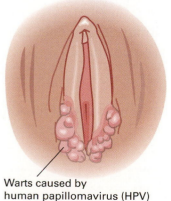

Warts caused by
human papillomavirus (HPV)

**Figure 18-15**  Genital warts.

of the uterine cavity and the scraping of the uterine wall to remove the fetus. As an alternative, the fetus may be removed by suction. This is also known as **vacuum aspiration**.

### Abruptio Placentae (ab-**RUP**-she-oh plah-**SEN**-tee)

Premature detachment of the placenta from the uterine wall resulting in hemorrhage and premature labor and ending in termination of the pregnancy.

### Infertility and Assisted Reproductive Therapy

Infertility is defined as not having the ability to get pregnant despite having unprotected sex for at least one year. **Assisted reproductive therapy** (ART) gives the highest chance of pregnancy for most couples. Three types of ART are described below.

*Fertility medications* Drugs that stimulate follicle development in the ovaries.

*In vitro fertilization* In vitro fertilization (IVF) is the most common technique. IVF involves removal of mature eggs from a woman, fertilizing the eggs with a man's sperm in a dish in a laboratory, and implanting the fertilized egg in the uterus. The hope is that the fertilized egg will attach to the uterine wall and continue to develop into a fetus until delivery. **In vitro** means in a glass, test tube, or dish.

*Artificial insemination* **Artificial insemination** (in-**sem**-ih-**NAY**-shun) is the introduction of sperm into the uterus by means other than sexual intercourse. This is performed during the ovulatory period of the menstrual cycle.

### Placenta Previa (**PREH**-vee-ah)

Placenta previa is the attachment of the placenta near the cervix uteri instead of high up on the uterine wall. This can cause hemorrhaging and premature labor that places mother and baby at risk. Cesarean section is necessary.

### Preeclampsia (**pree**-eh-**KLAMP**-see-ah) and Eclampsia

Preeclampsia is a condition that can occur after the twentieth week of pregnancy. It is characterized by hypertension, albuminuria (protein in the urine), and excessive edema. If left untreated, convulsion and coma might result, and the condition is then called **eclampsia**, which can be fatal. Treatment includes medication and delivery of the fetus.

### Premature Infant

A premature infant is one born before 37 weeks' gestation, which is more than three weeks before the due date.

### Stillbirth

A stillbirth (SB) is a fetus that has died in utero. Most common in full-term pregnancies.

## Uterine Inertia

Uterine inertia is the loss of uterine muscle contractions during labor.

## 18.7　Look-Alike and Sound-Alike Words

*Below is a list of look-alike and sound-alike words. Study the spelling and definitions of each set of words. Questions will follow in the Review Exercises.*

### TABLE 18-1　Look-Alike and Sound-Alike Words

| | |
|---|---|
| menorrhagia | excessive uterine bleeding during menstruation |
| menorrhalgia | painful menstruation |
| metrorrhagia | uterine bleeding at times other than at the regular menstrual period |
| perineal | pertaining to the perineum |
| peritoneal | pertaining to the peritoneum |
| peroneal | pertaining to the fibula or outer side of the leg |
| parametrium | connective tissue located beside the uterus |
| perimetrium | outermost wall of the uterus |

## 18.8　Review Exercises

### EXERCISE 18-1　Look-Alike and Sound-Alike Words

*Read the sentences carefully and circle the word in parentheses that correctly completes the meaning. Use Table 18-1 if it helps you.*

1. The patient was admitted with excessive menstrual bleeding. It was decided that a hysterectomy would be a permanent solution for her (**menorrhagia/ metrorrhagia**).

2. Dysmenorrhea and (**menorrhagia/menorrhalgia/metrorrhagia**) mean the same thing.

3. The third degree (**perineal/peritoneal/peroneal**) tear was a complication of delivery due to a very large fetal head.

4. The malignant cells have spread outside the uterine wall to the (**perimetrium/ parametrium**).

## EXERCISE 18-2  Matching Word Parts with Meaning

*I. Match the word part in Column A with its meaning in Column B.*

| | Column A | Column B |
|---|---|---|
| _____ | **1.** ante- | A. vulva |
| _____ | **2.** episio- | B. uterus |
| _____ | **3.** colp/o | C. binding; tying |
| _____ | **4.** gynec/o | D. month |
| _____ | **5.** salping/o | E. ovary |
| _____ | **6.** ligati/o | F. beginning |
| _____ | **7.** men/o | G. fallopian tubes |
| _____ | **8.** -arche | H. before |
| _____ | **9.** metr/o | I. woman |
| _____ | **10.** oophor/o | J. vagina |

*II. Match the word part in Column A with its meaning in Column B.*

| | Column A | Column B |
|---|---|---|
| _____ | **1.** -rrhaphy | A. none |
| _____ | **2.** nulli- | B. milk |
| _____ | **3.** lact/o | C. tilting |
| _____ | **4.** top/o | D. suture |
| _____ | **5.** mamm/o | E. breast |
| _____ | **6.** -gravida | F. to give birth |
| _____ | **7.** myc/o | G. pregnancy |
| _____ | **8.** -para | H. first |
| _____ | **9.** versi/o | I. place |
| _____ | **10.** primi- | J. fungus |

## EXERCISE 18-3  Matching–Anatomy

*Match the term in Column A with its description in Column B.*

| | Column A | Column B |
|---|---|---|
| _____ | **1.** estrogen | A. discharge of endometrial tissue |
| _____ | **2.** ovum | |
| _____ | **3.** fimbriae | B. neck of the uterus |
| _____ | **4.** cervix uteri | C. inner lining of the uterus |
| _____ | **5.** endometrium | D. part of the external genitalia |

_____ **6.** rectouterine pouch

_____ **7.** labium majora

_____ **8.** progesterone

_____ **9.** uterus

_____ **10.** menstruation

E. hormone responsible for the growth of blood vessels in the endometrium

F. egg

G. houses and protects the developing fetus

H. cul-de-sac of Douglas

I. hormone responsible for developing female secondary characteristics

J. portion of the fallopian tube

## EXERCISE 18-4 Matching—Pathology

_Match the following terms with its description that is written below. Not all terms are used._

metastasize _____

endometriosis _____

endometrial cancer _____

breast cancer _____

uterine prolapse _____

Chlamydia _____

**1.** ectopic endometrium _____

**2.** the spread of cancer from one organ to another _____

**3.** the most common cancer of the female reproductive system

_____

**4.** displacement of the uterus through the vaginal canal

_____

**5.** a sexually transmitted disease _____

## EXERCISE 18-5  Labeling—Female Reproductive Tract

*Using the body structures listed below, label Figure 18-16. Write your answer in the numbered spaces provided below, or if you prefer, on the diagram.*

cervix

fallopian tube

ovary

rectouterine pouch

urethra

urinary bladder

uterus

vagina

1. _____

2. _____

3. _____

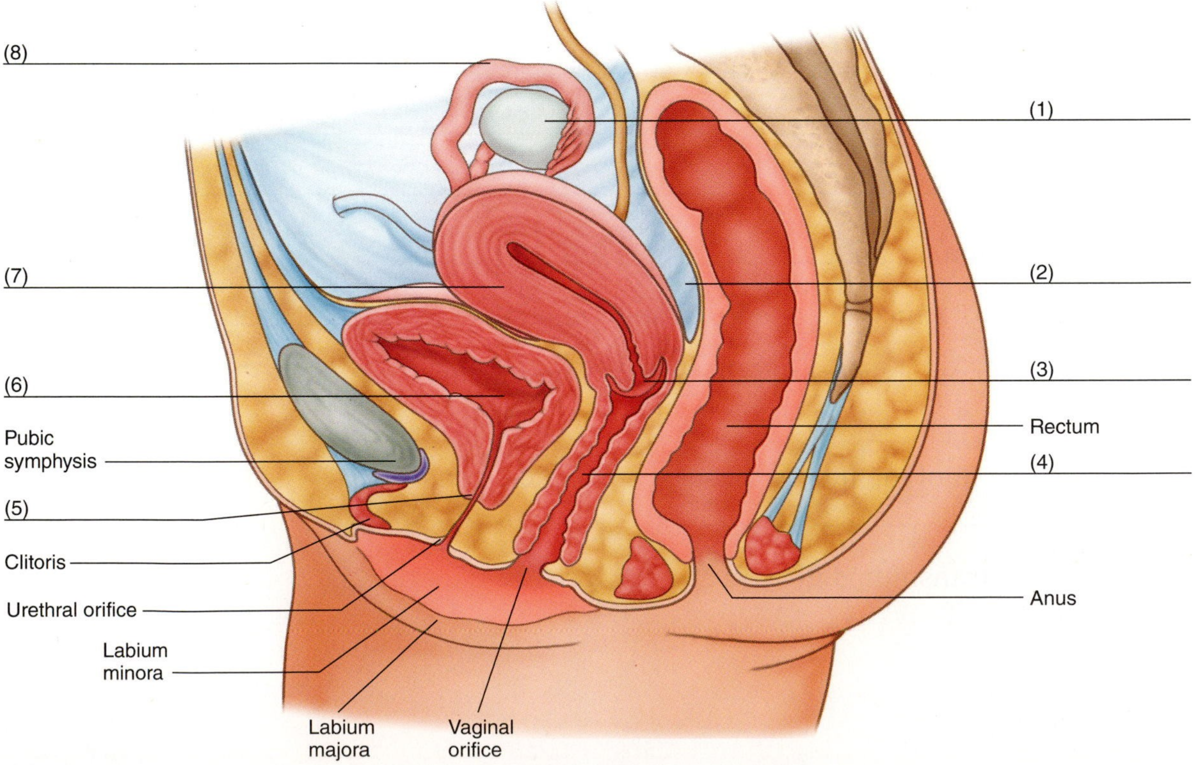

(8)

(7)

(6)

Pubic
symphysis

(5)

Clitoris

Urethral orifice

Labium
minora

Labium
majora

Vaginal
orifice

(1)

(2)

(3)

Rectum

(4)

Anus

**Figure 18-16** Major organs of the female reproductive system.

**4.** _____

**5.** _____

**6.** _____

**7.** _____

**8.** _____

## EXERCISE 18-6 Definitions—Anatomy

_Define the following terms:_

**1. estrogen** _____

**2. adnexa** _____

**3. myometrium** _____

**4. fertilization** _____

**5. lactiferous ducts** _____

**6. perimetrium** _____

**7. lactiferous sinus** _____

**8. ovulation** _____

**9. fetus** _____

**10. fundus of the uterus** _____

**11. puerperium** _____

**12. parturition** _____

**13. zygote** _____

**14. chorion** _____

**15. Apgar score** _____

## EXERCISE 18-7 Physiology

_Write one function for each of the following._

**1.** ovaries _____

**2.** fimbriae _____

**3.** Bartholin gland _____

**4.** mammary glands _____

5. amniotic fluid _____

6. progesterone _____

7. fallopian tubes _____

8. uterus _____

9. vagina _____

## EXERCISE 18-8  Definitions—Learning the Terms

*Define the following terms.*

1. **cervical polyp** _____

2. **colporrhaphy** _____

3. **episiotomy** _____

4. **fibroadenoma** _____

5. **salpingo-oophorectomy** _____

6. **gynecologist** _____

7. **labial** _____

8. **lactogenesis** _____

9. **tubal ligation** _____

10. **mastopexy** _____

11. **menorrhea** _____

12. **menorrhagia** _____

13. **metrorrhagia** _____

14. **hysterectomy** _____

15. **vaginomycosis** _____

16. **cystocele** _____

17. **hydrosalpinx** _____

18. **anteflexion** _____

19. **retroversion** _____

20. **cervicitis** _____

21. **multipara** _____

22. **amniocentesis** _____

## EXERCISE 18-9  Building Medical Words

*I. Use the combining form men/o to build medical words for the following definitions.*

**a.** no menstruation _____

**b.** painful menstruation _____

**c.** normal menstruation _____

**d.** excessive uterine bleeding during menstruation _____

*II. Use the combining form metr/o to build medical words for the following definitions.*

**a.** inner uterine wall _____

**b.** uterine bleeding at times other than regular menstrual periods

_____

**c.** muscular uterine wall _____

**d.** outermost wall of the uterus _____

*III. Use the suffix -gravida to build medical words for the following definitions.*

**a.** woman who has been pregnant two or more times

_____

**b.** woman who has never been pregnant _____

**c.** woman who is pregnant for the first time _____

## EXERCISE 18-10  Definitions in Context

*Define the bolded terms in the spaces provided. Use your medical dictionary if necessary.*

**1. Laparoscopic tubal ligation** was performed following delivery.

**a.** laparoscopic tubal ligation _____

**2.** At laparoscopy, the **uterus** was small and normal in appearance. Both **fallopian tubes** were normal in appearance. The fallopian tubes were clamped and **ligated**.

**b.** uterus _____

**c.** fallopian tubes _____

**d.** ligated _____

**3.** There was one area of **endometriosis** near the **fimbrial** aspect of the right fallopian tube.

**e.** endometriosis _____

**f.** fimbrial _____

**4.** On examination, the uterus was enlarged, and an **ultrasound** confirmed the presence of **fibroids**.

**g.** ultrasound _____

**h.** fibroids _____

## EXERCISE 18-11 Spelling

*Circle any words that are spelled incorrectly in the list below. Then correct the spelling in the space provided.*

**1.** menstration _____

**2.** Bartolin cyst _____

**3.** epiziorhaphy _____

**4.** dismenorrhea _____

**5.** pereniorrhaphy _____

**6.** rectroflection _____

**7.** endometriosis _____

**8.** sphylis _____

## EXERCISE 18-12 Short Answer—Pathology

*State whether the following sentences are true or false. If false, explain why.*

**1.** In stage IV breast cancer there is no lymph node involvement and there is no metastasis to distant organs. _____

**2.** Removal of the breast including the pectoral muscles and axillary lymph nodes is called a radical mastectomy. _____

**3.** A miscarriage is also known as a spontaneous abortion.
_____

**4.** Fertility medications stimulate the uterus to develop follicles.
_____

**5.** Eclampsia is a complication of pregnancy that may cause death.
_____

**6.** Uterine inertia is a complication of labor. _____

**7.** A primigravida is a woman who has given birth to a viable infant for the first time.
_____

**8.** The amnion is the inner lining of the placenta. _____

**9.** After a total hysterectomy a woman cannot produce estrogen and progesterone. _____

**10.** A zygote is a fertilized egg. _____

**11.** Syphilis is caused by *Treponema pallidum.* _____

**12.** Genital warts are caused by herpes simplex. _____

## Animations

Visit the companion website to view the videos on **Amniocentesis**; **Mastectomies**; and **Secondary Sex Characteristics**.

## 18.9  Pronunciation and Spelling

1. Listen to each word on the audio file provided in the Student Companion Website.

2. Spell each word in the space provided.

| Word | Pronunciation | Spelling |
|------|---------------|----------|
| adnexa | ad-**NECK**-sah | |
| amenorrhea | ah-**men**-oh-**REE**-ah | |
| areola | ah-**REE**-oh-lah | |
| cervicitis | **ser**-vih-**SIGH**-tis | |
| cervix uteri | **SER**-vicks **YOO**-ter-eye | |
| Chlamydia | klah-**MID**-ee-ah | |
| colporrhaphy | kohl-**POR**-ah-fee | |
| cul-de-sac of Douglas | **kuhl**-deh-sack of **DUG**-lass | |
| cystocele | **SIS**-toh-seel | |
| dysmenorrhea | **dis**-men-oh-**REE**-ah | |
| endometriosis | **en**-doh-**mee**-tree-**OH**-sis | |
| endometrium | **en**-doh-**MEE**-tree-um | |
| episiorrhaphy | eh-**piz**-ee-**OR**-ah-fee | |
| estrogen | **ES**-troh-jen | |

| Word | Pronunciation | Spelling |
|------|---------------|----------|
| **fallopian tubes** | fal-**LOH**-pee-an **TOOBZ** | |
| **fetus** | **FEE**-tus | |
| **genitalia** | **jen**-ih-**TAIL**-ee-ah | |
| **gynecologist** | **gye**-neh-**KOL**-oh-jist | |
| **hysterectomy** | **hiss**-ter-**ECK**-toh-mee | |
| **menstruation** | **men**-stroo-**AY**-shun | |
| **myometrium** | **my**-oh-**MEE**-tree-um | |
| **oophorrhagia** | oh-**off**-oh-**RAY**-jee-ah | |
| **parturition** | **par**-tyoo-**RISH**-un | |
| **obstetrician** | **ob**-steh-**TRIH**-shun | |
| **ovary** | **OH**-vah-ree | |
| **ovulation** | **ahv**-yoo-**LAY**-shun | |
| **ovum** | **OH**-vum | |
| **papillomavirus** | **pap**-ih-**LOH**-mah-**vye**-rus | |
| **perimetrium** | **per**-ih-**MEE**-tree-um | |
| **progesterone** | pro-**JES**-teh-rohn | |
| **retroflexion** | **ret**-roh-**FLECK**-shun | |
| **rectouterine pouch** | **reck**-toh-**YOO**-ter-in **POWCH** | |
| **salpingo-oophorectomy** | sal-**ping**-goh-oh-**off**-oh-**RECK**-toh-mee | |
| **syphilis** | **SIF**-ih-lis | |
| **uterine fibroids** | **YOO**-ter-in **FYE**-broidz | |
| **uterine inertia** | **YOO**-ter-in in-**ER**-shee-ah | |
| **uterovesical** | **yoo**-ter-oh-**VES**-ih-kal | |
| **uterus** | **YOO**-ter-us | |
| **vagina** | vah-**JIGH**-nah | |

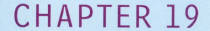

# Endocrine System

## Chapter Outline

## Learning Objectives

*After studying this chapter and completing the review exercises, you should be able to:*

1. Define endocrine glands and hormones.
2. Name the endocrine glands and the hormones they secrete.
3. Understand the function of these hormones in the body.
4. Describe the structure and location of the endocrine glands.
5. Pronounce, spell, define, and write the medical terms related to the endocrine system.
6. Describe common diseases related to the endocrine system.
7. Listen, read, and study so you can speak and write.

## Introduction

The endocrine (**EN**-doh-krin) system consists of several glands. You can see them in Figure 19-1. Glands are located in many areas of the body. They secrete powerful chemicals called **hormones** (**HOR**-mohnz) into the bloodstream. Hormones travel in the blood to various sites throughout

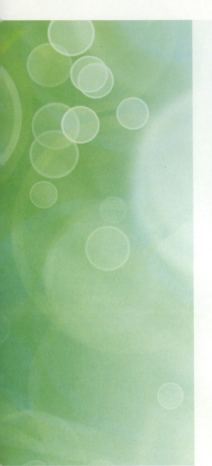

the body. They regulate organ function and keep the body in a balanced, normal state no matter what is happening outside it. This balance is called **homeostasis** (**hoh**-mee-oh-**STAY**-sis). One example of homeostasis is the regulation of body temperature. Hormones secreted by glands in the endocrine system maintain the body's normal temperature of about 98.6 degrees Fahrenheit (37 degrees Celsius) regardless of the outside temperature.

This chapter is organized under two major headings: **peripheral endocrine glands** and **central endocrine glands**. The peripheral endocrine glands are the **thyroid** (**THIGH**-royd), **parathyroids** (**par**-ah-**THIGH**-roydz), **adrenals** (ah-**DREE**-nalz), **pineal** (**PIN**-ee-al), **thymus** (**THIGH**-mus), and **pancreas** (**PAN**-kree-as). The first four have only one function: the production of hormones. The thymus produces hormones and functions in immunity. The pancreas also produces hormones and has important digestive functions. In this way, the thymus and pancreas are similar to other mixed-function organs, such as the kidneys, liver, ovaries, and testicles: They produce hormones as well as perform important work to maintain body function. The functions of these organs, except for the pancreas, have been taken up in their respective chapters.

There are only two central endocrine glands: the **pituitary** (pih-**TOO**-ih-**tar**-ee) gland and the **hypothalamus** (**high**-poh-**THAL**-ah-mus). They are both in the brain.

## 19.1  Glands of the Endocrine System

**PRACTICE FOR LEARNING: Glands of the Endocrine System**

Write the words below in the correct spaces on Figure 19-1. To help you, the number beside the word tells you where it goes on the figure. Be sure to pronounce each word as you write it. Repeat the pronunciation several times if you find the word hard to say.

1. pituitary (pih-**TOO**-ih-**tar**-ee) gland
2. hypothalamus (**high**-poh-**THAL**-ah-mus)
3. pineal (**PIN**-ee-al) gland
4. parathyroid (**par**-ah-**THIGH**-roid) gland
5. thymus (**THIGH**-mus) gland
6. ovaries (**OH**-vah-rees)
7. testicles (**TESS**-tih-kulz)
8. pancreas (**PAN**-kree-as)
9. adrenal (ah-**DREE**-nal) glands
10. thyroid (**THIGH**-royd) gland

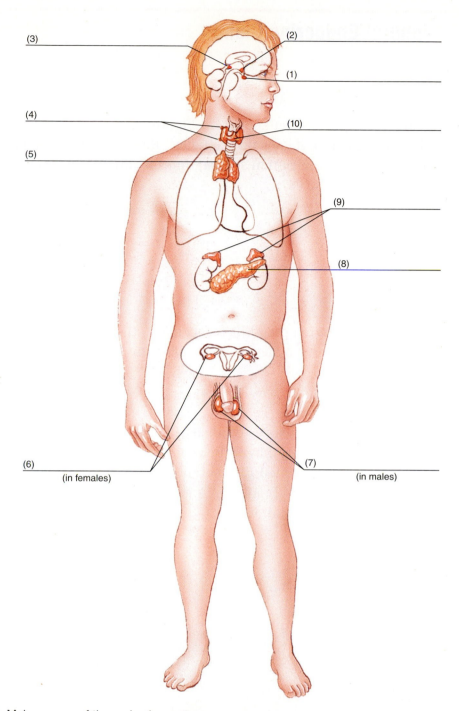

**Figure 19-1**  Major organs of the endocrine system.

## 19.2   Peripheral Endocrine Glands

### Thyroid Gland

**PRACTICE FOR LEARNING: Thyroid Gland**

Write the words below in the correct spaces on Figure 19-2. To help you, the number beside the word tells you where it goes on the figure. Be sure to pronounce each word as you write it. Repeat the pronunciation several times if you find the word hard to say.

1. thyroid gland
2. right lobe
3. left lobe
4. isthmus (**ISS**-mus)

### Location and Structure

Figure 19-2 illustrates the thyroid gland. It is located in the neck, below the larynx. It has right and left lobes connected by a structure called the **isthmus** (**ISS**-mus).

### Function

The thyroid secretes the hormones $T_3$ and $T_4$. $T_3$ is triiodothyronine (trigh-**eye**-oh-doh-**THIGH**-roh-nen). $T_4$ is thyroxine (thigh-**ROCK**-sin). Thyroxine is also spelled thyroxin. These hormones regulate how much energy is used by the body's cells to perform their functions. This is called the metabolic rate. Iodine must be consumed in order for the thyroid to produce $T_3$ and $T_4$. A goiter (enlarged thyroid) will result if there is insufficient iodine in the diet.

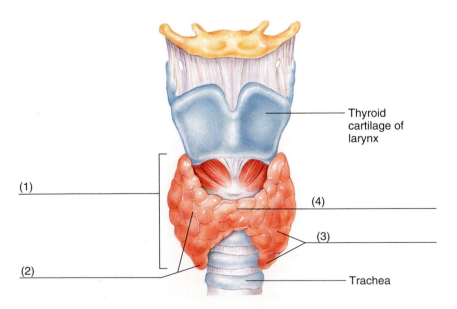

**Figure 19-2**  Thyroid gland.

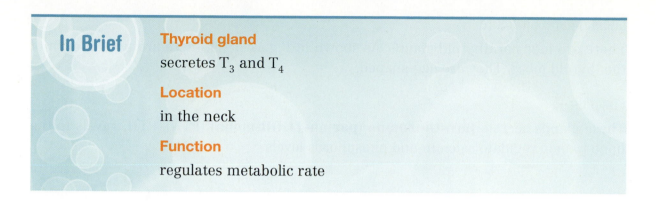

**In Brief**

**Thyroid gland**

secretes $T_3$ and $T_4$

**Location**

in the neck

**Function**

regulates metabolic rate

## Parathyroid Gland

PRACTICE FOR LEARNING: **Parathyroid Gland**

Write the words below in the correct spaces on Figure 19-3. To help you, the number beside the word tells you where it goes on the figure. Be sure to pronounce each word as you write it. Repeat the pronunciation several times if you find the word hard to say.

**1.** thyroid gland

**2.** parathyroid glands

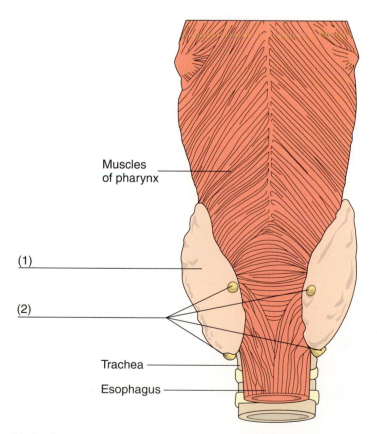

Muscles of pharynx

(1)

(2)

Trachea

Esophagus

**Figure 19-3**  Parathyroid glands.

### Location and Structure

There are four parathyroid glands. As shown in Figure 19-3, there are two on each of the thyroid lobes. They are egg-shaped.

### Function

These glands secrete **parathormone** (**par**-ah-**THOR**-mohn) (PTH). PTH travels to the bone to help regulate calcium and phosphorus levels.

**In Brief**

**Parathyroid gland**

secretes PTH

**Location**

embedded in the thyroid gland

**Function**

regulates calcium and phosphorus

## Thymus

### Location and Structure

The **thymus gland** (Figure 19-1) is located near the heart in the thoracic cavity. It consists of two lobes. Each lobe contains many smaller lobes called lobules (**LOB**-yoolz).

### Function

The thymus is both a lymphatic organ and an endocrine gland. As a lymphatic organ, the thymus protects the body from disease. As an endocrine gland, it secretes a hormone called **thymosin** (**THIGH**-moh-sin). Thymosin stimulates red bone marrow to produce T cells (T lymphocytes), which mature in the thymus gland.

**In Brief**

**Thymus**

secretes thymosin

**Location**

near the heart

**Function**

stimulates red bone marrow to produce T cells

## Adrenal Glands

**PRACTICE FOR LEARNING:** **Adrenal Glands**

Write the words below in the correct spaces on Figure 19-4. To help you, the number beside the word tells you where it goes on the figure. Be sure to pronounce each word as you write it. Repeat the pronunciation several times if you find the word hard to say.

1. adrenal (ah-**DREE**-nal) gland
2. adrenal cortex (**KOR**-tecks)
3. adrenal medulla (meh-**DULL**-ah)

### Location and Structure

The adrenal glands sit on top of the kidneys, as shown in Figure 19-4. The outer and inner portions of each adrenal gland are actually separate glands. The outer portion is the adrenal cortex. The inner portion is the adrenal medulla. These glands are different in structure and function.

### Function

The adrenal cortex secretes the following hormones: **aldosterone** (al-**DOS**-ter-ohn), **cortisol** (**KOR**-tih-sol), estrogen, and **androgen** (**AN**-droh-jen).

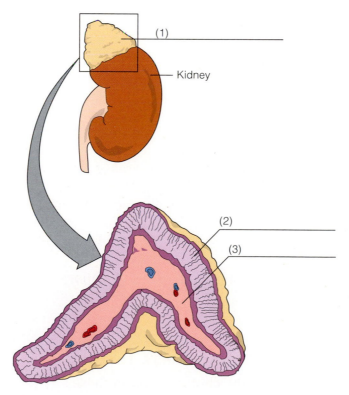

(1)

Kidney

(2)

(3)

**Figure 19-4**  Adrenal gland.

Aldosterone regulates sodium and potassium levels. Cortisol (hydrocortisone) has several important functions. It regulates our immune system. It also plays a key role in how carbohydrates, fats, and proteins are used by the body.

Estrogens and androgens are the sex hormones. They are secreted in very small amounts to maintain secondary female and male sex characteristics such as hair growth and muscle bulk. These sex hormones are secreted in larger amounts by the ovaries and testicles.

The adrenal medulla produces **adrenaline** (ah-**DREN**-ah-len) (epinephrine) and **noradrenaline** (**nor**-ah-**DREN**-ah-len) (norepinephrine). These are called the "flight-or-fight" hormones. If a person is frightened enough to run away or angry enough to fight, these hormones prepare the body for the physical exertion needed during these times.

## In Brief

**Adrenal cortex**

secretes aldosterone, cortisol, and sex hormones

**Location**

on top of the kidneys

**Function**

**aldosterone**

regulates sodium and potassium

**cortisol**

regulates immune system and plays a role in the metabolism of carbohydrates, fats, and proteins

**sex hormones**

regulate male and female secondary sexual characteristics

**Adrenal medulla**

secretes adrenaline (epinephrine) and noradrenaline (norepinephrine)

**Function**

epinephrine and norepinephrine prepare the body for times of stress and fear

## PRACTICE FOR LEARNING: Thyroid, Parathyroids, Thymus, Adrenals

Choose the correct answer from the choices in parentheses.

1. Aldosterone is secreted by the (adrenal cortex/parathyroid/adrenal medulla) gland.

2. ($T_4$/Parathormone/Cortisol) regulates the metabolic rate.

3. (Aldosterone/Parathormone/Cortisol) regulates blood calcium.

4. (Aldosterone/Cortisol/Estrogen) regulates sodium and potassium levels.

5. (Epinephrine/Cortisol) prepares the body for flight-or-fight.

6. (Parathormone/Aldosterone/$T_3$) is secreted by the thyroid gland.

7. (Epinephrine/Estrogen/$T_3$) is secreted by the adrenal cortex.

8. The adrenal medulla secretes (aldosterone/sex hormones/norepinephrine/cortisol).

9. (Thyroxine/Triiodothyronine/Thymosin) stimulates red bone marrow to produce T cells.

> Answers: 1. adrenal cortex. 2. $T_4$. 3. parathormone. 4. aldosterone. 5. epinephrine. 6. $T_3$. 7. estrogen. 8. norepinephrine. 9. thymosin.

## Pineal Gland

### Location and Structure

The **pineal** (**PIN**-ee-al) gland is shown in Figure 19-1. It looks like a pine cone and is located deep within the brain.

### Function

The pineal gland secretes **melatonin** (**mel**-ah-**TOH**-nin). This hormone plays a role in telling us when it is time to go to sleep and when it is time to wake up. It is also connected to mood. It may be involved in determining when we commence puberty and in regulating the ovarian cycles.

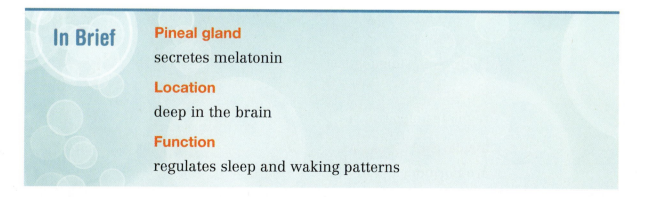

**In Brief**

**Pineal gland**
secretes melatonin

**Location**
deep in the brain

**Function**
regulates sleep and waking patterns

## Pancreas

### Location and Structure

As described in Chapter 11, the **pancreas** (**PAN**-kree-as) is a long, fish-shaped organ lying behind the stomach.

## Function

The pancreas has both digestive and endocrine functions. The digestive function involves the secretion of digestive enzymes to break down food.

The endocrine function involves cells in the pancreas called the **islets of Langerhans** (**LANG**-er-hanz). These islets are made up of **beta** and **alpha cells**. Beta cells produce and secrete the hormone **insulin** (**IN**-suh-lin), and alpha cells produce and secrete the hormone **glucagon** (**GLOO**-kah-gon).

When there is too much sugar in the body, insulin lowers blood glucose (sugar) by:

**1.** stimulating the absorption of glucose by body cells

**2.** converting glucose to **glycogen** (**GLYE**-koh-jen)

Glycogen is the storage form of glucose and is stored in the liver.

| glucose | insulin $\rightarrow$ | glycogen |
|---------|------------|----------|

The hormone glucagon increases blood sugar by converting glycogen back to glucose when the body requires energy to function.

| glycogen | glucagon $\rightarrow$ | glucose |
|----------|-------------|---------|

Insulin and glucagon work together to regulate the amount of glucose in the blood. This balancing process is called **homeostasis** (**hoh**-mee-oh-**STAY**-sis).

**In Brief**

**Pancreas**
secretes insulin and glucagon

**Location**
behind the stomach

**Function**
regulates blood sugar

**Insulin and glucagon**
are hormones

**Glycogen**
is the storage form of glucose

**PRACTICE FOR LEARNING: Pineal Gland and Pancreas**

Write the correct answers in the spaces provided.

**1.** Which hormone is secreted by the pineal gland?

_____

**2.** Which hormones are secreted by the pancreas?

_____

**3.** Name one function of the pineal gland.

_____

**4.** Name one function of the pancreatic hormones.

_____

**5.** Name the hormone that changes glucose to glycogen.

_____

**6.** Name the hormone that changes glycogen to glucose.

_____

**7.** Which is a hormone? Glucose, glycogen, or glucagon?

_____

> **Answers:  1. melatonin. 2. insulin and glucagon. 3. regulates sleep and waking patterns; it is also connected to moods. 4. regulates blood sugar levels. 5. insulin. 6. glucagon. 7. glucagon.**

## 19.3  Central Endocrine Glands

### Pituitary Gland

#### Location and Structure

The pituitary gland, also known as the **hypophysis** (high-**POF**-eh-sis), is about the size of a pea. It is located at the base of the brain. It hangs from the hypothalamus by a stalk called the **infundibulum** (in-fun-**DIB**-yoo-lum). This is illustrated in Figure 19-5.

The pituitary gland has two lobes: anterior and posterior.

#### Function

The anterior lobe of the pituitary gland secretes several hormones. Many of these hormones stimulate other glands to secrete their own hormones or, in the case of the breasts, milk. Because these hormones stimulate other glands, their names often end in the suffix -**tropic** (**TROH**-pick), which means "to nourish" or "to stimulate." Following is a list of these hormones. (See also Figure 19-6.)

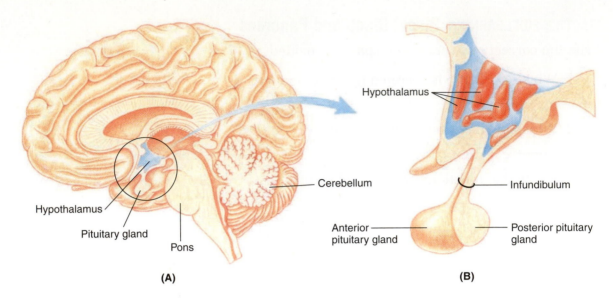

**Figure 19-5** (A) Hypothalamus. (B) Pituitary gland.

1. **Adrenocorticotropic** (ah-**dree**-noh-**kor**-tih-koh-**TROH**-pick) hormone (ACTH) stimulates the adrenal cortex.

2. **Growth hormone** (GH), or **somatotropic** (**soh**-mah-toh-**TROH**-pick) **hormone** (STH), stimulates growth in all body cells.

3. **Thyroid-stimulating hormone** (TSH), or **thyrotropic** (**thigh**-roh-**TROH**-pick) **hormone**, stimulates the thyroid gland.

4. **Gonadotropic** (**goh**-nah-doh-**TROH**-pick) **hormones** stimulate the gonads (ovaries and testicles). There are three gonadotropic hormones: **follicle-stimulating hormone** (FSH) and **luteinizing** (**LOO**-tee-in-**eye**-zing) **hormone** (LH) in the female, and **interstitial cell-stimulating hormone** (ICSH) in the male. FSH stimulates the monthly development of the egg in the follicle. LH triggers ovulation in females. ICSH regulates testosterone secretion.

5. **Prolactin** (proh-**LACK**-tin) (PRL), or **lactogenic hormone** (LTH), stimulates and maintains the secretion of breast milk.

6. **Melanocyte-stimulating hormone** (MSH) stimulates the skin to produce melanocytes.

**In Brief**

**Anterior pituitary**
secretes ACTH, GH, TSH, FSH, LH, ICSH, PRL, MSH

**Posterior pituitary**
secretes ADH and OXT

**Location**
deep in the brain

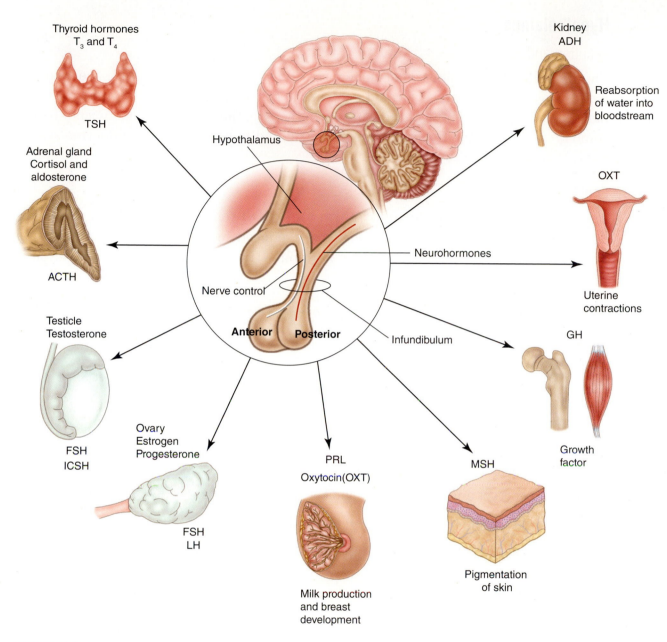

Thyroid hormones
T$_3$ and T$_4$

TSH

Adrenal gland
Cortisol and
aldosterone

ACTH

Testicle
Testosterone

FSH
ICSH

Ovary
Estrogen
Progesterone

FSH
LH

Hypothalamus

Nerve control

**Anterior**   **Posterior**

Neurohormones

Infundibulum

PRL
Oxytocin(OXT)

Milk production
and breast
development

MSH

Pigmentation
of skin

Kidney
ADH

Reabsorption
of water into
bloodstream

OXT

Uterine
contractions

GH

Growth
factor

**Figure 19-6** The pituitary gland secretes hormones that stimulate the activity of other endocrine glands. Abbreviations used in this figure are defined in Table 19-1.

The **posterior lobe of the pituitary** is an extension of the hypothalamus. It stores and secretes two hormones produced by the hypothalamus:

1. Antidiuretic (**an**-tih-**dye**-yoo-**RET**-ick) hormone (ADH). It prevents excessive loss of water.

2. Oxytocin (**ock**-see-**TOH**-sin) (OXT). It stimulates uterine contractions during labor, maintains labor during childbirth, and causes the production of milk from the mammary glands.

## Hypothalamus

### Location and Structure

The hypothalamus is illustrated in Figure 19-5. It works together with the pituitary gland. The hypothalamus is located deep in the central brain, below the thalamus. It is made up of neurons. Some of the neurons in the hypothalamus produce hormones and some do not. Thus, the hypothalamus is considered to be part of the endocrine system as well as the nervous system.

### Function

The hypothalamus produces **neurohormones** (**NOO**-roh-**hor**-monz). They are called neurohormones because the hormones are produced by neurons. The hypothalamus produces oxytocin and the antidiuretic hormone. These neurohormones are stored in the posterior pituitary (Figure 19-6).

**In Brief**

**Hypothalamus**

produces the antidiuretic hormone and oxytocin

**Location**

deep in the brain, under the thalamus

### PRACTICE FOR LEARNING: Pituitary Gland and Hypothalamus

Choose the correct answer from the choices in parentheses.

1. The (hypothalamus/pituitary gland) produces oxytocin.
2. FSH and LH are (thyroid-stimulating hormones/adrenocorticotropic hormones/ gonadotropic hormones).
3. The hormone responsible for milk production is (antidiuretic hormone/ prolactin/oxytocin/gonadotropic hormone).
4. The adrenocorticotropic hormone is secreted by the (adrenal gland/posterior pituitary gland/anterior pituitary gland).
5. The thyroid-stimulating hormone is secreted by the (thyroid gland/anterior pituitary gland/posterior pituitary gland).
6. ADH is produced by the (hypothalamus/posterior pituitary gland/anterior pituitary gland) and stored in the (hypothalamus/posterior pituitary gland/ anterior pituitary gland).
7. Gonadotropic hormones stimulate the (thyroid gland/adrenal cortex/ovaries/ adrenal medulla).

Answers: 1. hypothalamus. 2. gonadotropic. 3. prolactin. 4. anterior pituitary gland. 5. anterior pituitary gland. 6. hypothalamus; posterior pituitary gland. 7. ovaries.

## 19.4 Abbreviations of Major Hormones

Hormones are commonly indicated by abbreviations. Table 19-1 lists the major hormones and their abbreviations.

### TABLE 19-1 Abbreviations of Major Hormones

| | |
|---|---|
| adrenocorticotropic hormone | ACTH |
| antidiuretic hormone | ADH |
| follicle-stimulating hormone | FSH |
| growth hormone | GH |
| interstitial cell-stimulating hormone | ICSH |
| lactogenic hormone | LTH |
| luteinizing hormone | LH |
| oxytocin | OXT |
| parathormone | PTH |
| prolactin | PRL |
| somatotropic hormone | STH |
| thyroid-stimulating hormone | TSH |
| thyroxine | $T_4$ |
| triiodothyronine | $T_3$ |

## 19.5 New Roots, Suffixes, and Prefixes

| ROOT | MEANING |
|---|---|
| calc/o | calcium |
| gonad/o | gonads (ovaries, testicles) |
| kal/o | potassium |
| natr/o | sodium |
| parathyroid/o | parathyroid |
| pituitar/o | pituitary gland |
| somat/o | body |

| SUFFIX | MEANING |
|---|---|
| -dipsia | thirst |
| -gen | producing; produced by |

## 19.6  Learning the Terms

Following these steps will make it easier for you to learn medical terms:

1. Pronounce the term repeatedly until it is easy for you.
2. Write it down. Ensure the spelling is correct.
3. Also write the definition. If possible, relate the word to a word, thought, or picture that will help you remember it.
4. Analyze the term with the method taught in this text.

### Roots

| ROOT acr/o | | MEANING extremity; top |
|---|---|---|
| Term | Term Analysis | Definition |
| acromegaly (**ack**-roh-**MEG**-ah-lee) | -megaly = enlargement | enlargement of many skeletal structures, particularly the extremities |

| ROOT adrenal/o | | MEANING adrenal gland |
|---|---|---|
| Term | Term Analysis | Definition |
| adrenalitis (ah-**dree**-nal-**EYE**-tiss) | -itis = inflammation | inflammation of the adrenal gland |

| ROOT andr/o | | MEANING male |
|---|---|---|
| Term | Term Analysis | Definition |
| androgen (**AN**-droh-jen) | -gen = producing | substance producing male characteristics; an example is testosterone. |

| ROOT crin/o | | MEANING to secrete |
|---|---|---|
| *Term* | *Term Analysis* | *Definition* |
| endocrinologist (**en**-doh-krih-**NOL**-oh-jist) | -logist = specialist<br>endo- = within | specialist in the study of the diagnosis and treatment of diseases of the endocrine glands and their hormonal secretions |

| ROOT estr/o | | MEANING female |
|---|---|---|
| *Term* | *Term Analysis* | *Definition* |
| estrogen (**ESS**-troh-jen) | -gen = producing | female sex hormone |

| ROOT gluc/o; glyc/o | | MEANING glucose; sugar |
|---|---|---|
| *Term* | *Term Analysis* | *Definition* |
| glucogenesis (**gloo**-koh-**JEN**-eh-sis) | -genesis = production | production of glucose |
| glycolysis (glye-**KOL**-ih-sis) | -lysis = breakdown; separation; destruction | breakdown of sugars |

| ROOT glycogen/o | | MEANING glycogen |
|---|---|---|
| *Term* | *Term Analysis* | *Definition* |
| glycogenolysis (**glye**-koh-jeh-**NOL**-ih-sis) | -lysis = breakdown | breakdown of glycogen to form glucose |

| ROOT home/o | | MEANING same |
|---|---|---|
| *Term* | *Term Analysis* | *Definition* |
| homeostasis (**hoh**-mee-oh-**STAY**-sis) | -stasis = standing; stable | a balanced, yet sometimes varied state |

**Note:** The function of the endocrine system is to regulate hormonal balance. It secretes more hormones when needed and fewer when there is an excess. In this way, a balance (homeostasis) is maintained.

| ROOT<br>pituitar/o | | MEANING<br>pituitary gland |
|---|---|---|
| *Term* | *Term Analysis* | *Definition* |
| hyperpituitarism<br>(**high**-per-pih-**TOO**-ih-tahr-izm) | -ism = process; condition | condition of excess secretion of pituitary hormones |

| ROOT<br>thyr/o; thyroid/o | | MEANING<br>thyroid gland |
|---|---|---|
| *Term* | *Term Analysis* | *Definition* |
| euthyroid<br>(yoo-**THIGH**-royd) | -oid = resembling<br>eu- = good; normal | normal thyroid gland |
| hyperthyroidism<br>(**high**-per-**THIGH**-royd-izm) | -ism = condition; process<br>hyper- = excessive | condition characterized by excessive secretion of thyroid hormones |

## Suffixes

| SUFFIX<br>-tropic; -trophic | | MEANING<br>nourish; stimulate |
|---|---|---|
| *Term* | *Term Analysis* | *Definition* |
| adrenocorticotropic hormone<br>(ah-**dree**-noh-**kor**-tih-koh-**TROH**-pick) | adren/o = adrenal gland<br>cortic/o = cortex; outer layer | chemical secreted by the anterior pituitary that stimulates the adrenal cortex to secrete its own hormones |
| gonadotropic hormone<br>(**goh**-nah-doh-**TROH**-pick) | gonad/o = gonads; sex glands (ovaries and testicles) | chemicals secreted by the anterior pituitary that stimulates the ovaries or testicles to secrete their own hormones |
| **Note:** Examples of gonadotropic hormones are LH, FSH, and ICSH. | | |
| somatotropic hormone<br>(**soh**-mah-toh-**TROH**-pick) | somat/o = body | chemical secreted by the anterior pituitary that stimulates the growth in all body cells; growth hormone |

## Prefixes

| PREFIX hyper- | | MEANING increase; excessive |
|---|---|---|
| Term | Term Analysis | Definition |
| hypercalcemia (**high**-per-kal-**SEE**-mee-ah) | -emia = blood condition calc/o = calcium | excessive calcium in the blood |
| hyperkalemia (**high**-per-kal-**EE**-mee-ah) | -emia = blood condition kal/o = potassium | excessive potassium in the blood |
| hyperglycemia (**high**-per-gligh-**SEE**-mee-ah) | -emia = blood condition glyc/o = sugar | excessive sugar in the blood |

| PREFIX hypo- | | MEANING decrease; deficient |
|---|---|---|
| Term | Term Analysis | Definition |
| hyponatremia (**high**-poh-nah-**TREE**-mee-ah) | -emia = blood condition natr/o = sodium | decreased sodium in the blood |
| hypoparathyroidism (**high**-poh-**par**-ah-**THIGH**-roid-izm) | -ism = process; condition parathyroid/o = parathyroid | condition characterized by decreased secretions of the parathyroid hormone |
| hypopituitarism (**high**-poh-pih-**TOO**-ih-tar-izm) | -ism = process; condition pituitar/o = pituitary gland | condition characterized by decreased secretion of pituitary hormones |
| panhypopituitarism (pan-**high**-poh-pih-**TOO**-ih-tar-izm) | -ism = condition; process pan- = all pituitar/o = pituitary gland | condition characterized by deficiency of **all** pituitary hormones |

| PREFIX poly- | | MEANING many; much |
|---|---|---|
| Term | Term Analysis | Definition |
| polydipsia (**pol**-ee-**DIP**-see-ah) | -dipsia = thirst | excessive thirst |
| polyuria (**pol**-ee-**YOO**-ree-ah) | -uria = urination | excessive urination |

**Note:** Polydipsia and polyuria are symptoms of diabetes mellitus.

## 19.7 Pathology

### Hypersecretion and Hyposecretion of Hormones from the Endocrine Glands

Hypersecretion (excess secretion) and hyposecretion (inadequate secretion) may indicate pathology. Often, hypersecretion is caused by the growth of a tumor on the gland. Hyposecretion can indicate congenital absence of the gland, tumors large enough to take over the gland, and infections. In addition, both hypersecretion and hyposecretion can be caused by autoimmune conditions (conditions in which the body turns against itself, thereby causing the disease).

### Major Abnormalities Caused by Hypersecretion and Hyposecretion of Endocrine Glands

#### Pituitary Gland

#### Hypersecretion of Growth Hormone

- **Acromegaly** in adults occurs after bones have stopped growing; there is enlargement of many skeletal structures, particularly the extremities.
- **Gigantism** in children occurs before the bones have stopped growing; there is abnormal growth in height, muscles, and organs.

#### Hyposecretion of Growth Hormone

- **Pituitary dwarfism** is a deficiency of growth hormone in childhood and results in an abnormally small but well-proportioned individual.

#### Hyposecretion of ADH

- **Diabetes insipidus** (**dye**-ah-**BEE**-teez in-**SIP**-ih-duss) is the deficiency of ADH resulting in polyuria, polydipsia, and severe chemical imbalance.

#### Hyposecretion of oxytocin

- **Uterine inertia** is the loss of uterine muscle contraction during labor.

#### Thyroid Gland

#### Hyperthyroidism

- **Graves disease** includes hyperthyroidism, goiter, and exophthalmia. Hyperthyroidism is excessive secretion of the thyroid hormones. It enlarges the thyroid gland (goiter) and has an effect on the tissues behind the eyeball, which pushes the eye outward (exophthalmia). Exophthalmia is also known as exophthalmos or exophthalmus. Graves disease is an autoimmune disorder.

Antibodies that normally protect the body attack the thyroid gland. This causes increased secretion of the thyroid hormone.

## Hypothyroidism

- **Cretinism** (**KRET**-in-izm) is hyposecretion of the thyroid hormone in infancy or during fetal development, causing low metabolic rate and reduced activity, physical growth, and mental growth.
- **Myxedema** (**micks**-eh-**DEE**-mah) is hyposecretion of thyroid hormone in adulthood, causing a slowing of the metabolic rate, weight gain, and slow movement.

## Parathyroid Gland

### Hyperparathyroidism

- Increased secretion of parathormone results in excessive bone loss, which, over time, can lead to pathological fractures and urinary stones.

### Hypoparathyroidism

- Reduced levels of PTH causes hypocalcemia and hypocalciuria. This reduced calcium can lead to severe muscle spasms, a condition called tetany (**TET**-ah-nee).

## Pancreas

### Hyperinsulinism

- Increased insulin causes hypoglycemia. This results in the lack of glucose to body cells, particularly the brain, causing disorientation, unconsciousness, or death due to insulin shock.

### Hypoinsulinism

**Diabetes mellitus** (**dye**-ah-**BEE**-teez **MEL**-ih-tus) (DM) is a disease in which the body is unable to use sugar to produce energy. One cause is insufficient insulin secreted from the pancreas. Another is the production of ineffective insulin. When either of these occurs, sugar is unable to move from the blood into body cells, where it is normally used to produce energy. The result is abnormally high levels of blood glucose. This is called **hyperglycemia**. It is a major symptom of diabetes. Other symptoms include polydipsia, polyuria, and polyphagia.

When the body does not have enough glucose, it will break down fats and proteins for fuel. Over a long period of time, this results in the buildup of toxic wastes called **ketones** (**KEE**-tohnz). The condition is called **ketoacidosis** (**kee**-toh-**ass**-ih-**DOH**-sis). The excess sugars and ketones in the blood cause many long-term complications of DM including retinopathy, which can cause blindness; neuropathy, which can cause numbness and tingling; and arteriosclerosis, which can cause heart attacks and gangrene of the lower extremities. Gestational diabetes can occur during pregnancy. However, blood glucose levels usually fall back to normal after delivery.

There are two major types of diabetes:

- Type 1 is an abrupt end to insulin production, often before the age of 25. The pancreatic cells do not produce enough insulin. This is thought to be due to an autoimmune reaction. Treatment involves regular injections of insulin.
- Type 2 is a reduction in insulin production, often after the age of 40. Genetic factors and obesity play a role in the majority of the cases. Being overweight requires the pancreas to work harder to produce more insulin. Over time, the pancreatic cells secrete less insulin. Treatment includes diet, exercise, weight loss, and if necessary, oral hypoglycemics or insulin.

## Adrenal Gland

- Hypersecretion of cortisol results in obesity and puffy appearance due to changes in carbohydrate and protein breakdown.
- Hypersecretion of epinephrine and norepinephrine causes hypertension, hyperglycemia, nervousness, and sweating. Complete exhaustion occurs.
- Hypersecretion of aldosterone causes abnormal imbalance of electrolytes (sodium, potassium, calcium, magnesium).
- Hyposecretion of aldosterone and cortisol cause Addison disease. Weakness, tiredness, dark pigmentation, and hypotension result.

## 19.8  Look-Alike and Sound-Alike Words

*Below is a list of look-alike and sound-alike words. Study the spelling and definitions of each set of words. Questions will follow in the Review Exercises.*

### TABLE 19-2  Look-Alike and Sound-Alike Words

| | |
|---|---|
| hyper- | increase; excessive |
| hypo- | decrease; deficient |
| glycogenesis | production of glycogen |
| glucogenesis | production of glucose |
| hyperkalemia | excessive potassium in the blood |
| hypercalcemia | excessive calcium in the blood |
| polyuria | excessive urination |
| polyurea | a chemical substance used as a protective coating in severe environments |
| pancreas | a fish-like gland situated behind the stomach |
| pancrease | a drug used to replace enzyme function in the pancreas |

## 19.9 Review Exercises

### EXERCISE 19-1 Look-Alike and Sound-Alike Words

*Read the sentences carefully and circle the word in parentheses that correctly completes the meaning. Use Table 19-2 if it helps you.*

1. A tumor growing on the pituitary gland reducing hormone secretion is (**hyperpituitarism/hypopituitarism**).

2. The medical term for production of glucose is (**glycogenesis/glucogenesis/ glycolysis/glucolysis**).

3. Reduced levels of parathormone causes (**hypocalcemia/hypokalemia**).

4. A common symptom of diabetes mellitus is (**polyurea/polyuria**).

5. You can take a course in (**polyurea/polyuria**) coating.

6. The (**pancreas/pancrease**) is an organ that secretes digestive enzymes and hormones.

### EXERCISE 19-2 Matching Word Parts with Meaning

*Match the word part in Column A with its meaning in Column B.*

| | Column A | Column B |
|---|---|---|
| _____ | 1. home/o | A. male |
| _____ | 2. estr/o | B. sugar |
| _____ | 3. crin/o | C. female |
| _____ | 4. natr/o | D. sodium |
| _____ | 5. acr/o | E. thirst |
| _____ | 6. -tropic | F. potassium |
| _____ | 7. glyc/o | G. secrete |
| _____ | 8. kal/o | H. same |
| _____ | 9. andr/o | I. extremity |
| _____ | 10. -dipsia | J. nourishment |

## EXERCISE 19-3 Short Answers

*I. Match the hormone with its endocrine gland (listed immediately below). The glands can be used more than once.*

**a.** adrenal cortex

**b.** adrenal medulla

**c.** anterior pituitary

**d.** pancreas

**e.** posterior pituitary

**f.** thyroid

**1.** aldosterone _____

**2.** antidiuretic hormone _____

**3.** $T_3$ _____

**4.** cortisol _____

**5.** epinephrine _____

**6.** glucagon _____

**7.** follicle-stimulating hormone _____

**8.** insulin _____

**9.** prolactin _____

**10.** norepinephrine _____

*II. Match the hormone with its function (listed immediately below). One function can be used more than once.*

**a.** plays a key role in the body's response to stress

**b.** prevents excess loss of fluid

**c.** regulates blood calcium and phosphorus

**d.** regulates blood glucose levels

**e.** regulates metabolic rate

**f.** regulates sodium and potassium levels

**g.** stimulates the adrenal cortex

**h.** stimulates the development of the gonads

**i.** stimulates uterine contractions

**1.** adrenocorticotropic hormone

_____

**2.** oxytocin

_____

**3.** T$_4$

_____

**4.** parathormone

_____

**5.** aldosterone

_____

**6.** cortisol

_____

**7.** insulin

_____

**8.** glucagon

_____

**9.** antidiuretic hormone

_____

**10.** follicle-stimulating hormone

_____

## EXERCISE 19-4 Pathology

_I. Answer the following questions on diabetes mellitus._

**1.** Write one common symptom of diabetes mellitus.

_____

**2.** Why is glucose important to body cells?

_____

**3.** Define _ketones_.

_____

**4.** What is the cause of diabetes mellitus?

_____

**5.** Define *type 1 diabetes.*

_____

_____

**6.** Define *type 2 diabetes.*

_____

_____

*II. Select the correct answer and write it in the space provided.*

**1.** Hypersecretion of the growth hormone in children causes

_____.

   acromegaly     gigantism

**2.** Hyposecretion of ADH causes _____.

   diabetes mellitus     diabetes insipidus

**3.** Hypothyroidism in adults is _____.

   Graves disease     cretinism     myxedema

**4.** Hyperparathyroidism results in _____.

   fractures     tetany     hypocalciuria

**5.** Hypoinsulinism causes _____.

   diabetes mellitus     diabetes insipidus

**6.** A patient with a diagnosis of hypersecretion of cortisol exhibits

_____.

   darkened pigmentation     puffy appearance

## EXERCISE 19-5   Definitions

*Define the following terms:*

**1. tropic hormones** _____

**2. neurohormones** _____

**3. homeostasis** _____

**4. acromegaly** _____

**5. glycolysis** _____

   **6. euthyroid** _____

   **7. polydipsia** _____

   **8. glucogenesis** _____

   **9. estrogen** _____

**10. hyperkalemia** _____

## EXERCISE 19-6  Building Medical Words

*I. Using the suffix -emia, build the medical word meaning*

   **a.** excessive calcium in the blood _____

   **b.** excessive blood sugar _____

   **c.** decreased sodium in the blood _____

   **d.** excessive potassium in the blood _____

*II. Using the suffix -tropic, build the medical word meaning*

   **a.** stimulating the adrenal cortex _____

   **b.** stimulating the gonads _____

## EXERCISE 19-7  Definitions in Context

*Define the bolded terms in the spaces provided. Use your medical dictionary if necessary.*

   **1.** A 34-year-old was referred for **hyperthyroidism**. The patient was first found to
   be hyperthyroid one year ago. He has all the classic symptoms of **Graves disease**,
   including **goiter**, **exophthalmia**, and weakness.

   **a.** hyperthyroidism _____

   **b.** Graves disease _____

   **c.** goiter _____

   **d.** exophthalmia _____

   **2.** Three days after admission, the diagnosis of **adrenal insufficiency** was confirmed.
   Apparently, **hypopituitarism** was ruled out.

   **e.** adrenal insufficiency _____

   **f.** hypopituitarism _____

**3.** This elderly patient was admitted because of a slowly growing mass in the right lobe of his **thyroid**. A **thyroid scan** showed regions of a nonfunctioning thyroid. Thyroid function was within normal limits. **Biopsy** of the thyroid confirmed a **benign adenoma**.

**g.** thyroid _____

**h.** thyroid scan _____

**i.** biopsy _____

**j.** benign adenoma _____

### EXERCISE 19-8  Labeling

*Using the body structures listed below, label Figure 19-7. Write your answer on the numbered spaces provided below or, if you prefer, on the diagram.*

adrenal glands _____

hypothalamus _____

ovaries _____

pancreas _____

parathyroid gland _____

pineal gland _____

pituitary gland _____

testicles _____

thymus gland _____

thyroid gland _____

1. _____

2. _____

3. _____

4. _____

5. _____

6. _____

7. _____

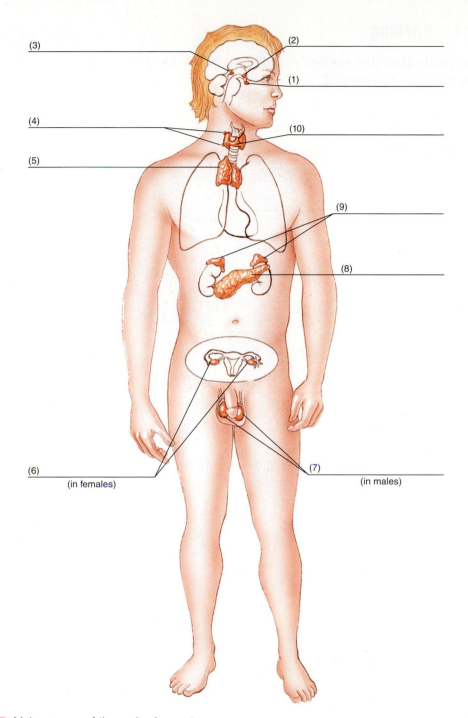

**Figure 19-7**  Major organs of the endocrine system.

8. _____

9. _____

10. _____

**EXERCISE 19-9  Spelling**

*Circle any words that are spelled incorrectly in the list below. Then correct the spelling in the space provided.*

1. antidiretic _____

2. lutienizing _____

3. aldosterone _____

4. pancrease _____

5. diabetis _____

6. cortisal _____

7. hypopituitarism _____

8. homeostasis _____

9. hyperkalemia _____

10. polydipsia _____

**EXERCISE 19-10  Abbreviations**

*Write the meaning of the following abbreviations on the space provided.*

1. ACTH _____

2. $T_3$ _____

3. ADH _____

4. $T_4$ _____

5. FSH _____

6. TSH _____

7. GH _____

8. STH _____

9. PRL _____

10. ICSH _____

11. PTH _____

12. LH _____

## Animations

Visit the companion website to view the videos on the **Endocrine System**; **Dual Role of the Pancreas**; and **Diabetic Retinopathy.**

## 19.10 Pronunciation and Spelling

*Listen, read, and study, so you can speak and write.*

**1.** Listen to each word on the audio file provided in the Student Companion Website.

**2.** Spell each word in the space provided.

| Word | Pronunciation | Spelling |
|------|---------------|----------|
| acromegaly | **ack**-roh-**MEG**-ah-lee | |
| adrenocorticotropic hormone | ah-**dree**-noh-**kor**-tih-koh-**TROH**-pick | |
| aldosterone | al-**DOS**-ter-ohn | |
| androgen | **AN**-droh-jen | |
| antidiuretic | **an**-tih-dye-yoo-**RET**-ick | |
| cortisol | **KOR**-tih-sol | |
| endocrine | **EN**-doh-krin | |
| endocrinologist | **en**-doh-krih-**NOL**-oh-jist | |
| estrogen | **ESS**-troh-jen | |
| euthyroid | yoo-**THIGH**-royd | |
| glucagon | **GLOO**-kah-gon | |
| glycolysis | glye-**KOL**-ih-sis | |
| homeostasis | **hoh**-mee-oh-**STAY**-sis | |
| hormones | **HOR**-mohnz | |
| hypercalcemia | **high**-per-kal-**SEE**-mee-ah | |
| hyperglycemia | **high**-per-glye-**SEE**-mee-ah | |
| hyperkalemia | **high**-per-kah-**LEE**-mee-ah | |
| hyperthyroidism | **high**-per-**THIGH**-royd-izm | |
| hyponatremia | **high**-poh-nah-**TREE**-mee-ah | |

| Word | Pronunciation | Spelling |
|---|---|---|
| hypopituitarism | **high**-poh-pih-**TOO**-ih-tar-izm | |
| hypothalamus | **high**-poh-**THAL**-ah-mus | |
| insulin | **IN**-suh-lin | |
| isthmus | **ISS**-mus | |
| oxytocin | **ock**-see-**TOH**-sin | |
| pancreas | **PAN**-kree-as | |
| panhypopituitarism | pan-**high**-poh-pih-**TOO**-ih-tar-izm | |
| parathyroid | **par**-ah-**THIGH**-roydz | |
| pineal | **PIN**-ee-al | |
| pituitary | pih-**TOO**-ih-**tar**-ee | |
| polydipsia | **pol**-ee-**DIP**-see-ah | |
| polyuria | **pol**-ee-**YOO**-ree-ah | |
| thymus | **THIGH**-mus | |
| thyroid | **THIGH**-royd | |
| thyroxine | thigh-**ROCK**-sin | |
| triiodothyronine | trigh-**eye**-oh-doh-**THIGH**-roh-**nen** | |

# APPENDIX A

# Pronunciations

It is very important that you know how to pronounce the medical terms you learn. If you cannot pronounce a term, it will be difficult for you to remember how to spell it, and accurate spelling is very important. However, the proper pronunciation of a medical term is not always obvious. Therefore, all difficult terms in the first appearance are followed by a common pronunciation.

The system of pronunciation used is quite simple. Each term is re-spelled using combinations of letters that are commonly known to have a particular sound. For instance when *tion* appears in a word, the pronunciation will be written *shun*. The long "u" sound is made with *yoo*. So the word "cute" would be written as *kyoot*. Long "i," as in the word "hi," is usually written as *eye*. However, that is confusing in some words, and so sometimes the letters *ey* or *igh* are used instead. The goal is to provide an easy guide to pronunciation that fits the particular word. Further examples are listed in Table A-1.

The syllables in the pronunciations are separated by hyphens (-). The most strongly emphasized syllable is written bold type with capital letters (e.g., **BOLD**). Any syllable with secondary emphasis is written in bold but without capitals (e.g., **bold**). To help you put this all together, here are a few examples.

### TABLE A-1 Pronunciation of Medical Terms

| | |
|---|---|
| **a** in *at* = **ah** | |
| **a** in *rain* = **ay** | |
| **e** in *pet* = **eh** | |
| **e** in *meet* = **ee** | |
| **i** in *skin* = **ih** | |
| **i** in *pie* = **eye, ey,** or **igh** | |
| **o** in *of* = **uh** | |
| **o** in *boat* = **oh** | |
| **o** in *boot* = **oo** | |
| **u** in *under* = **uh** | |
| **u** in *cute* = **yoo** | |
| **tion** = **shun** | |

# APPENDIX B

# Plurals

Plurals are formed in various ways, depending on which letters are at the end of a term. Following are examples of how to change a specific singular ending to its plural form.

To form the plural of singular terms ending in *is*, change the *i* to an *e*, as shown in the following examples:

| SINGULAR | PLURAL |
|---|---|
| diagnosis<br>(dye-ag-**NOH**-sis) | diagnoses<br>(dye-ag-**NOH**-seez) |
| pelvis<br>(**PEL**-vis) | pelves<br>(**PEL**-veez) |
| neurosis<br>(noo-**ROH**-sis) | neuroses<br>(noo-**ROH**-seez) |

To form the plural of many singular words ending in *us*, change the *us* to an *i*, as shown in the following examples:

| SINGULAR | PLURAL |
|---|---|
| bronchus<br>(**BRONG**-kus) | bronchi<br>(**BRONG**-kye) |
| bacillus<br>(bah-**SILL**-us) | bacilli<br>(bah-**SILL**-eye) |
| calculus<br>(**KAL**-kyoo-lus) | calculi<br>(**KAL**-kyoo-lye) |
| embolus<br>(**EM**-boh-lus) | emboli<br>(**EM**-boh-lye) |

There are a few exceptions. For example, the plural of *virus* (**VYE**-rus) is *viruses* (**VYE**-rus-ez), and the plural of *sinus* (**SIGH**-nus) is *sinuses* (**SIGH**-nus-ez).

The plural of singular words ending in *a* is formed by adding an *e* to the word, as shown in the following examples. Modifiers in Latin must agree with the noun. For example, the plural of *vena cava* is *venae cavae*.

| SINGULAR | PLURAL |
|---|---|
| sclera<br>(**SKLEHR**-ah) | sclerae<br>(**SKLEHR**-ee) |
| scapula<br>(**SKAP**-yoo-lah) | scapulae<br>(**SKAP**-yoo-lee) |
| vena cava<br>(**VEE**-nah **CAV**-ah) | venae cavae<br>(**VEE**-nee **CAV**-ee) |

Singular terms ending in *um* are pluralized by changing the *um* to an *a*, as shown in the following examples:

| SINGULAR | PLURAL |
|---|---|
| acetabulum<br>(ass-eh-**TAB**-yoo-lum) | acetabula<br>(ass-eh-**TAB**-yoo-lah) |
| capitulum<br>(kah-**PIT**-yoo-lum) | capitula<br>(kah-**PIT**-yoo-lah) |
| septum<br>(**SEP**-tum) | septa<br>(**SEP**-tah) |
| diverticulum<br>(dye-ver-**TICK**-yoo-lum) | diverticula<br>(dye-ver-**TICK**-yoo-lah) |

To form the plural of singular words ending in *ix* or *ex*, change the *ix* or *ex* to *ices*, as shown in the following examples:

| SINGULAR | PLURAL |
|---|---|
| calix<br>(**KAY**-licks) | calices<br>(**KAY**-lih-seez) |
| cervix<br>(**SER**-vicks) | cervices<br>(**SER**-vih-seez) |
| index<br>(**IN**-decks) | indices<br>(**IN**-dih-seez) |
| varix<br>(**VAR**-icks) | varices<br>(**VAR**-ih-seez) |

Singular words ending in *oma* are made plural by the addition of *ta* or *s*, as shown in the following examples:

| SINGULAR | PLURAL |
|---|---|
| adenoma<br>(ad-eh-**NOH**-mah) | adenomata<br>(ad-eh-no-**MAT**-ah)<br><br>or<br><br>adenomas<br>(ad-eh-**NOH**-mahz) |
| carcinoma<br>(kar-sih-**NOH**-mah) | carcinomata<br>(kar-sin-oh-**MAT**-ah)<br><br>or<br><br>carcinomas<br>(kar-sin-**OH**-mahz) |
| fibroma<br>(figh-**BROH**-mah) | fibromata<br>(figh-broh-**MAT**-ah)<br><br>or<br><br>fibromas<br>(figh-**BROH**-mahz) |

To form the plural of singular words ending in *nx*, change the *x* to *g* and add *es*, as shown in the following examples:

| SINGULAR | PLURAL |
|---|---|
| larynx<br>(**LAR**-inks) | larynges<br>(**LAR**-in-jeez) |
| phalanx<br>(**FAH**-lanks) | phalanges<br>(fah-**LAN**-jeez) |

To form the plural of singular words ending in *on*, change the *on* to an *a* or simply add an *s,* as shown in the following example:

| SINGULAR | PLURAL |
|---|---|
| ganglion<br>(**GANG**-glee-on) | ganglia<br>(**GANG**-glee-ah)<br><br>or<br><br>ganglions<br>(**GANG**-glee-onz) |

To form the plural of singular words ending in *ax*, change the *ax* to *aces*, as shown in the following example:

| SINGULAR | PLURAL |
|---|---|
| **thorax** (**THOR**-acks) | **thoraces** (**THOR**-ah-sees) |

# APPENDIX C

# Word Part to Definition

| WORD PART | DEFINITION | WORD PART | DEFINITION |
|-----------|------------|-----------|------------|
| **A** | | **an/o** | anus |
| **a(n)-** | inadequate; no; not; lack of | **ana-** | apart; up |
| **ab-** | away from | **andr/o** | male; man |
| **abdomin/o** | abdomen | **angi/o** | vessel |
| **-ac** | pertaining to | **anis/o** | unequal size |
| **acetabul/o** | acetabulum; hip socket | **ankyl/o** | fusion of parts; stiffening; bent; crooked |
| **acr/o** | extremity; top | **ante-** | before |
| **acromi/o** | acromion | **anter/o** | front |
| **ad-** | toward | **anti-** | against |
| **aden/o** | gland | **aort/o** | aorta |
| **adenoid/o** | adenoids | **append/o** | appendix |
| **adip/o** | fat | **aque/o** | water |
| **adren/o** | adrenal gland | **-ar** | pertaining to |
| **adrenal/o** | adrenal gland | **-arche** | beginning |
| **aer/o** | air | **arteri/o** | artery |
| **against** | contra- | **arthr/o** | joint |
| **-aise** | ease | **articul/o** | joint |
| **-al** | pertaining to | **-ary** | pertaining to |
| **albin/o** | white | **-assay** | analysis of a mixture to identify its contents |
| **albumin/o** | albumin (a blood protein) | **-asthenia** | no strength |
| **-algia** | pain | **atel/o** | incomplete; imperfect |
| **all/o** | referring to another | **ather/o** | fatty debris; fatty plaque |
| **alveol/o** | air sacs; alveolus | **atri/o** | atrium (upper chambers of the heart) |
| **ambly/o** | dull; dim | **audi/o** | hearing |
| **ametr/o** | out of proportion | **audit/o** | hearing |
| **amni/o** | amnion; sac in which the fetus lies in the uterus | **aur/o** | ear |
| **-an** | pertaining to | | |

| WORD PART | DEFINITION |
|---|---|
| auto- | self |
| axill/o | armpit |

## B

| WORD PART | DEFINITION |
|---|---|
| bacteri/o | bacteria |
| balan/o | glans penis |
| bil/i | bile |
| bilirubin/o | bilirubin (a bile pigment) |
| bi/o | life |
| -blast | immature; growing thing |
| blephar/o | eyelid |
| brachi/o | arm |
| brady- | slow |
| bronch/o | bronchus |
| bronchi/o | bronchus |
| bronchiol/o | bronchioles; small bronchi |
| bucc/o | cheek |
| burs/o | bursa (sac filled with synovial fluid located around joints) |

## C

| WORD PART | DEFINITION |
|---|---|
| cac/o | bad |
| calc/o | calcium |
| calcane/o | heel |
| calic/o; calyc/o | calix/calyx |
| -capnia | carbon dioxide |
| capsul/o | capsule |
| carcin/o | cancer; cancerous |
| cardi/o | heart |
| carp/o | wrist |
| cartilagin/o | cartilage |
| catheter/o | something inserted |
| caud/o | tail |
| caus/o | burning |
| cec/o | cecum |
| -cele | hernia (protrusion or displacement of an organ from the structure that normally contains it) |
| cellul/o | cell |

| WORD PART | DEFINITION |
|---|---|
| -centesis | surgical puncture to remove fluid |
| cephal/o | head |
| cerebell/o | cerebellum |
| cerebr/o | brain |
| cervic/o | cervix; neck; neck of uterus; cervix uteri |
| -chalasia | relaxation |
| cheil/o | lips |
| chem/o | drug |
| chol/e | bile; gall |
| cholangi/o | bile ducts |
| cholecyst/o | gallbladder |
| choledoch/o | common bile duct |
| cholesterol/o | cholesterol |
| chondr/o | cartilage |
| chori/o | choroid |
| chrom/o | color |
| -cidal | to kill |
| cili/o | hair |
| cis/o | to cut |
| -clasis | surgical fracture or refracture |
| -clast | breakdown |
| clavicul/o | clavicle; collarbone |
| -cle | small |
| -clonus | turmoil; violent action |
| -clysis | washing; irrigation |
| coagulati/o | to condense; to clot |
| -coccus | berry-shaped |
| coccyg/o | coccyx; tailbone |
| cochle/o | cochlea |
| col/o | colon; large intestine |
| colon/o | colon |
| colp/o | vagina |
| coni/o | dust |
| conjunctiv/o | conjunctiva |
| constrict/o | to draw together |
| -continence | to stop |
| contra- | against |

| WORD PART | DEFINITION |
|-----------|------------|
| -conus | cone-shaped |
| core/o | pupil |
| corne/o | cornea |
| coron/o | crown |
| corpor/o | body |
| cortic/o | cortex; outer covering; outer layer |
| cost/o | rib |
| crani/o | skull |
| crin/o | to secrete |
| -crine | to secrete |
| -crit | separate |
| cry/o | cold |
| crypt/o | hidden |
| culd/o | cul-de-sac |
| -cusis | hearing |
| cutane/o | skin |
| cyan/o | blue |
| cycl/o | ciliary body |
| -cyesis | pregnancy |
| cyst/o | bladder; sac |
| cyt/o | cell |
| -cyte | cell |
| -cytosis | slight increase in the number of cells; condition of cells |

## D

| WORD PART | DEFINITION |
|-----------|------------|
| dacry/o | tears; lacrimal duct |
| de- | lack of; removal |
| dent/o | tooth |
| derm/o | skin |
| -derma | skin |
| dermat/o | skin |
| -dermis | skin |
| -desis | surgical binding; surgical fusion |
| di- | two |
| dia- | complete; through |
| diaphor/e | profuse sweating |

| WORD PART | DEFINITION |
|-----------|------------|
| dilat/o | dilation; dilatation; to expand; widen |
| dipl/o | double |
| -dipsia | thirst |
| don/o | donate |
| dors/o | back |
| dorsi- | back |
| -drome | to run |
| duct/o | to draw |
| duoden/o | duodenum (proximal portion of small intestine) |
| dur/o | dura mater (outermost membrane surrounding the brain) |
| -dynia | pain |
| dys- | bad; difficult; painful; poor |

## E

| WORD PART | DEFINITION |
|-----------|------------|
| e- | out; outside; outward; without |
| -eal | pertaining to |
| -ear | pertaining to |
| ec- | out |
| ech/o | sound |
| -ectasis | dilation; dilatation; stretching |
| -ectomy | excision; surgical removal |
| -edema | accumulation of fluid; swelling |
| electr/o | electric |
| -emesis | vomit; vomiting |
| -emia | blood condition |
| emmetr/o | in proper measure |
| en- | inward |
| encephal/o | brain |
| endo- | with; within |
| enter/o | small intestine |
| epi- | above; on; upon |
| epididym/o | epididymis |
| episi/o | vulva; external genitalia; pudendum |

| WORD PART | DEFINITION |
|---|---|
| epitheli/o | covering |
| -er | specialist; one who specializes; specialist in the study of |
| erythemat/o | red |
| erythem/o | red |
| erythr/o | red |
| eso- | inward |
| esophag/o | esophagus |
| -esthesia | sensation |
| estr/o | female |
| ethm/o | ethmoid bone; sieve |
| eu- | normal; good |
| ex- | out; outside; outward |
| exo- | out; outside; outward |
| extra- | out; outside; outward |

## F

| WORD PART | DEFINITION |
|---|---|
| faci/o | face |
| fasci/o | fascia |
| femor/o | femur; thigh bone |
| fibr/o | fibers; fibrous tissue |
| fibul/o | fibula |
| flex/o | bend |
| -flux | flow |
| front/o | frontal bone |

## G

| WORD PART | DEFINITION |
|---|---|
| galact/o | milk |
| gastr/o | stomach |
| -gen | producing; produced by |
| -genesis | production; formation; development |
| -genic | producing; produced by |
| -genous | produced by |
| gingiv/o | gums |
| glen/o | socket; pit; glenoid cavity |
| gli/o | glue |
| glomerul/o | glomerulus |
| gloss/o | tongue |

| WORD PART | DEFINITION |
|---|---|
| gluc/o | sugar |
| glyc/o | sugar |
| glycogen/o | glycogen (storage form of sugar) |
| -gnosis | knowledge |
| gonad/o | gonads; sex glands |
| goni/o | angle (especially of the anterior chamber) |
| -grade | to step; to go |
| -gram | record; writing |
| granul/o | granules |
| -graph | instrument used to record |
| -graphy | process of recording; producing images |
| -gravida | pregnancy |
| gynec/o | female; woman |

## H

| WORD PART | DEFINITION |
|---|---|
| hem/o | blood |
| hemat/o | blood |
| hemi- | half |
| hepat/o | liver |
| herni/o | hernia |
| -hexia | habit |
| hiat/o | hiatus, opening |
| hidr/o | sweat |
| hist/o | tissue |
| histi/o | tissue |
| home/o | same; constant |
| humer/o | humerus; upper arm |
| hydr/o | water |
| hyper- | abnormal increase; above; above normal; excessive |
| hypo- | abnormal decrease; below; below normal; under |
| hyster/o | uterus |

## I

| WORD PART | DEFINITION |
|---|---|
| -ia | condition; state of |
| -iasis | abnormal condition; process |

| WORD PART | DEFINITION |
|---|---|
| iatr/o | physician |
| -ic | pertaining to |
| -ician | specialist; one who specializes; expert |
| idi/o | one's own; distinct; individual |
| ile/o | ileum (distal portion of the small intestine) |
| ili/o | hip |
| -immune | immunity; safe |
| immun/o | immunity; safe |
| in- | no; not; in; into |
| -ine | pertaining to |
| infer/o | below; downward |
| infra- | below; under |
| inguin/o | groin |
| insulin/o | insulin |
| inter- | between |
| intestin/o | intestine |
| intra- | within |
| -ion | process |
| -ior | pertaining to |
| ir/o | iris |
| irid/o | iris |
| is/o | equal |
| isch/o | hold back |
| ischi/o | ischium (posterior portion of the hip bone) |
| -ism | condition; process; state of |
| -ist | specialist; one who specializes; specialist in the study of |
| -itis | inflammation (the redness, swelling, heat, and pain that occur when the body protects itself from injury) |
| -ium | structure |

**J**

| WORD PART | DEFINITION |
|---|---|
| jejun/o | jejunum (medial portion of small intestine) |

**K**

| WORD PART | DEFINITION |
|---|---|
| kal/o | potassium |
| kerat/o | cornea; hard; horn-like |
| keratin/o | hard; horn-like |
| -kines | movement |
| kinesi/o | movement |
| -kinesia | movement; motion |
| -kinesis | movement; motion |
| kyph/o | humpback |

**L**

| WORD PART | DEFINITION |
|---|---|
| labi/o | lip |
| labyrinth/o | inner ear; labyrinth |
| lacrim/o | lacrimal apparatus; tears |
| lact/o | milk |
| lapar/o | abdominal wall; abdomen |
| later/o | side |
| laryng/o | larynx; voice box |
| lei/o | smooth |
| -lepsy | seizure |
| leuk/o | white |
| ligati/o | binding; tying |
| lingu/o | tongue |
| lip/o | fat |
| lipid/o | fat |
| -listhesis | slipping |
| -lith | calculus; stone |
| lith/o | stone |
| lob/o | lobe |
| -logist | specialist; one who specializes; specialist in the study of |
| -logy | study of; process of study |
| lord/o | swayback |
| lumb/o | lower back; loins |
| -luxation | dislocation |
| lymph/o | lymph (clear, watery fluid) |
| lymphaden/o | lymph glands; lymph nodes |

| WORD PART | DEFINITION |
|-----------|------------|
| lymphangi/o | lymph vessels |
| -lysis | breakdown; destruction; separate; separation |
| -lytic | pertaining to destruction, separation, or breakdown |

## M

| WORD PART | DEFINITION |
|-----------|------------|
| magnet/o | magnet |
| -malacia | softening |
| malleol/o | malleolus (bony projection on the distal aspects of the tibia and fibula) |
| mamm/o | breast |
| mandibul/o | mandible; lower jaw |
| mast/o | breast |
| maxill/o | maxilla; upper jaw |
| meat/o | meatus |
| medi/o | middle |
| medull/o | marrow; medulla; inner portion of an organ |
| megal/o | large |
| -megaly | enlargement |
| melan/o | black |
| men/o | menses; menstruation; month |
| ment/o | mind |
| mening/o | membrane; meninges |
| meso- | middle |
| meta- | beyond |
| metacarp/o | metacarpals (bones of the hand) |
| metatars/o | metatarsals (bones of the foot) |
| -meter | instrument used to measure |
| metr/o | uterus |
| -metrist | one who measures |
| -metry | process of measuring; to measure; measurement |
| mi/o | contraction; less |
| mono- | one |
| -mortem | death |

| WORD PART | DEFINITION |
|-----------|------------|
| muc/o | mucus (a bodily secretion, of the mucous membrane, sometimes sticky and frequently thick) |
| multi- | multiple |
| muscul/o | muscle |
| my/o | muscle |
| myc/o | fungus |
| mydri/o | dilation; dilatation; wide |
| -myein | to shut |
| myel/o | bone marrow; spinal cord |
| myelin/o | myelin sheath |
| myos/o | muscle |
| myring/o | tympanic membrane; eardrum |

## N

| WORD PART | DEFINITION |
|-----------|------------|
| narc/o | stupor |
| nas/o | nose |
| nat/o | birth |
| natr/o | sodium |
| necr/o | death |
| neo- | new |
| nephr/o | kidney |
| neur/o | nerve |
| noct/o | night |
| norm/o | normal |
| nulli- | none |
| nyct/o | night |

## O

| WORD PART | DEFINITION |
|-----------|------------|
| o/o | egg |
| occipit/o | occiput (back part of the head) |
| ocul/o | eye |
| odont/o | teeth; tooth |
| -oid | resembling |
| -ole | small |
| olecran/o | elbow; olecranon |

| WORD PART | DEFINITION | WORD PART | DEFINITION |
|---|---|---|---|
| oligo- | deficient; few; scanty | path/o | disease |
| -oma | mass; tumor | -pathy | disease |
| onych/o | nail | -pause | stoppage; cessation |
| oophor/o | ovary | pector/o | chest |
| ophthalm/o | eye | pedicul/o | lice |
| -opia | visual condition; vision | ped/o | child |
| -opsia | visual condition; vision | pelv/i | pelvis |
| -opsy | to view | pelv/o | pelvis |
| -opt/o | vision; sight | -penia | decrease; deficiency |
| -or | one who; person or thing that does something | -pepsia | digestion |
| | | peri- | around |
| or/o | mouth | perine/o | perineum |
| orchi/o | testicle; testis | peritone/o | peritoneum |
| orchid/o | testicle; testis | -pexy | surgical fixation |
| orex/i | appetite | phac/o | lens |
| ortho- | straight | -phagia | swallow; to eat |
| -ory | pertaining to | phalang/o | phalanx (one of three bones making up each finger or toe) |
| -ose | pertaining to | | |
| -osis | abnormal condition | phall/o | penis |
| oste/o | bone | pharmac/o | drug |
| ot/o | ear | pharyng/o | pharynx; throat |
| -ous | pertaining to | -phasia | speech |
| ov/o | egg | phleb/o | vein |
| ovari/o | ovary | -phobia | fear; irrational fear |
| ox/o | oxygen | -phonia | voice |
| oxy- | quick; sharp | -phoresis | transmission; carry |
| | | phot/o | light |
| | | phren/o | diaphragm |
| **P** | | physi/o | nature |
| | | -physis | to grow |
| palpebr/o | eyelid | pil/o | hair |
| pan- | all | pine/o | pineal gland |
| pancreat/o | pancreas | pituitar/o | pituitary gland |
| papill/o | nipple-like; optic disc | -plakia | patches |
| para- | abnormal; beside; near | -plasia | development; formation |
| -para | give birth; part with child | -plasm | development; formation |
| parathyroid/o | parathyroid gland | -plasty | surgical repair or reconstruction |
| pariet/o | parietal bone; wall | | |
| -partum | labor; delivery; childbirth | | |
| patell/o | patella; kneecap | | |

| WORD PART | DEFINITION | WORD PART | DEFINITION |
|-----------|-----------|-----------|-----------|
| -plegia | paralysis (loss or impairment of motor function) | **Q** | |
| pleur/o | pleura; pleural cavity | quadri- | four |
| -pnea | breathing | **R** | |
| pneum/o | air; respiration; lungs | radi/o | x-ray; radius (one of the bones of the lower arm) |
| pneumat/o | air; respiration; lungs | radicul/o | nerve roots |
| pneumon/o | lungs | ras/o | scrape |
| -poiesis | production; manufacture; formation | re- | back |
| -poietin | a hormone that stimulates the production of blood cells | rect/o | rectum |
| | | ren/o | kidney |
| poikil/o | variation; irregular | reticul/o | network |
| poli/o | gray matter | retin/o | retina |
| poly- | many | retro- | backward; back; behind |
| -porosis | porous | rhabd/o | rod-shaped; striped; striated |
| post- | after | | |
| poster/o | back | rhin/o | nose |
| -potence | power | rhythm/o | rhythm |
| practition/o | practice | -rrhage | bursting forth |
| -prandial | meal | -rrhagia | bursting forth |
| presby- | old age | -rrhaphy | suture; sew |
| primi- | first | -rrhea | flow; discharge |
| pro- | before | -rrhexis | rupture |
| proct/o | rectum | | |
| pronati/o | pronation | **S** | |
| prostat/o | prostate; prostate gland | sacr/o | sacrum |
| proxim/o | near; close | salping/o | eustachian tube; fallopian tubes; uterine tubes |
| pseudo- | false | | |
| -ptosis | downward displacement; drooping; falling; prolapse; sagging | -salpinx | fallopian tubes; uterine tubes |
| | | sarc/o | flesh |
| -ptysis | spitting | -sarcoma | malignant tumor of connective tissue |
| pub/o | pubis (portion of the hip bone) | | |
| pulmon/o | lungs | scapul/o | scapula |
| pupill/o | pupil | -schisis | cleft; splitting |
| py/o | pus | scint/i | spark |
| pyel/o | renal pelvis (upper dilated portion of the ureter) | scler/o | hardening |
| | | -sclerosis | hardening |
| pylor/o | pylorus (distal portion of the stomach); pyloric sphincter | scoli/o | curved; crooked |

| WORD PART | DEFINITION |
|---|---|
| -scope | instrument used to visually examine (a body cavity or organ) |
| -scopy | process of visually examining (a body cavity or organ) |
| seb/o | sebum |
| sect/o | to cut |
| secundi- | second |
| semi- | half |
| septic/o | infection |
| sial/o | saliva |
| sialaden/o | salivary glands |
| sigmoid/o | sigmoid colon |
| sinus/o | sinuses |
| -sis | condition; state of |
| skelet/o | skeleton |
| somat/o | body |
| son/o | sound |
| -spadias | opening; split |
| -spasm | sudden, involuntary contraction |
| sperm/o | spermatozoa; sperm; seminal fluid |
| spermat/o | spermatozoa; sperm |
| sphen/o | sphenoid bone; wedge |
| spin/o | backbone; spine; spinal column; vertebral column |
| spir/o | breathing |
| splen/o | spleen |
| spondyl/o | vertebra; backbone; spinal column; spine |
| -sphyxia | pulse |
| staped/o | stapes |
| staphyl/o | resembling a bunch of grapes |
| -stasis | stable; stoppage; stopping; controlling |
| steat/o | fat |
| -stenosis | narrowing; stricture |
| stern/o | sternum; breastbone |

| WORD PART | DEFINITION |
|---|---|
| steth/o | chest |
| -stitial | to place |
| stom/o | mouth |
| strept/o | twisted |
| stomat/o | mouth |
| -stomy | new opening |
| sub- | under |
| super/o | above; toward the head |
| supra- | above; beyond; excessive |
| sym- | together; with |
| synovi/o | synovium; synovial membrane |

**T**

| WORD PART | DEFINITION |
|---|---|
| tachy- | fast |
| -taxia | order |
| tele- | distant |
| tempor/o | temporal bone |
| ten/o | tendon |
| tend/o | tendon |
| tendin/o | tendon |
| tenosynovi/o | tendon sheath (covering of a tendon) |
| tens/o | stretch |
| tensi/o | tension |
| test/o | testicle; testis |
| testicul/o | testicle; testis |
| tetra- | four |
| thalam/o | thalamus |
| thel/o | nipple |
| -therapy | treatment |
| -thermy | heat |
| thorac/o | chest; thorax |
| -thorax | chest |
| thromb/o | clot |
| thym/o | thymus gland |
| thyr/o | thyroid gland; shield |
| thyroid/o | thyroid gland; shield |
| tibi/o | tibia; shin |

| WORD PART | DEFINITION | WORD PART | DEFINITION |
|---|---|---|---|
| -tic | pertaining to | -uria | urine; urination |
| -tocia | labor | urin/o | urine |
| -tocin | labor | ur/o | urinary tract; urine; urination |
| tom/o | to cut | -us | condition; thing |
| -tome | instrument used to cut | uter/o | uterus |
| -tomy | to cut; incise; process of cutting; incision | uve/o | uvea (includes the choroid, ciliary body, and iris) |
| ton/o | tension | | |
| tonsill/o | tonsils | **V** | |
| top/o | place | vagin/o | vagina |
| tox/o | poison | valvul/o | valve |
| trabecul/o | trabecula (strands of connective tissue) | varic/o | varicose vein; dilated, twisted vein |
| trache/o | trachea; windpipe | vas/o | vas deferens; vessel |
| trans- | across | vascul/o | vessel |
| trigon/o | trigone | ven/o | vein |
| -tripsy | crushing | ventr/o | front |
| -trophy | nourishment; growth | ventricul/o | ventricle (lower chambers of the heart) |
| -tropia | turning | | |
| -tropic; -trophic | nourish; stimulate | versi/o | turning; tilting; tipping |
| -tropion | turning | vertebr/o | vertebra |
| tub/o | fallopian tube | vesic/o | bladder |
| tympan/o | tympanic membrane; eardrum | viscer/o | internal organs |
| | | vitre/o | glasslike; gel-like |
| **U** | | vulv/o | vulva; external genitalia; pudendum |
| -ule | small | | |
| uln/o | ulna (one of the bones of the lower arm) | **X** | |
| ultra- | excess; beyond | xer/o | dry |
| -um | structure | xiph/o | sword |
| ungu/o | nail | **Y** | |
| ure/o | urea (end product of protein break down) | -y | process; condition |
| ureter/o | ureters | **Z** | |
| urethr/o | urethra | zygomat/o | cheekbone |

# APPENDIX D

# Definition to Word Part

| DEFINITION | WORD PART | DEFINITION | WORD PART |
|------------|-----------|------------|-----------|
| **A** | | angle (especially of the anterior chamber) | **goni/o** |
| abdomen | **abdomin/o; lapar/o** | anus | **an/o** |
| abdominal wall | **lapar/o** | aorta | **aort/o** |
| abnormal | **para-** | apart | **ana-** |
| abnormal condition | **-iasis; -osis** | appendix | **append/o** |
| abnormal increase | **hyper-** | appetite | **orex/i** |
| above | **epi-; hyper-; super/o; supra-** | arm | **brachi/o** |
| | | armpit | **axill/o** |
| accumulation of a fluid | **-edema** | around | **circum-; peri-** |
| | | artery | **arteri/o** |
| acetabulum | **acetabul/o** | aspiration | **-centesis** |
| acromion | **acromi/o** | atrium | **atri/o** |
| across | **trans-** | away from | **ab-** |
| adenoids | **adenoid/o** | | |
| adrenal gland | **adren/o; adrenal/o** | **B** | |
| after | **post-** | back | **dorsi-; dors/o; poster/o; re-; retro-** |
| against | **anti-; contra-** | | |
| air | **aer/o; pneum/o; pneumat/o** | back part of the head (occiput) | **occipit/o** |
| air sacs | **alveol/o** | backbone | **spin/o** |
| albumin (a blood protein) | **albumin/o** | backward | **retro-** |
| all | **pan-** | bacteria | **bacteri/o** |
| alveolus | **alveol/o** | bad | **dys-; cac/o** |
| amnion | **amni/o** | bear (to) | **-para** |
| analysis of a mixture to identify its contents | **-assay** | before | **ante-; pro-** |
| | | beginning | **-arche** |

511

| DEFINITION | WORD PART | DEFINITION | WORD PART |
|---|---|---|---|
| behind | **retro-** | **C** | |
| below | **hypo-; infer/o; infra-;** | calcium | **calci/o; calc/o** |
| | **sub-** | calculus | **-lith** |
| | | calix; calyx | **calic/o; calyc/o** |
| below normal | **hypo-** | cancer | **carcin/o** |
| bend | **flex/o** | cancerous | **carcin/o** |
| bent | **ankyl/o** | capsule | **capsul/o** |
| berry-shaped | **-coccus** | carbon dioxide | **-capnia** |
| beside | **para-** | carry | **-phoresis** |
| between | **inter-** | cartilage | **cartilagin/o;** |
| beyond | **meta-; supra-; ultra-** | | **chondr/o** |
| | | cecum | **cec/o** |
| bile | **bil/i; chol/e** | cell | **cellul/o; cyt/o;** |
| bile vessel | **cholangi/o** | | **-cyte** |
| bilirubin (a bile pigment) | **bilirubin/o** | cerebellum | **cerebell/o** |
| binding | **ligati/o** | cervix | **cervic/o** |
| birth | **nat/o** | cervix uteri | **cervic/o** |
| black | **melan/o** | cessation | **-pause** |
| bladder | **cyst/o; vesic/o** | cheek | **bucc/o** |
| blood | **hem/o; hemat/o** | cheekbone | **zygomat/o** |
| blood condition | **-emia** | chest | **pector/o; steth/o;** |
| blue | **cyan/o** | | **thorac/o;** |
| body | **corpor/o; somat/o** | | **-thorax** |
| | | child | **ped/o** |
| bone | **osse/o; oste/o** | childbirth | **-partum** |
| bone marrow | **myel/o** | cholesterol | **cholesterol/o** |
| bony projection on the distal aspects of the tibia and fibula | **malleol/o** | choroid | **chori/o** |
| | | ciliary body | **cycl/o** |
| brain | **cerebr/o; encephal/o** | clavicle | **clavicul/o** |
| | | clear, watery fluid | **lymph/o** |
| breakdown | **-clast; -lysis** | cleft | **-schisis** |
| breast | **mamm/o; mast/o** | close | **proxim/o** |
| breastbone | **stern/o** | clot | **thromb/o** |
| breathing | **-pnea; spir/o** | clot (to) | **coagulati/o** |
| bronchioles | **bronchiol/o** | coccyx | **coccyg/o** |
| bronchus | **bronchi/o; bronch/o** | cochlea | **cochle/o** |
| | | cold | **cry/o** |
| burning | **caus/o** | collarbone | **clavicul/o** |
| bursa | **burs/o** | colon | **col/o; colon/o** |
| bursting forth | **-rrhage; -rrhagia** | | |

| DEFINITION | WORD PART | DEFINITION | WORD PART |
|---|---|---|---|
| color | **chrom/o** | discharge | **-rrhea** |
| common bile duct | **choledoch/o** | disease | **path/o;** |
| complete | **dia-** | | **-pathy** |
| condense (to) | **coagulati/o** | dislocation | **-luxation** |
| condition | **-ia; -ism; -sis** | displacement | **-cele** |
| condition of cells | **-cytosis** | distant | **tele-** |
| cone-shaped | **-conus** | distinct | **idi/o** |
| constant | **home/o** | donates | **don/o** |
| contraction | **mi/o** | double | **dipl/o** |
| controlling | **-stasis** | downward | **infer/o** |
| cornea | **corne/o; kerat/o** | downward displacement | **-ptosis** |
| cortex | **cortic/o** | draw (to) | **duct/o** |
| covering | **epitheli/o** | draw together (to) | **constrict/o** |
| covering of a tendon | **tenosynovi/o** | drooping | **-ptosis** |
| crooked | **ankyl/o; scoli/o** | drug | **pharmac/o;** |
| crown | **coron/o** | | **chem/o** |
| crushing | **-tripsy** | dry | **xer/o** |
| cul-de-sac | **culd/o** | dull | **ambly/o** |
| curved | **scoli/o** | duodenum (proximal portion of small intestine) | **duoden/o** |
| cut (to) | **cis/o; sect/o; tom/o; -tomy** | dura mater (outer-most membrane surrounding the brain) | **dur/o** |

## D

| death | **necr/o; -mortem** |
|---|---|
| decrease | **hypo-; -penia** |
| deficiency | **-penia** |
| deficient | **oligo-** |
| delivery | **-partum** |
| destruction | **-lysis** |
| development | **-plasia; -plasm; -genesis** |
| diaphragm | **phren/o** |
| difficult | **dys-** |
| digestion | **-pepsia** |
| dilated, twisted vein | **varic/o** |
| dilation (dilatation) | **dilat/o; -ectasis; mydri/o** |
| dim | **ambly/o** |

## E

| ear | **aur/o; ot/o** |
|---|---|
| eardrum | **myring/o; tympan/o** |
| ease | **-aise** |
| eat (to) | **-phagia** |
| egg | **o/o; ov/o** |
| elbow | **olecran/o** |
| electric | **electr/o** |
| enlargement | **-megaly** |
| epididymis | **epididym/o** |
| equal | **is/o** |
| esophagus | **esophag/o** |
| ethmoid bone | **ethm/o** |
| eustachian tube | **salping/o** |
| excess | **ultra-** |

| DEFINITION | WORD PART | DEFINITION | WORD PART |
|---|---|---|---|
| excessive | hyper-; supra- | formed in | -genic |
| excision | -ectomy | four | quadri-; tetra- |
| expand (to) | dilat/o | front | anter/o; ventr/o |
| expert | -ician | | |
| external genitalia | episi/o; vulv/o | frontal bone | front/o |
| extremity | acr/o | fungus | myc/o |
| eye | ocul/o; ophthalm/o | fusion of parts | ankyl/o |
| eyelid | blephar/o; palpebr/o | **G** | |
| | | gall | chol/e |
| **F** | | gallbladder | cholecyst/o |
| face | faci/o | gel-like | vitre/o |
| falling | -ptosis | give birth | -para |
| fallopian tube | salping/o; -salpinx; tub/o | gland | aden/o |
| | | glans penis (tip of penis) | balan/o |
| false | pseudo- | glasslike | vitre/o |
| fascia (band of tissue surrounding a muscle) | fasci/o | glenoid cavity | glen/o |
| | | glomerulus | glomerul/o |
| fast | tachy- | glycogen (storage form of sugar) | glycogen/o |
| fat | adip/o; lip/o; lipid/o; steat/o | go (to) | -grade |
| | | gonads | gonad/o |
| fatty debris | ather/o | good | eu- |
| fatty plaque | ather/o | granules | granul/o |
| fear | -phobia | gray matter | poli/o |
| female | estr/o; gynec/o | groin | inguin/o |
| femur | femor/o | grow (to) | -physis |
| few | oligo- | growing thing | -blast |
| fibers | fibr/o | growth | -trophy |
| fibrous tissue | fibr/o | gums | gingiv/o |
| fibula | fibul/o | | |
| first | primi- | **H** | |
| flesh | sarc/o | habit | -hexia |
| flow | -flux; -rrhea | hair | cili/o; pil/o |
| formation | -genesis; -plasia; -plasm -poiesis | half | hemi-; semi- |
| | | hard | kerat/o; keratin/o |
| | | hardening | -sclerosis; scler/o |

| DEFINITION | WORD PART | DEFINITION | WORD PART |
|---|---|---|---|
| head | cephal/o | inner ear | labyrinth/o |
| hearing | audi/o; -cusis | instrument used to cut | -tome |
| heart | cardi/o | instrument used to measure | -meter |
| heat | -thermy | instrument used to record | -graph |
| heel | calcane/o | instrument used to visually examine a body cavity or organ | -scope |
| hernia (protrusion or displacement of an organ from the structure that normally contains it) | -cele; herni/o | insulin | insulin/o |
| | | internal organ | viscer/o |
| hiatus | hiat/o | intestine | intestin/o |
| hidden | crypt/o | inward | en-; eso- |
| hip | ili/o | iris | irid/o; ir/o |
| hip socket | acetabul/o | irrational fear | -phobia |
| hold back | isch/o | irregular | poikil/o |
| hormone that stimulates the production of blood cells | -poietin | irrigation | -clysis |
| | | ischium | ischi/o |
| horn-like | kerat/o; keratin/o | **J** | |
| humerus | humer/o | jejunum (medial portion of small intestine) | jejun/o |
| humpback | kyph/o | joint | arthr/o; articul/o |

**I**

| | | | |
|---|---|---|---|
| ileum (distal portion of the small intestine) | ile/o | **K** | |
| | | kidney | nephr/o; ren/o |
| immature | -blast | kill (to) | -cidal |
| immunity | immun/o; -immune | kneecap | patell/o |
| | | knowledge | -gnosis |
| imperfect | atel/o | | |
| in; into | in- | **L** | |
| in proper measure | emmetr/o | labor | -partum; -tocia; -tocin |
| inadequate | a(n)- | | |
| incise | -tomy | labyrinth | labyrinth/o |
| incision | -tomy | lack of | de- |
| incomplete | atel/o | lacrimal apparatus | lacrim/o |
| individual | idi/o | lacrimal duct | dacry/o |
| infection | septic/o | large | megal/o |
| inflammation (redness, swelling, heat, and pain that occur when the body protects itself from injury) | -itis | large intestine | col/o |
| | | larynx | laryng/o |
| | | lens | phac/o; phak/o |
| | | less | mi/o |

| DEFINITION | WORD PART | DEFINITION | WORD PART |
|---|---|---|---|
| lice | pedicul/o | membrane | mening/o |
| life | bi/o | meninges | mening/o |
| light | phot/o | menses | men/o |
| lips | cheil/o; labi/o | menstruation | men/o |
| little bronchi | bronchiol/o | metacarpals (bones of the hand) | metacarp/o |
| liver | hepat/o | | |
| lobe | lob/o | metatarsals (bones of the foot) | metatars/o |
| loins | lumb/o | | |
| loss or impairment of motor function | -plegia | middle | medi/o; meso- |
| | | milk | galact/o; lact/o |
| lower back | lumb/o | mind | ment/o |
| lower jaw | mandibul/o | month | men/o |
| lungs | pneum/o | motion | -kinesia; -kinesis |
| | pneumon/o; pneumat/o | mouth | or/o; stomat/o; stom/o |
| | pulmon/o | movement | -kinesia; -kinesis; -kines |
| lymph (clear, watery fluid) | lymph/o | | |
| lymph gland | lymphaden/o | mucus (a bodily secretion, of the mucous membrane, sometimes sticky and frequently thick) | muc/o |
| lymph node | lymphaden/o | | |
| lymph vessel | lymphangi/o | | |

## M

| | | | |
|---|---|---|---|
| | | multiple | multi- |
| magnet | magnet/o | muscle | muscul/o; myos/o |
| male | andr/o | | |
| malignant tumor of connective tissue | -sarcoma | myelin sheath | myelin/o |

## N

| | | | |
|---|---|---|---|
| malleolus | malleol/o | nail | onych/o; ungu/o |
| man | andr/o | narrowing | -stenosis |
| mandible | mandibul/o | nature | physi/o |
| manufacture | -poiesis | near | proxim/o; para- |
| many | poly-; multi- | neck | cervic/o |
| marrow | medull/o | neck of uterus | cervic/o |
| mass | -oma | nerve | neur/o |
| maxilla | maxill/o | nerve roots | radicul/o |
| meal | -prandial | network | reticul/o |
| measurement | -metry | new opening | -stomy |
| measure (to) | -metry | night | noct/o; nyct/o |
| meatus | meat/o | nipple | thel/o |
| medulla | medull/o | | |

| DEFINITION | WORD PART | DEFINITION | WORD PART |
|---|---|---|---|
| nipple-like | **papill/o** | pancreas | **pancreat/o** |
| no | **a(n)-; in-** | paralysis | **-plegia** |
| no strength | **-asthenia** | parathyroid gland | **parathyroid/o** |
| none | **nulli-** | parietal bone | **pariet/o** |
| normal | **eu-; norm/o** | part with child | **-para** |
| nose | **nas/o; rhin/o** | patches | **-plakia** |
| not | **a(n)-; in-** | patella | **patell/o** |
| nourish, stimulate | **-tropic; -trophic** | pelvis | **pelv/i; pelv/o** |
| nourishment | **-trophy** | penis | **phall/o** |
| | | perineum | **perine/o** |
| | | peritoneum | **peritone/o** |

**O**

| | | person or thing that does something | **-or** |
|---|---|---|---|
| occiput (back part of the head) | **occipit/o** | pertaining to | **-ac; -al; -an; -ar; -ary;** |
| old age | **presby-** | | **-eal; -ear; -ic; ine;** |
| olecranon | **olecran/o** | | **-ior; -or; -ory;** |
| on | **epi-** | | **-ose; -ous; -tic** |
| one | **mono-** | | |
| one's own | **idi/o** | | |
| one who | **-or** | | |
| one who measures | **-metrist** | pertaining to breakdown; destruction, or separation, | **-lytic** |
| one who specializes; specialist | **-logist; -ician; -er; -or; -ist** | | |
| opening | **-spadias; hiat/o** | phalanges (one of three bones making up each finger or toe) | **phalang/o** |
| optic disc | **papill/o** | | |
| order | **-taxia** | pharynx | **pharyng/o** |
| out | **e-; ec-; ex-; exo-; extra-** | physician | **iatr/o** |
| | | pineal gland | **pine/o** |
| outer layer | **cortic/o** | pit | **glen/o** |
| out of proportion | **ametr/o** | pituitary gland | **pituitar/o** |
| outside | **e-; ec-; ex-; exo-; extra-** | place | **top/o** |
| | | place (to) | **-stitial** |
| outward | **e-; ec-; ex-; exo-; extra-** | pleura | **pleur/o** |
| | | pleural cavity | **pleur/o** |
| ovary | **oophor/o; ovari/o** | poison | **tox/o** |
| oxygen | **ox/o** | poor | **dys-** |
| | | porous | **-porosis** |

**P**

| | | posterior portion of the hip bone | **ischi/o** |
|---|---|---|---|
| pain | **-algia; -dynia** | | |
| painful | **dys-** | potassium | **kal/o** |

| DEFINITION | WORD PART | DEFINITION | WORD PART |
|---|---|---|---|
| power | -potence | record | -gram |
| practice | practition/o | rectum | proct/o; rect/o |
| pregnancy | -cyesis; -gravida | red | erythemat/o; erythem/o; erythr/o; |
| process | -iasis; -ion; -ism; -y | referring to another | all/o |
| process of cutting | -tomy | relaxation | -chalasis |
| process of measuring | -metry | removal | de- |
| process of producing images | -graphy | renal pelvis | pyel/o |
| | | resembling | -oid |
| process of recording | -graphy | resembling a bunch of grapes | staphyl/o |
| process of study | -logy | | |
| process of visually examining a body cavity or organ | -scopy | respiration | pneumat/o; pneum/o |
| produced by | -gen -genic; -genous | retina | retin/o |
| | | rhythm | rhythm/o |
| producing | -gen; -genic | rib | cost/o |
| production | -genesis; -poiesis | rod-shaped | rhabd/o |
| | | run (to) | -drome |
| profuse sweating | diaphor/e | rupture | -rrhexis |
| prolapse | -ptosis | | |
| pronation | pronati/o | **S** | |
| prostate | prostat/o | sac | cyst/o |
| protrusion | -cele | sac filled with synovial fluid located around joints | burs/o |
| pubis (a portion of the hip bone) | pub/o | sac in which the fetus lies in the uterus | amni/o |
| pudendum | episi/o; vulv/o | sacrum | sacr/o |
| pulse | -sphyxia | safe | immunity; -immune |
| pupil | core/o; pupill/o | | |
| pus | py/o | sagging | -ptosis |
| pyloric sphincter | pylor/o | saliva | sial/o |
| pylorus | pylor/o | salivary gland | sialaden/o |
| | | same | home/o |
| **Q** | | scanty | oligo- |
| quick | oxy- | scapula | scapul/o |
| | | scrape | ras/o |
| **R** | | sebum | seb/o |
| radius (bone of lower arm) | radi/o | second | secundi- |
| reconstruction | -plasty | | |

| DEFINITION | WORD PART | DEFINITION | WORD PART |
|---|---|---|---|
| secrete (to) | crin/o; -crine | spark | scint/i |
| seizure | -lepsy | specialist; specialist in the study of | -ician; -logist; -er; -or; -ist |
| self | auto- | | |
| seminal fluid | sperm/o; spermat/o | speech | -phasia |
| | | spermatozoa (sperm) | sperm/o; spermat/o |
| sensation | -esthesia | | |
| separate | -crit; -lysis | sphenoid bone | sphen/o |
| sew | -rrhaphy | spinal column | spin/o |
| sex glands | gonad/o | spinal cord | myel/o |
| sharp | oxy- | spine | spin/o |
| shield | thyr/o; thyroid/o | spitting | -ptysis |
| shin | tibi/o | spleen | splen/o |
| shut (to) | -myein | split | -spadias |
| side | later/o | splitting | -schisis |
| sieve | ethm/o | stable | -stasis |
| sight | opt/o | standing | -stasis |
| sigmoid colon | sigmoid/o | stapes | staped/o |
| sinuses | sinus/o | state of | -ia; -ism; -sis |
| skeleton | skelet/o | step (to) | -grade |
| skin | cutane/o; derm/o; -derma; dermat/o; -dermis | sternum | stern/o |
| | | stiffening | ankyl/o |
| | | stimulate | -tropic |
| | | stomach | gastr/o |
| | | stone | -lith; lith/o |
| skull | crani/o | stop (to) | -continence |
| slight increase in the number of cells | -cytosis | stoppage; stopping | -pause; -stasis |
| | | straight | ortho- |
| slipping | -listhesis | stretching | -ectasis |
| slow | brady- | striated | rhabd/o |
| small | -ole; -ule; -cle | stricture | -stenosis |
| small bronchial tubes | bronchiol/o | striped | rhabd/o |
| small intestine | enter/o | structure | -ium; -um |
| smooth | lei/o | study of | -logy |
| socket | glen/o | stupor | narc/o |
| sodium | natr/o | sudden, involuntary contraction | -spasm |
| softening | -malacia | | |
| something inserted | catheter/o | sugar | gluc/o; glyc/o |
| sound | ech/o; son/o | supination | supinati/o |

| DEFINITION | WORD PART | DEFINITION | WORD PART |
|---|---|---|---|
| surgical binding | -desis | thyroid gland | thyr/o; thyroid/o |
| surgical fixation | -pexy | tibia | tibi/o |
| surgical fracture | -clasis | tilting | versi/o |
| surgical fusion | -desis | tip of penis | balan/o |
| surgical puncture to remove fluid | -centesis | tipping | versi/o |
| | | tissue | hist/o; histi/o |
| surgical reconstruction | -plasty | together | sym- |
| surgical refracture | -clasis | tone | ton/o |
| surgical removal | -ectomy | tongue | gloss/o; lingu/o |
| surgical repair | -plasty | tonsil | tonsill/o |
| suture (to sew) | -rrhaphy | tooth | dent/o; odont/o |
| swallow | -phagia | top | acr/o |
| swayback | lord/o | toward | ad- |
| sweat | hidr/o | toward the head | super/o |
| sword | xiph/o | trabecula (strands of connective tissue) | trabecul/o |
| synovial membrane | synovi/o | | |
| synovium | synovi/o | trachea | trache/o |
| | | transmission | -phoresis |
| **T** | | treatment | -therapy |
| tail | caud/o | trigone | trigon/o |
| tailbone | coccyg/o | tube | tub/o |
| tears | dacry/o; lacrim/o | tumor | -oma |
| teeth | odont/o | turmoil | -clonus |
| temporal bone | tempor/o | turning | -tropia; -tropion; versi/o |
| tendon | tend/o; tendin/o | | |
| tendon sheath | tenosynovi/o | twisted | strept/o |
| tension | tensi/o; ton/o | two | di- |
| testicle | orchi/o; orchid/o; test/o; testicul/o | tying | ligati/o |
| | | tympanic membrane | tympan/o; myring/o |
| testis | orchi/o; orchid/o; test/o; testicul/o | | |
| | | **U** | |
| thalamus | thalam/o | ulna (bone of lower arm) | uln/o |
| thigh bone | femor/o | umbilicus | umbilic/o |
| thing | -us | under | hypo-; sub-; infra- |
| thirst | -dipsia | | |
| thorax | thorac/o | unequal | anis/o |
| throat | pharyng/o | up | ana- |
| thymus gland | thym/o | upon | epi- |

| DEFINITION | WORD PART | DEFINITION | WORD PART |
|---|---|---|---|
| upper arm | **humer/o** | view (to) | **-opsy** |
| upper dilated portion of the ureter | **pyel/o** | violent action | **-clonus** |
| | | vision | **-opia; -opsia; opt/o** |
| upper jaw | **maxill/o** | | |
| urea (end product of protein breakdown) | **ure/o** | visual condition | **-opia; -opsia** |
| | | voice | **-phonia** |
| ureter | **ureter/o** | voice box | **laryng/o** |
| urethra | **urethr/o** | vomit | **-emesis** |
| urinary tract | **ur/o** | vulva | **episi/o; vulv/o** |
| urination | **ur/o; -uria** | | |
| urine | **ur/o; -uria; urin/o** | **W** | |
| | | wall | **pariet/o** |
| uterine tube | **salping/o; -salpinx** | washing | **-clysis** |
| | | water | **aque/o; hydr/o** |
| uterus | **uter/o; hyster/o; metr/o** | | |
| | | wedge | **sphen/o** |
| uvea | **uve/o** | white | **albin/o; leuk/o** |
| | | wide | **mydri/o** |
| **V** | | widen | **dilat/o** |
| vagina | **colp/o; vagin/o** | windpipe | **trache/o** |
| valve | **valvul/o** | with | **endo-; sym-** |
| variation | **poikil/o** | within | **endo-; infra-; intra-** |
| varicose vein | **varic/o** | | |
| vas deferens | **vas/o** | without | **e-** |
| vein | **phleb/o; ven/o** | woman | **gynec/o** |
| ventricle (lower chambers of the heart) | **ventricul/o** | wrist | **carp/o** |
| | | writing | **-gram** |
| vertebra; vertebral column | **vertebr/o; spin/o spondyl/o** | **X** | |
| vessel | **angi/o; vas/o; vascul/o** | x-rays | **radi/o** |

# APPENDIX E

# Abbreviations, Acronyms, and Symbols

## A

| | |
|---|---|
| $^{99m}Tc$ | technetium 99m |
| AAT | alpha$_1$ antitrypsin |
| Ab | antibody |
| ABG | arterial blood gases |
| ABR | auditory brainstem response |
| ACh | acetylcholine |
| ACL | anterior cruciate ligament |
| ACTH | adrenocorticotropic hormone |
| AD | Alzheimer disease; right ear |
| ADH | antidiuretic hormone |
| AED | automatic external defibrillator |
| AF; A-fib | atrial fibrillation |
| AFB | acid-fast bacillus |
| Ag | antigen |
| AIDS | acquired immunodeficiency syndrome |
| ALOC | altered levels of consciousness |
| ALP | alkaline phosphatase |
| ALS | amyotrophic lateral sclerosis |
| ALT | alanine transaminase |
| AM; a.m. | morning |
| AMD | age-related macular degeneration |
| ANA | antinuclear antibody |
| AP | anteroposterior |

| | |
|---|---|
| aPTT | activated partial thromboplastin time |
| ARF | acute renal failure |
| ART | assisted reproductive therapy |
| AS | left ear |
| AST | aspartate transaminase |
| ATP | adenosine triphosphate |
| AV | atrioventricular |

## B

| | |
|---|---|
| BBB | blood-brain barrier |
| BM | bowel movement |
| BP | blood pressure |
| BPH | benign prostatic hypertrophy |
| BRCA1; BRCA2 | breast cancer genes |
| BSE | breast self-examination |
| BSO | bilateral salpingo-oophorectomy |
| BUN | blood urea nitrogen |

## C

| | |
|---|---|
| C | cervical |
| C&S | culture and sensitivity |
| Ca | calcium |
| CABG | coronary artery bypass graft |
| CAD | coronary artery disease |
| CAPD | continual ambulatory peritoneal dialysis |

| | |
|---|---|
| CBC | complete blood count |
| CBD | common bile duct |
| CD | Crohn disease |
| CF | cystic fibrosis |
| CHD | coronary heart disease |
| CHF | congestive heart failure |
| CHO | carbohydrate |
| mCi | millicurie |
| µCi | microcurie |
| CK | creatine kinase |
| CNS | central nervous system |
| CO$_2$ | carbon dioxide |
| COPD | chronic obstructive pulmonary disease |
| CPAP | continuous positive airway pressure |
| CPK | creatine phosphokinase |
| CPR | cardiopulmonary resuscitation |
| CRF | chronic renal failure |
| CRP | C-reactive protein |
| CS | cesarean section |
| CSF | cerebrospinal fluid |
| CT | computed tomography |
| CTS | carpal tunnel syndrome |
| CVA | cerebrovascular accident |
| CVS | cardiovascular system; chorionic villus sampling |
| CXR | chest x-ray |

**D**

| | |
|---|---|
| D | dorsal |
| D&C | dilation and curettage |
| dB | decibels |
| DCIS | ductal carcinoma in situ |
| DI | diagnostic imagining; diabetes insipidus |
| dL | deciliter |
| DM | diabetes mellitus |
| DNA | deoxyribonucleic acid |
| DRE | digital rectal exam |
| Dx | diagnosis |

**E**

| | |
|---|---|
| EBV | Epstein-Barr virus |
| ECCE | extracapsular cataract extraction |
| ECG; EKG | electrocardiogram |
| EDB | estimated date of birth |
| EECP | enhanced external counterpulsation |
| EEG | electroencephalography |
| EENT | eyes, ears, nose, and throat |
| ENT | ears, nose, throat |
| ELISA | enzyme-linked immunosorbent assay |
| EMG | electromyography |
| endo | endoscopy |
| ENT | ears, nose, and throat |
| EOM | extraocular muscles |
| ER | emergency room |
| ERCP | endoscopic retrograde cholangiopancreatography |
| ERS | endoscopic retrograde sphincterotomy |
| ESL | extracorporeal shockwave lithotripsy |
| ESR | erythrocyte sedimentation rate |
| ESRD | end-stage renal disease |
| EUA | examination under anesthesia |
| EXU | excretory urogram |

**F**

| | |
|---|---|
| FB | foreign body |
| FBS | fasting blood glucose |
| FEV$_1$ | forced expiratory volume |

| | | | | |
|---|---|---|---|---|
| **FSH** | follicle-stimulating hormone | | **HPV** | human papillomavirus |
| **FVC** | forced vital capacity | | **H$_p$SA** | *Helicobacter pylori* stool antigen |
| | | | **HSV** | herpes simplex virus |
| **G** | | | **Hz** | Hertz |
| **G** | gram | | | |
| **mg** | microgram | | **I** | |
| **G** | gravida; pregnancy | | **IBS** | irritable bowel syndrome |
| **G1, G2, G3** | first, second, third pregnancy | | **ICD** | implantable cardioverter-defibrillator |
| **GB** | gallbladder | | | |
| **GERD** | gastroesophageal reflux disease | | **I&D** | incision and drainage |
| **GGT** | gamma-glutamyl transpeptidase | | **ICSH** | interstitial cell-stimulating hormone |
| **GH** | growth hormone | | **ICU** | intensive care unit |
| **GI** | gastrointestinal | | **IDD** | insulin-dependent diabetes |
| **GIT** | gastrointestinal tract | | **IDDM** | insulin-dependent diabetes mellitus |
| **GTT** | glucose tolerance test | | | |
| **GU** | genitourinary | | **Ig** | immunoglobulin |
| | | | **IM** | intramuscular |
| **H** | | | **IOL** | intraocular lens |
| | | | **IOP** | intraocular pressure |
| **HAV** | hepatitis A virus | | **IP** | interphalangeal |
| **HBV** | hepatitis B virus | | **IPD** | intermittent peritoneal dialysis |
| **HCG** | human chorionic gonadotrophin | | **IPPA** | inspection, palpation, percussion, and auscultation |
| **HCT** | hematocrit | | | |
| **HCV** | hepatitis C virus | | **IPPB** | intermittent positive pressure breathing |
| **HD** | hemodialysis; Hodgkin disease | | **IUD** | intrauterine device |
| **HDL** | high density lipoprotein | | **IV** | intravenous |
| **HDN** | hemolytic disease of the newborn | | **IVC** | inferior vena cava |
| | | | **IVF** | in vitro fertilization |
| **HEENT** | head, eyes, ears, nose, and throat | | **IVP** | intravenous pyelogram |
| | | | **IVU** | intravenous urography |
| **HF** | heart failure | | | |
| **Hgb, Hb** | hemoglobin | | **K** | |
| **HGH** | human growth hormone | | **KKUB** | kidney, kidney, ureter, bladder |
| **HIV** | human immunodeficiency virus | | **KUB** | kidney, ureter, bladder |

## L

| | |
|---|---|
| L | lumbar; liter |
| LAP | leucine aminopeptidase |
| LAVH | laparoscopic assisted vaginal hysterectomy |
| lb | pound |
| LASEK | laser assisted subepithelial keratectomy |
| LASIK | laser assisted in-situ keratomileusis |
| LBBB | left bundle branch block |
| LCIS | lobular carcinoma in situ |
| LDH | lactate dehydrogenase |
| LDL | low density lipoprotein |
| LEEP | loop electrocautery excision procedure |
| LES | lower esophageal sphincter |
| LFT | liver function tests |
| LH | luteinizing hormone |
| LLQ | left lower quadrant |
| LNMP | last normal menstrual period |
| LOC | level of consciousness |
| LP | lumbar puncture |
| LRT | lower respiratory tract |
| LTH | lactogenic hormone |
| LUQ | left upper quadrant |
| LUTS | lower urinary tract symptoms |

## M

| | |
|---|---|
| m | meter; milli |
| MA | mental age |
| MBJ | muscles, bones, and joints |
| mcg | microgram |
| mcL | microliter |
| MCP | metacarpophalangeal |
| MD | muscular dystrophy |
| mEq | milliequivalent |

| | |
|---|---|
| mg | milligram (1/1000 gram) |
| mg% | milligram percent |
| mg/dL | milligrams per deciliter |
| Mg | magnesium |
| MG | myasthenia gravis |
| MI | myocardial infarction |
| mL | milliliter |
| mm | millimeter (1/1000 meter) |
| mm Hg; mmHg | millimeters of mercury |
| mμ | millimicron (1/1000 micron) |
| mmol | millimole |
| MRI | magnetic resonance imaging |
| MRSA | methicillin-resistant *Staphylococcus aureus* |
| MS | multiple sclerosis |
| MSH | melanocyte stimulating hormone |
| MSS | musculoskeletal system |
| MUGA | multiple-gated acquisition scan (of heart) |

## N

| | |
|---|---|
| NAD | no appreciable disease |
| NB | newborn |
| ng | nanogram |
| NG | nasogastric |
| NHL | non-Hodgkin lymphoma |
| NOS | not otherwise specified |
| NS | nervous system |
| NSAID | nonsteroidal anti-inflammatory drugs |
| NTP | normal temperature and pulse |
| NYD | not yet diagnosed |

## O

| | |
|---|---|
| $O_2$ | oxygen |
| OA | Osteoarthritis |

| | | | | |
|---|---|---|---|---|
| **OB/GYN** | Obstetrics and Gynecology | | **PMN** | polymorphonuclear |
| **OD** | overdose; right eye; oculus dexter | | **PNS** | peripheral nervous system |
| **ORIF** | open reduction and internal fixation | | **PPD** | purified protein derivative |
| | | | **PRL** | prolactin |
| **OS** | left eye; oculus sinister | | **PSA** | prostatic-specific antigen |
| **os** | opening bone | | **PT** | prothrombin time |
| **OSS** | organs of special sense | | **PTA** | prior to admission |
| **OXT** | oxytocin | | **PTC** | percutaneous transhepatic cholangiography |
| **oz** | ounce | | **PTH** | parathormone |
| | | | **PYO** | pyrexia of unknown origin |

**P**

| | | | | |
|---|---|---|---|---|
| **P** | -para (given birth); pulse; phosphorus | | **R** | |
| **P1, P2, P3** | given birth 1, 2, or 3 times | | **R** | respiration |
| **PA** | posteroanterior | | **RA** | rheumatoid arthritis |
| **PaCO₂** | partial pressure of carbon dioxide | | **RBBB** | right bundle branch block |
| | | | **RBC** | red blood cell |
| **PaO₂** | partial pressure of oxygen | | **RDS** | respiratory distress syndrome |
| **PCL** | posterior cruciate ligament | | **RF** | rheumatoid factors |
| **PCP** | *Pneumocystis carinii* | | **Rh** | rhesus |
| **PD** | Parkinson disease; peritoneal dialysis | | **RIA** | radioimmunoassay |
| **PEEP** | positive end-expiratory pressure | | **RICE** | rest, ice, compression, elevation |
| **PERRLA** | pupils equal, round, react to light and accommodation | | **RLQ** | right lower quadrant |
| | | | **ROM** | range of motion |
| **PET** | positron-emission tomography | | **RP** | retrograde pyelogram |
| | | | **RS** | respiratory system |
| **PFT** | pulmonary function test | | **RUQ** | right upper quadrant |
| **pH** | a measure of the alkalinity or acidity of a substance | | | |
| **physio** | physiotherapy | | **S** | |
| **PID** | pelvic inflammatory disease | | **S** | sacral |
| **PIP** | proximal interphalangeal (joint) | | **S** | second |
| | | | **SAP** | serum alkaline phosphatase |
| **PM; p.m.** | afternoon | | **SB** | stillbirth |
| **PMI** | point of maximum impulse; point of maximum intensity | | **SIADH** | syndrome of inappropriate antidiuretic hormone |
| | | | **SLR** | straight leg raising |

The P header notation represents partial pressures: $PaCO_2$ is the partial pressure of carbon dioxide and $PaO_2$ is the partial pressure of oxygen.

| | |
|---|---|
| **SOB** | shortness of breath |
| **sp gr** | specific gravity |
| **stat** | immediately |
| **STD** | sexually transmitted disease |
| **STH** | somatotropic hormone |
| **STI** | sexually transmitted infection |
| **SVC** | superior vena cava |

## T

| | |
|---|---|
| **T** | thoracic; temperature |
| **T&A** | tonsillectomy and adenoidectomy |
| **TB** | tuberculosis |
| **T$_3$** | triiodothyronine |
| **T$_4$** | thyroxine; thyroxin |
| **TAH** | total abdominal hysterectomy |
| **TAH-BSO** | total abdominal hysterectomy and bilateral salpingo-oophorectomy |
| **TFT** | thyroid function test |
| **TIA** | transient ischemic attack |
| **TLC** | tender loving care |
| **TM** | tympanic membrane |
| **TMJ** | temporomandibular joint |
| **TPR** | temperature, pulse, and respiration |
| **TRUS** | transrectal ultrasound |
| **TSH** | thyroid-stimulating hormone |
| **TUP** | transurethral prostatectomy |
| **TUR** | transurethral resection |
| **TURP** | transurethral resection of prostate |
| **Tx** | treatment |

## U

| | |
|---|---|
| **UA** | urinalysis |
| **URT** | upper respiratory tract |
| **US** | ultrasound |
| **UTI** | urinary tract infection |

## V

| | |
|---|---|
| **VD** | vomiting and diarrhea; venereal disease |
| **V/Q scan** | ventilation/perfusion scan (Q stands for quotient) |
| **VF; V-fib** | ventricular fibrillation |

## W

| | |
|---|---|
| **WBC** | white blood cell |
| **Wt** | weight |

## Symbols

| | |
|---|---|
| $=$ | equal |
| $\neq$ | unequal |
| $+$ | plus; positive |
| $-$ | minus; negative |
| $\uparrow$ | above; increase |
| $\downarrow$ | below; decrease |
| ♂ | male |
| ♀ | female |
| $>$ | is greater than |
| $<$ | is less than |
| % | percent |
| $:$ | ratio |
| ' | foot |
| " | inches |
| $\bar{c}$ | with |
| $\bar{s}$ | without |
| # | pound |

# Glossary of Diagnostic Tests

## A

**abdominal x-ray:** x-ray of the kidneys, ureters, and bladder (KUB) without the use of contrast medium. Also known as **flat plate of abdomen**.

**Achilles jerk; ankle jerk:** a test in which a tap on the Achilles tendon causes plantar flexion of the foot.

**allergy testing:** skin tests that show the body's response to foreign substances (antigens).

**anteroposterior (AP) view:** x-rays enter the body from the front to the back.

**antiglobulin test (Coombs' test) (KOOMZ):** laboratory test used to detect abnormal antibodies on the surface of red blood cells.

**antinuclear antibody (ANA):** a blood test used to detect unusual antibodies called antinuclear antibodies, which cause tissue damage and are an indicator of autoimmune disease.

**arterial blood gases (ABG):** a laboratory test that measures the amount of oxygen and carbon dioxide in the blood.

**arthroscopy:** a surgical method of looking into a joint without making a large incision. A small incision is made near the joint and an arthroscope is inserted. The arthroscope has a video camera attached, which allows the surgeon to view the entire joint cavity. Surgery is performed by inserting surgical instruments into additional small incisions. Recovery time is minimal and hospital stay is reduced.

**aspiration biopsy:** tissue is removed without a surgical incision. A needle is placed into tissue such as bone marrow, and the material is aspirated (withdrawn) into the needle. The tissue is then examined.

**audiometry:** a test that measures hearing ability.

**auditory brainstem response (ABR):** a test that helps determine the cause of hearing loss by measuring nervous impulses to the brainstem after the cochlea is stimulated by sound.

## B

**Babinski** (bah-**BIN**-skee) **reflex:** dorsiflexion (backward flexion) of the toes when the sole of the foot is stimulated. This is a normal response in newborns and infants but it indicates nerve dysfunction in others.

**barium enema:** barium is placed into the rectum as a contrast medium followed by x-rays of the large bowel.

**barium studies:** an x-ray procedure used to diagnose digestive-tract problems. Barium sulfate is used as a contrast medium. As barium settles in the organs, it will appear white on the x-ray film.

**barium swallow:** barium is taken by mouth, followed by x-rays of the pharynx and esophagus.

**biopsy:** removal of a piece of tissue for examination under a microscope.

**bleeding time:** a test used to measure the time it takes for bleeding to stop following a small puncture wound to the skin.

**blood glucose levels:** a test used to determine the amount of glucose (sugar) in the blood. It is also known as serum glucose level. The amount of glucose in the blood is expressed as milligrams per deciliter (mg/dL). Normal blood glucose level is 70 to 100 mg/dL.

**blood urea nitrogen (BUN):** a test that measures the amount of urea in the blood. Urea is a waste product that is carried in the blood to the kidney, where it is filtered by the nephrons and excreted in urine.

**bone scan:** a picture of the bone is produced using a special camera after the patient has been injected with radioactive phosphate. The radioactive phosphate is picked up by the diseased bone and shows up as dark areas called *hot spots* on the scan.

**breath test:** a procedure used to diagnose ulcers caused by the bacteria *Helicobacter pylori.*

# C

**cardiac count:** a catheter is inserted into a vein in the arm or femur and pushed upward into the heart. An x-ray of the blood vessels of the heart (angiocardiography) is performed at the same time as the catheterization so that the placement of the catheter can be monitored. Diagnostic information such as levels of oxygen and carbon dioxide, or indicators of coronary artery disease and disorders of the heart valves, is obtained.

**cardiac enzymes:** a test for myocardial infarction by measuring cardiac enzymes such as creatine phosphokinase (CPK) and lactate dehydrogenase (LDH). During a myocardial infarction, the damaged cells release CPK and LDH into the bloodstream. High levels of these enzymes in the blood are a good indicator of myocardial infarction.

**Cardiolite scan:** this test uses a radiopharmaceutical, known as a tracer, to produce images of the heart muscle. An exercise test is used with it to diagnose coronary heart disease. While the patient is exercising on a treadmill, the tracer is injected into a vein in the arm. The tracer travels through the blood, to the coronary arteries, and is picked up by the heart muscle. Healthy areas of the heart that have sufficient blood supply pick up the tracer immediately and appear as *hot spots* on the scan. Areas that do not have sufficient blood supply pick up the tracer slowly and appear as *cold spots* on the scan.

**catheter:** a tube-shaped, flexible, surgical instrument that can be inserted into a body cavity for the withdrawal or introduction of fluid.

**catheterization:** the process of passing a catheter into a body cavity.

**centesis:** surgical puncture to remove excess fluid or to remove fluid for diagnostic purposes. The type of centesis is named after its location. Abdominocentesis (abdomen). Arthrocentesis (joint). Cardiocentesis (heart).

**chest x-ray:** an image is taken of the internal structures of the chest. The pictures can be taken in different body positions.

**cholangiography:** x-ray of the bile ducts following injection of a contrast medium.

**coagulation time:** measurement of the time it takes blood to clot in a test tube. Also known as clotting time.

**cold spot:** a term used to describe areas on a scan where there is low uptake into the tissues of a radioactive substance that has been injected into the body.

**colposcopy** (kol-**POS**-koh-pee): process of visually examining the vagina and cervix using a special magnifying device called a colposcope.

**complete blood count (CBC):** a general screening test during routine physical examinations. Several tests are done on a sample of blood including hematocrit, hemoglobin, white blood cell count, and platelet count.

**computed tomography** (kom-**PYOO**-ted toh-**MOG**-rah-fee): a procedure utilizing an x-ray beam passing through a body part. The beam visually cuts the part into many slices at various depths. This information is computer analyzed and a series of pictures is assembled into one image of the part. CT scans allow for clearer visualization than conventional x-ray. Common body parts studied in this fashion include the brain, abdomen, kidneys, and chest. Abbreviation: **CT scan**.

**c-reactive protein (CRP):** the liver produces CRP only when there is an inflammatory process within the body. This test is performed to diagnose inflammation within the body.

**contrast medium:** a dye that is placed into the patient's body to improve the visibility of an x-ray.

**count:** any test that involves the calculation of the total number of something in a sample.

**creatine kinase (CK); creatine phosphokinase (CPK):** a laboratory test to evaluate the levels of CPK in the blood. CPK is an enzyme found in cardiac and skeletal muscle tissue. When muscle is damaged, the cells release CPK. CPK spills into the blood, elevating normal blood levels.

**creatinine clearance:** a test of blood and urine to assess kidney function. It measures the kidney's ability to clear creatinine from the blood. Creatinine is a waste product produced by the breakdown of creatine (a protein found in muscle). Creatinine is excreted in the urine.

**culture:** a method of identifying bacteria. Microorganisms or living tissue cells are placed in an environment that stimulates growth. As the microorganism multiplies, it can be easily identified.

**culture and sensitivity (C&S):** a test to measure a microorganism's sensitivity to antibiotics. The microorganism is cultured and exposed to various antibiotics. The antibiotic that is most effective in killing the microorganism is the one used to treat the patient.

**culture specimen:** a sample of microorganisms or living tissue cells taken from an area of the body for laboratory examination. Culture specimens can be taken from sputum (mucus and other material brought up through the respiratory tract), blood, urine, throat, cervix uteri, and stool.

**cystoscopy:** visual examination of the bladder using a cystoscope. The cystoscope is placed through the urethra and into the bladder with or without anesthetic. A tiny camera inside the cystoscope shows the inside of the organs on a television monitor. Other instruments can be used with the cystoscope to perform biopsies, remove calculi, or burn (cauterize) abnormal tissue.

# D

**differential; white blood cell differential:** a count of each different type of white blood cell (eosinophils, basophils, neutrophils, lymphocytes, and monocytes).

**digital rectal exam (DRE):** palpation (feeling) of the prostate and other structures by placing a gloved finger through the anal canal and into the rectum.

**dilation and curettage** (dye-**LAY**-shun and kyoo-reh-**TAZH**): a surgical procedure used to determine the cause of uterine bleeding or other conditions. The cervical opening is widened with an instrument called a dilator. This is followed by the insertion of a second instrument called a **curet** (kyoo-**RET**), which has jagged edges on one side. The curet is used to scrape the endometrial lining from the uterine wall so that it may be examined. Abbreviation: **D&C.**

**Doppler** (**DOP**-ler) **ultrasound:** the use of ultrasound to measure the speed and direction of blood flow through a blood vessel.

**drawer test:** a test to determine the stability of the anterior and posterior cruciate ligaments that support and stabilize the knee joint.

# E

**echocardiography:** a procedure that produces an image of the heart using ultrasound waves.

**electrocardiography (ECG; EKG):** a measurement of the electrical activity of the heart. The record produced is called an electrocardiogram. It is a *snapshot* of how well the conduction system is working.

**electrocochleography** (ee-leck-troh-kock-lee-**OG**-rah-fee): a process for recording the electrical activity of the cochlea.

**electroencephalography** (ee-leck-troh-en-sef-ah-**LOG**-rah-fee): a procedure used to record the electrical impulses of the brain. Abbre. **EEG.**

**electrolytes:** substances capable of producing an electrical charge. They are found in blood, body tissues, and urine. They are important in muscle and nerve function. Examples include calcium, sodium, potassium, chloride, and magnesium.

**electromyography** (ee-leck-troh-my-**OG**-rah-fee): a procedure used to record the electrical impulses produced by a muscle when it is at rest and when it is moving. This is done by inserting tiny needle electrodes into the muscle. Abbreviation: **EMG.**

**electrophoresis:** a test on blood or urine that utilizes an electrical current to separate proteins in a mixture. This allows different protein components and quantities to be determined.

**ELISA (enzyme-linked immunosorbent assay):** blood test to screen patients for antibodies to HIV.

**endoscope:** any instrument utilizing a narrow flexible tube with a tiny video camera attached to view inside body organs and cavities. Endoscopes are named using the root of the organ or cavity being viewed. Examples include *gastroscope*, instrument used to view the inside of the stomach; *bronchoscope*, instrument used to view the inside of the bronchus; *laparoscope*, instrument used to view the inside of the abdominal cavity; and *cystoscope*, instrument used to view the bladder.

**endoscopic retrograde cholangiopancreatography (ERCP):** the bile ducts and pancreas are studied using an endoscope. The endoscope is inserted through the mouth, into the stomach, and into the duodenum. A contrast medium is introduced through the endoscope. It flows backward (retrograde) and highlights the biliary ducts and pancreas. X-rays are taken.

**endoscopy:** the process of visually examining a body cavity or organ using an instrument called an endoscope. Biopsies and tissue repair can also be done by inserting cutting devices through the endoscope. Endoscopies are named using the root of the organ or cavity being viewed.

**enzymes:** proteins within cells that act as a catalyst in chemical reactions.

**erythrocyte count:** see red blood cell count.

**erythrocyte sedimentation rate (ESR):** a test that measures the time it takes for red blood cells to settle out of plasma to the bottom of a test tube.

**excretory urography (EXU):** examination of the kidneys, ureters, and bladder following injection of a contrast medium into a vein. Also known as **intravenous urography** (IVU) or **intravenous pyelography** (IVP).

**exercise stress test:** an electrocardiogram obtained while the patient is exercising.

**exophthalmometry:** the process of measuring the forward protrusion of the eyeball as seen in exophthalmia.

## F

**fasting blood sugar (FBS):** laboratory test that measures blood glucose levels after the patient has fasted for at least eight hours.

**fluoroscopy** (floo-**ROSS**-kah-pee): an x-ray of moving structures, such as the movement of substances through the digestive tract. The image is produced on a fluorescent screen rather than on a single x-ray film. This procedure has the advantage of allowing observation of structures as they move. Fluoroscopy is used with barium studies to observe how well barium flows through the gastrointestinal tract.

**frozen section:** during surgery, a piece of tissue is removed and quickly frozen for microscopic examination. Frozen sections are done when a quick diagnosis is needed to eliminate the need for two operations, one for diagnosis and one for treatment.

**funduscopy** (fun-**DOS**-ka-pee): the process of visually examining the interior of the eye. Also known as **ophthalmoscopy** (**ahf**-thal-**MOS**-koh-pee).

## G

**gastric analysis:** contents of the stomach are analyzed for acid levels, appearance, and volume.

**Gleason score:** a grading system for prostatic cancer. A grade of 1 to 5 is assigned based upon the microscopic appearance of the abnormal prostatic growth. Grade 1 is less severe, grade 5 more severe cancer indication. Also known as Gleason grade.

**glucose tolerance test (GTT):** a test that monitors the body's ability to utilize glucose after a measured amount of a sweet drink has been taken by the patient. The blood sugar is measured before and after the drink. Blood sugar should return to normal after three hours.

**glycated hemoglobin test:** a test that measures the amount of glucose attached to hemoglobin. The more glucose attached to hemoglobin, the higher the blood glucose level.

## H

**Heaf test:** see tuberculin skin test.

**hematocrit (HCT):** a laboratory test to determine the percentage of erythrocytes per volume of blood.

**hemoccult** (hee-moh-**KULT**) **test:** an examination of stool for blood. It is called a hemoccult (*hem/o* blood; *occult* hidden) because the blood is difficult to see. A small amount of stool is placed on a special hemoccult card. Guaiac (**GWEE**-ack), a special substance, is then added to the stool to reveal any hidden blood.

**hemoglobin (Hgb, Hb):** a test to determine the total amount of hemoglobin in a sample of blood.

**HIDA scan:** a procedure used to produce an image of the liver, gallbladder, and biliary ducts following injection of radiopharmaceutical into a vein. The radiopharmaceutical travels to the liver and is excreted by the biliary ducts. It is traced by a special scanner that takes the images.

**Holter monitor:** an electrocardiogram taken while the patient is going about a typical daily routine.

**hot spot:** a term used to identify areas on a scan where there is high uptake into the tissue of the radiopharmaceutical that has been injected into the body.

## I

**immunoelectrophoresis** (ih-myoo-noh-ee-leck-troh-for-**EE**-sis): a procedure utilizing an electric current to identify and measure immunoglobulins in a sample of blood. Immunoglobulins are proteins that function as antibodies. Under normal conditions, they are present in the blood in predictable amounts. They are classified into IgG, IgA, IgM, IgD, and IgE.

## J

**jerk:** a sudden, involuntary response to a stimulus; a sudden reflex.

## K

**knee jerk:** see reflex, patellar.

## L

**laparoscopy** (**lap**-eh-**ROSS**-keh-pee): process of viewing the inside of the abdomen using a laparoscope that is passed through a small incision in the abdominal wall.

**lateral decubitus view:** an x-ray position; x-rays enter the body from the side while the patient is lying down.

**lateral view:** an x-ray position; x-rays enter the body from either the right or left side of the chest.

**leukocyte count:** see white blood cell count.

**lipid tests:** a measurement of the amount of lipids (fats) in a sample of blood. Types of lipids are cholesterol, triglycerides, phospholipids, high-density lipoprotein, and low-density lipoproteins.

**liver function tests (LFTs):** a group of blood tests measuring the level of liver enzymes in the blood. These enzymes are normally in hepatic cells but are released when the liver is diseased or damaged. ALT, AST, ALP, and LDH are some of the more common enzymes. The enzymes are known by their abbreviations. Look at the Abbreviation Glossary for the meanings of these abbreviations.

**lumbar puncture (LP); spinal tap:** an examination of the cerebrospinal fluid for microorganisms or blood. A needle is inserted into the subarachnoid space below the third lumbar vertebra. Cerebrospinal fluid is withdrawn and analyzed.

**lung perfusion and ventilation scan:** a type of nuclear medicine test that produces an image of blood and air flow to the lungs. A radiopharmaceutical is injected into a vein and eventually settles in the arterioles of the lungs. A special camera is used to detect the radiopharmaceutical, and a series of pictures are made of the thorax. These pictures are seen on a special screen called an oscilloscope. A normal scan will show even distribution of the radiopharmaceutical throughout the lungs. An abnormal scan will show no radiopharmaceutical, which suggests decreased blood flow to that part of the lung.

**lymphangiography:** an x-ray of the lymphatic system following injection of a contrast medium into the feet. A fluoroscope (a type of x-ray that displays movement onto a television monitor) is used. The flow of the contrast medium is followed as it travels from the feet upward toward the abdomen. Once the dye has been completely injected, x-rays are taken of the lymphatic system.

**lymphoscintography** (**lim**-foh-sin-**TIG**-grah-fee): a type of nuclear imaging process that records the lymphatic vessels or lymph nodes to detect metastatic tumors, lymphedema, or lymph node blockage.

## M

**magnetic resonance imaging (MRI):** a picture of a body structure produced by the use of electromagnetic energy rather than conventional x-ray, ultrasound, or radioactive substances. No contrast medium is used. MRIs provide clear pictures of soft-tissue abnormalities such as edema and tumors.

**mammography:** process of taking x-rays of the breast.

**Mantoux test:** see tuberculin skin test.

**MUGA scan (multiple-gated acquisition scan):** an image is produced of the heart muscle following injection of technetium 99m ($^{99m}$Tc), a radioactive substance. It can provide information on blood flow through the heart and how well the ventricles pump blood out of the heart.

**myelography:** x-ray of the spinal cord following injection of a contrast media into the subarachnoid space.

# O

**oblique view:** an x-ray position; x-rays enter the body on a slant in order to visualize behind structures.

**ophthalmoscopy:** see **funduscopy**.

**otoscopy (oh-TOSS-kah-pee):** the process of viewing the middle and inner ear using an otoscope. Video otoscopy is a recent advancement providing color images of the ear that can be copied and enlarged.

# P

**Pap smear:** a laboratory test that allows examination of cells from the cervix uteri for disease, especially cancerous cells.

**patch test:** a test in which a small amount of a substance called an **allergen (AL-er-jen)** is placed on the skin and covered with a patch. If the patient is sensitive to the allergen, there will be an allergic reaction. The patient will develop a raised, itchy bump called a **wheal (WEEL)**. A wheal looks like a mosquito bite. It may be redder or paler than the surrounding skin.

**patellar reflex:** extension of the lower leg when the area below the patella (kneecap) is tapped; also called knee jerk.

**pelvic ultrasound:** the use of ultrasound to obtain an image of the abdomen and pelvis. This procedure is used during pregnancy to assess fetal size and development as well as placental location. As well, ovarian tumors and other pelvic masses can be detected using ultrasound.

**percutaneous transhepatic cholangiography (PTC):** the bile ducts undergo an x-ray exam following injection of a contrast medium through the skin and into the liver.

**plantar reflex:** toes curl under when the sole of the foot (plantar aspect) is stroked.

**platelet count:** a test that measures the number of platelets in a sample of blood. The normal value is 150,000 to 400,000 per microliter of blood.

**positron emission tomography (POZ-ee-tron ee-MISH-un toh-MOG-rah-fee) (PET scan):** a procedure in which a picture is taken of internal body structures to study how cells function in certain body areas. A radioactive substance is injected into a vein and traced as it travels through the body. PET scans are helpful in diagnosing and treating such diseases as cancer, Alzheimer, schizophrenia, and stroke.

**posteroanterior(PA) view:** x-rays enter the body from back to front.

**prostate-specific antigen (PSA):** a test to determine the level of PSA in the blood. PSA is a protein produced by the prostate gland. PSA is removed from the body in semen, although a small amount enters the bloodstream and can be measured. An elevated PSA level may indicate prostatic cancer, benign prostatic hypertrophy, or prostatitis.

**prothrombin time (PT):** a laboratory test that measures the time it takes for a clot to form.

**pulmonary arteriography:** a procedure in which images of the pulmonary blood vessels are taken following injection of a contrast medium into the vascular system.

**pulmonary function test (PFT):** a series of tests on lung performance using a spirometer, an instrument to record breathing ability. It measures total lung capacity (TLC), which is the total volume of air the lungs can hold. Some of the test measurements are obtained by normal, quiet breathing, and other tests require forced inhalation or exhalation.

**pulse oximetry** (**PULSS**-ock-**SIM**-eh-tree): a procedure used to measure the percentage of hemoglobin saturated with oxygen. An instrument called an oximeter (ock-**SIM**-eh-ter) is used. It has a probe that attaches to the patient's fingertip. The probe is linked to a computerized unit. The probe emits a light that is absorbed by hemoglobin in various degrees, depending upon the amount of oxygen present. The computerized unit can then calculate the percentage of hemoglobin that is oxygenated.

**punch biopsy:** a circular piece of tissue is removed with a sharp instrument.

# R

**radioactive iodine uptake:** a test used to assess thyroid function. Radioactive iodine is taken orally. Eventually, it is taken up by the thyroid. A high uptake of radioactive iodine indicates too much thyroxine is being produced.

**radioimmunoassay (RIA):** a test used to identify antibodies the immune system has formed in response to the presence of antigens.

**radiopharmaceutical:** a radioactive substance combined with a chemical that is easily absorbed by the target organ.

**range of motion (ROM):** an assessment of the degree to which a joint can be moved in any direction, including adduction, abduction, flexion, extension, dorsiflexion, and plantar flexion. Range is measured in degrees. Limited joint movement may be 55 degrees, or full-range movement, 360 degrees.

**red blood cell count (RBC):** a test that measures the number of red blood cells in a sample of blood. The normal value is 4.7 to 6.1 million cells per microliter for men and 4.2 to 5.4 million cells per microliter for women.

**red blood cell morphology:** a study of red blood cells to determine abnormalities of size, shape, color, and structure.

**reflex:** a sudden, involuntary response to a stimulus.

**refraction test:** a common test used to study the bending of light rays as they pass through the eye, in order to clearly identify errors of refraction. The unit of measurement of the refractive power of the lens is diopter (dye-**OP**-ter).

**retrograde urography:** an x-ray of the urinary structures following injection of a contrast medium into the bladder through the urethra. The contrast medium flows backward (retrograde) highlighting urinary structures.

**rheumatoid factors (RF):** proteins present in the blood of patients with rheumatoid arthritis.

**Romberg** (**ROM**-bergz) **sign:** swaying or loss of balance when the patient is asked to stand erect with the feet together and the eyes closed. Indicates nerve dysfunction.

# S

**scan (nuclear medicine):** an image of a body organ is taken after a radiopharmaceutical has been introduced into the body. The radiopharmaceutical is known as a tracer. The tracer travels through the bloodstream to the body organ being studied. An area where there is high uptake of the radiopharmaceutical is known as a *hot spot.* An area where there is little or no uptake of the radiopharmaceutical is called a *cold spot*. The tracer gives off small amounts of radiation that is detected using a special camera (gamma camera). Images of the radioactivity are produced. The image is called a scan. Scans are commonly taken on bone, brain, liver, lung, thyroid, and heart.

**scratch test:** test to identify substances a person is allergic to. Potential allergens are applied to scratches made on the skin surface. If there is an allergic reaction, the patient will develop a raised, red area on the skin.

**scrotal transillumination:** a bright light is held behind the scrotum. A scrotum filled with watery fluid will shine red because the light will pass through it. More solid abnormalities such as testicular tumors are seen as dark shadows because the light will not pass through.

**semen analysis:** a laboratory test to evaluate infertility. Semen is collected in a specimen container and analyzed microscopically. The sperm in the semen is counted and examined for size, shape, and mobility. Semen is examined for pH (balance of acids and bases), thickness, appearance, and volume.

**serum alkaline phosphatase (SAP):** a blood test used to measure the levels of alkaline phosphatase, which is important in the building of new bone.

**serum calcium (Ca) and serum phosphorus (P):** measurement of calcium or phosphorus in the blood (serum).

**shave biopsy:** tissue that extends above the level of its surroundings is removed with a **scalpel** (**SKAL**-pel), a sharp knife.

**skeletal x-ray:** x-ray of the bone without the use of a contrast medium. The bone shows up clearly as a white object against a black background.

**small bowel series:** barium is taken by mouth, followed by x-rays of the small bowel (duodenum, jejunum, and ileum).

**smear:** a laboratory test used to identify microorganisms. The specimen is placed on a slide and stained using the **Gram stain** method. The Gram stain will highlight the microorganism so that it is visible and can be identified.

**spirometry** (speye-**ROM**-eh-tree): the process of measuring breathing ability using a spirometer.

**stool analysis:** an examination of stool (feces) to identify fats, microorganisms, occult (hidden) blood, and other abnormal substances.

# T

**thallium scan:** an image of the heart and its blood vessels is obtained following injection of a radioactive substance that includes thallium-201. Normal myocardial tissue absorbs the radioactive substance while diseased tissue does not.

**thrombocyte count:** see platelet count.

**thyroid function test (TFT):** this laboratory test measures thyroxine, triiodothyronine, and thyroid-stimulating hormone in the blood.

**tine test:** see tuberculin skin test.

**transillumination** (**tranz**-ih-loo-mih-**NAY**-shun): passing light through body tissues for the purpose of examining the part.

**transrectal ultrasound (TRUS):** the use of ultrasound to produce an image of the prostate. The well-lubricated transducer (instrument that emits the sound waves) is inserted into the rectum. An image is produced as the transducer is moved along the prostate.

**transvaginal ultrasound:** a procedure in which the transducer (instrument that emits the sound waves) is placed inside the vagina. The echogram is clearer and the details are sharper.

**tuberculin skin test:** tuberculin such as *PPD* (purified protein derivative of *mycobacterium tuberculosis*) is injected intradermally. This is called the *Mantoux test*. Another method is to apply the tuberculin to the skin. This is done by making many punctures in the skin. These are called the *Heaf* and *tine tests*. An inflammatory reaction will occur if the patient is sensitive to the tuberculin. This causes the localized area of skin to become red and swollen. This positive reaction means the persons has prior or present contact with *Mycobacterium tuberculosis*.

**tuning fork test:** a vibrating tuning fork is placed against the bones of the skull sending vibrations that can be heard if there is no hearing loss. Types include Weber and Rinne (**RIN**-ay).

**tympanometry** (tym-pah-**NOM**-eh-tree): measures how well sound can pass through the eardrum to the middle ear.

## U

**ultrasound/ultrasonography (US):** an image is produced using high frequency sound waves rather than x-rays, magnetic fields, or radioisotopes. An instrument called a transducer passes sound waves through the organ. These waves are reflected back from the organ and recorded on an oscilloscope (special screen). Because tissues of different density will be reflected at different rates, an image is formed. No contrast medium is placed into the body. The record of the ultrasound is called an echogram or sonogram.

**upper gastrointestinal series:** barium is taken by mouth, followed by x-rays of the upper digestive tract, from the pharynx to the ileum.

**uric acid:** a measurement of uric acid in the urine. Uric acid is a waste product of protein breakdown that is removed from the body in the urine. High amounts of uric acid in the urine can cause kidney stones.

**urinalysis** (yoo-rih-**NAL**-ih-sis) **(UA):** laboratory urinalysis of urine. It is one of the most common tests performed to evaluate the general health of a person. This test includes macroscopic (seen with the naked eye) observations of the urine and microscopic (seen with the help of a microscope) observations. The urine is analyzed for the presence of such elements as albumin (a protein), bacteria, bilirubin, blood, ketones, glucose, pus, white blood cells, and casts (clumps of cellular matter that have formed as if in a mold). The color, pH (balance between acids and bases), and specific gravity (the amount of wastes, minerals, and other substances) are also noted in urine.

**urinary catheterization:** insertion of a catheter into the urethra for the removal of urine.

## V

**visual acuity** (ah-**KYOO**-eh-tee): a noninvasive method of judging how good the patient's eyesight is. A **Snellen** (**SNEL**-en) chart is used. This chart contains different letters of different sizes. The patient stands 20 feet from the chart, covers one eye, and reads each letter. How well the patient sees the letters is an indication of visual acuity. It is measured as a fraction; 20/20 vision is normal.

**visual fields:** a noninvasive test used to examine the patient's peripheral vision.

**voiding cystography** (sis-**TOG**-raf-fee): a procedure in which x-rays of the bladder and urethra are taken while the patient is voiding. A contrast medium is placed directly into the urinary structures.

## W

**Western Block:** a blood test to screen patients for antibodies to HIV.

**white blood cell count (WBC):** a test used to measure the number of white blood cells in a sample of blood. The normal value is 5000 to 10000 cells per microliter of blood.

## X

**x-ray:** an image taken of internal structures using x-rays.

# INDEX